Respiratory Medicine

Series Editor:
Sharon I.S. Rounds

For further volumes:
http://www.springer.com/series/7665

Jeremy B. Richards • Renee D. Stapleton

Editors

Non-Pulmonary Complications of Critical Care

A Clinical Guide

Humana Press

Editors
Jeremy B. Richards
Division of Pulmonary,
   Critical Care and Sleep Medicine
Harvard Medical School
Beth Israel Deaconess Medical Center
Boston, MA, USA

Renee D. Stapleton
Pulmonary and Critical Care
University of Vermont
   College of Medicine
Burlington, VT, USA

ISSN 2197-7372   ISSN 2197-7380 (electronic)
ISBN 978-1-4939-0872-1   ISBN 978-1-4939-0873-8 (eBook)
DOI 10.1007/978-1-4939-0873-8
Springer New York Heidelberg Dordrecht London

Library of Congress Control Number: 2014939024

Printed on acid-free paper

Humana Press is a brand of Springer
Springer is part of Springer Science+Business Media (www.springer.com)

Preface

Complications of critical illness, both iatrogenic and non-iatrogenic, are common in the intensive care unit (ICU) and can lead to increased morbidity and mortality. Thus, it is extremely important to understand the nature of complications and how to best prevent and treat them when caring for critically ill patients. The first six chapters of this book thoroughly discuss these complications and are organized by organ system (cardiac, renal, neurologic, hematologic, gastrointestinal, and nutritional/endocrinologic). These chapters are followed by a chapter focusing on procedural complications. Finally, the book concludes with a chapter on preventing complications with meticulous supportive care and systems-based considerations in the ICU. Drug-related complications are mentioned throughout the book in relevant chapters. The topics covered in this book will help readers gain understanding of when to anticipate and how to prevent a wide array of potential complications of critical illness. When complications are encountered, these chapters also include detailed information on diagnosis, management, and prognostication.

We wish to thank the series editor, Dr. Sharon Rounds, for allowing us the opportunity to develop this volume and participate in the series. We are also grateful to the contributing authors for their time and effort in writing clear and concise chapters. Finally, we would like to thank Flora Kim, the developmental editor at Springer, whose assistance and dedication throughout the publication process helped to produce an excellent book.

Boston, MA, USA   Jeremy B. Richards, M.D., M.A.
Burlington, VT, USA   Renee D. Stapleton, M.D., Ph.D.

Contents

1 **Cardiovascular Complications**.. 1
   Ryan D. Clouser and Gilman Allen

2 **Renal Complications**... 19
   Elizabeth J. Lechner and Michael G. Risbano

3 **Neurologic Complications** 45
   John P. Kress

4 **Hematologic Complications** 61
   Ralitza Martin, Annette Esper, and Greg S. Martin

5 **Gastrointestinal Complications** 105
   Preeti Dhar and Eddy Fan

6 **Non-pulmonary Infectious Complications**............................. 135
   Pamela Paufler and Robert Kempainen

7 **Nutritional and Endocrinologic Complications** 165
   Eoin Slattery, Dong Wook Kim, and David S. Seres

8 **Procedural Complications**... 187
   Başak Çoruh, Amy E. Morris, and Patricia A. Kritek

9 **Preventing Complications: Consistent Meticulous
   Supportive Care in the ICU** 213
   Benjamin A. Bonneton, Serkan Senkal, and Ognjen Gajic

Index... 227

Contributors

Gilman Allen, M.D. Division of Pulmonary and Critical Care, University of Vermont, Burlington, VT, USA

Benjamin A. Bonneton, M.D. Division of Pulmonary and Critical Care Medicine, Mayo Clinic, Rochester, MN, USA

Ryan D. Clouser, D.O. Division of Pulmonary and Critical Care, University of Vermont, Burlington, VT, USA

Başak Çoruh, M.D. Division of Pulmonary and Critical Care Medicine, University of Washington, Seattle, WA, USA

Preeti Dhar, M.D. Interdepartmental Division of Critical Care, University of Toronto, Toronto, ON, Canada

Annette Esper, M.D., M.Sc. Division of Pulmonary, Allergy and Critical Care Medicine, Grady Memorial Hospital, Emory University, Atlanta, GA, USA

Eddy Fan, M.D., Ph.D. Interdepartmental Division of Critical Care, Mount Sinai Hospital, University of Toronto, Toronto, ON, Canada

Ognjen Gajic, M.D. Division of Pulmonary and Critical Care Medicine, College of Medicine, Mayo Clinic, Rochester, MN, USA

Robert Kempainen, M.D. Division of Pulmonary and Critical Care Medicine, Hennepin County Medical Center, University of Minnesota School of Medicine, Minneapolis, MN, USA

Dong Wook Kim, M.D. Nutrition and Weight Management Center, Boston Medical Center, Boston University of Medicine, Boston, MA, USA

John P. Kress, M.D. Section of Pulmonary and Critical Care, Department of Medicine, University of Chicago, Chicago, IL, USA

Patricia A. Kritek, M.D., EdM. Division of Pulmonary and Critical Care Medicine, University of Washington, Seattle, WA, USA

Elizabeth J. Lechner, M.D. Pulmonary and Critical Care Medicine, University of Pittsburgh Medical Center, Pittsburgh, PA, USA

Greg S. Martin, M.D., M.Sc. Division of Pulmonary, Allergy and Critical Care, Emory University School of Medicine, Atlanta, GA, USA

Ralitza Martin, M.D. Division of Pulmonary, Allergy and Critical Care, Emory University School of Medicine, Atlanta, GA, USA

Amy E. Morris, M.D. Division of Pulmonary and Critical Care Medicine, University of Washington, Seattle, WA, USA

Pamela Paufler, M.D. Division of Pulmonary and Critical Care Medicine, Hennepin County Medical Center, Minneapolis, MN, USA

Michael G. Risbano, M.D., M.A., F.C.C.P. Division of Pulmonary, Allergy and Critical Care Medicine, University of Pittsburgh Medical Center, CLC Pulmonary Hypertension Clinic, Pittsburgh, PA, USA

Serkan Senkal, M.D. Division of Pulmonary and Critical Care Medicine, Mayo Clinic, Rochester, MN, USA

David S. Seres, M.D., Sc.M., P.N.S. College of Physicians and Surgeons and Institute of Human Nutrition, Columbia University, New York, NY, USA

Medical Nutrition and Nutrition Support Service, Division of Preventative Medicine and Nutrition, Department of Medicine, Columbia University Medical Center, New York, NY, USA

Eoin Slattery, M.D. Division of Preventative Medicine and Nutrition, Department of Medicine, Columbia University Medical Center, New York, NY, USA

Chapter 1
Cardiovascular Complications

Ryan D. Clouser and Gilman Allen

Abstract Cardiovascular complications are a common occurrence while caring for the critically ill patient. Problems such as atrial fibrillation (A fib), acute myocardial infarction, cardiac arrest, cardiac tamponade, and ventricular fibrillation are not uncommon in critical illness. Treatment of these conditions should be focused on prompt organized assessment and care to ensure rapid stabilization of the patient. Treatment of A fib should be focused on conversion back to sinus rhythm in some instances versus rate control with nodal blocking agents. Care of acute myocardial infarction requires determination for the need of invasive management versus medical management, as well as antiplatelet medications and systemic anticoagulation. Cardiac arrest should be treated with cardiopulmonary resuscitation and provision of rapid defibrillation for shockable causes of cardiac arrest. Echocardiography should be considered to aid in diagnosis during rapid deterioration of patients. Selected patients who have return of spontaneous circulation post arrest should be quickly evaluated for utility of targeted temperature management in order to attenuate the systemic and neurologic effects of post resuscitation syndrome.

Keywords Atrial fibrillation • Cardiac arrest • Post resuscitation syndrome • Cardiac tamponade • Ventricular fibrillation • Ventricular tachycardia • Myocardial infarction

R.D. Clouser, D.O. (✉)
Division of Pulmonary and Critical Care, University of Vermont,
89 Beaumont Avenue, Given Bldg. D208, Burlington, VT 05405, USA
e-mail: ryan.clouser@vtmednet.org

G. Allen, M.D.
Division of Pulmonary and Critical Care, University of Vermont,
HSRF 220, 149 Beaumont Avenue, Burlington, VT 05405-0075, USA
e-mail: gil.allen@uvm.edu

J.B. Richards and R.D. Stapleton (eds.), *Non-Pulmonary Complications of Critical Care:*
A Clinical Guide, Respiratory Medicine, DOI 10.1007/978-1-4939-0873-8_1,
© Springer Science+Business Media New York 2014

Introduction

It is common for clinicians to be faced with a host of cardiovascular complications of critical illness while treating patients in the Intensive Care Unit (ICU). Even in patients admitted to the ICU for non-cardiac primary issues, acute cardiac complications often arise, requiring rapid clinical assessment and response. In this chapter we review the pathogenesis and evidence-based management of common cardiac complications of critical illness.

Atrial Fibrillation

Atrial fibrillation (A fib) is the most common arrhythmia experienced in the ICU [1] and it is often exacerbated by conditions commonly encountered in the ICU, such as acute myocardial ischemia, cardiac surgery, severe sepsis, shock, hypovolemia, and pulmonary emboli. A recent retrospective review of a large database of critical care units in California hospitals assessed the risk of A fib and its associated risks in the setting of severe sepsis. The study found that new onset A fib occurred far more frequently in hospitalized patients with severe sepsis than in those without severe sepsis [2].

General management of A fib depends on the stability of the patient. Loss of the atrial component of cardiac output can, in many cases, be an inciting event that leads to cardiogenic shock or exacerbation of other forms of shock. As a result of compromised diastolic filling, a rapid ventricular response to A fib or flutter can also lead to diastolic dysfunction and acute pulmonary edema, with subsequent respiratory failure. Any unstable patient with new onset rapid A fib should be considered a candidate for direct current cardioversion to sinus rhythm as quickly as possible. Cardioversion must include provision of some form of sedation and analgesia (with airway protection, as indicated) prior to delivery of percutaneous electricity to the patient.

For the hemodynamically stable patient with A fib and rapid ventricular response, it is important to first review the patient's past medical history and determine whether the patient is chronically in A fib, in which case conversion to sinus rhythm (either by pharmacotherapy or cardioversion) is unlikely to be maintained. In the case of chronic A fib, it is more sensible to shift one's focus to pharmacologic rate control with beta blockers, calcium channel blockers, or even digoxin (Table 1.1).

Table 1.1 Agents for management of atrial fibrillation

Amiodarone	150 mg loading dose, continuous infusion 1 mg/h × 8 h then 0.5 mg/h
Metoprolol	2.5–5 mg IV
Esmolol	0.5 mg/kg loading dose, 309825 continuous infusion 0.05 mg/kg to 0.3 mg/kg/min
Diltiazem	10–20 mg loading dose, continuous infusion 5–20 mg/h
Digoxin	0.5 mg IV load, 0.25 mg every 6 h × 2 doses, then 0.125 mg daily
Magnesium	37 mg/kg bolus followed by 25 mg/kg/h for 24 h

In the critically ill patient with new onset A fib, pharmacologic conversion to sinus rhythm has been extensively studied. The rates of conversion to sinus rhythm with amiodarone administration ranges between 50 and 70 % within 12 h of initiation of the drug, and about a 50 % stable conversion rate by 24 h [3, 4]. One study found that magnesium (37 mg/kg bolus followed by 25 mg/kg/h for 24 h) actually achieved a higher rate of conversion to sinus rhythm compared to amiodarone (77 versus 50 % at 24 h) [4], but this finding has not been replicated elsewhere. Conversion rates to sinus rhythm have also been reported with more traditional rate-controlling drugs, such as esmolol and diltiazem. Conversion rates were found to be higher with esmolol than with diltiazem (68 versus 33 %), but both agents were equally efficacious at rate control [5].

Aside from rate control, it is important to consider the risk of stroke and need for anticoagulation in a patient with either chronic or acute A fib in the ICU. The decision to provide systemic anticoagulation is often complicated in the critically ill, particularly following recent trauma or surgery, or in the setting of gastrointestinal bleeding, hematological malignancy, or disseminated intravascular coagulation (DIC) from sepsis. Thus, the risks and benefits should be weighed carefully, specifically taking into account the daily risk of thromboembolic complications (including cerebrovascular accidents) attributable to A fib. One important consideration is the presence of severe sepsis at the time of diagnosis of new onset A fib. New onset A fib in severe sepsis is associated with a six-fold higher incidence of ischemic stroke compared to patients without severe sepsis [2], and this should be factored into any decision regarding anti-coagulation for A fib in ICU patients.

Myocardial Infarction

Non-ST Elevation Myocardial Infarction

Non-ST elevation myocardial infarction (NSTEMI) and/or ST elevation myocardial infarction (STEMI) are common in the ICU setting. NSTEMI may be the reason for admission to the ICU when associated with refractory chest pain, pulmonary edema or acute respiratory failure, but can also be associated with or occur during the clinical course of other critical illnesses (such as severe sepsis). Clinical signs and symptoms of NSTEMI can be difficult to ascertain in intubated and sedated ICU patients. Early signs of NSTEMI include chest pain and/or pressure, which can often radiate into the jaw or left arm. An intubated and sedated patient may not be aware of or be able to report these symptoms to clinicians.

Diagnostic workup of acute coronary syndromes such as NSTEMI is dependent on the presence of symptoms and classic electrocardiogram (ECG) changes. The astute intensivist may note ST changes on continuous telemetry monitoring, but a 12-lead ECG should always be obtained as soon as concern for myocardial ischemia is entertained. ECG findings consistent with NSTEMI include ST depression of

>1–2 mm, typically in contiguous leads that correspond with one of the main coronary artery territories. Inversion of T waves is also a worrisome marker for ischemia but not nearly as sensitive or specific as deep ST depression [6]. Cardiac biomarkers are also an important part of the workup for NSTEMI and should be sent as soon as possible. Troponin assays, which are very sensitive, will become elevated within hours of active myocardial ischemia and should be followed serially until they peak. Continued elevation or rising of cardiac troponin should raise serious concern for ongoing myocardial necrosis and infarction.

There are numerous potential causes of NSTEMI in critically ill patients. The most common and classic cause of NSTEMI is the development of non-occlusive arterial thrombus within a coronary artery which leads to a mismatch in myocardial oxygen supply and Verbose and unnecessary demand. This pathophysiologic mechanism explains why critically ill patients are at increased risk for NSTEMI: myocardial oxygen demand is higher in the critically ill. This process is initiated by the rupture of an unstable coronary plaque within a native coronary vessel. The rupture of the plaque leads to activation of platelets and the coagulation cascade, which can progress to further myocardial injury as coagulation and platelet plugs form within the vessel lumen, decreasing vascular luminal diameter and decreasing myocardial oxygen delivery (in the setting of increased myocardial oxygen demand).

Other potential causes of NSTEMI in the ICU setting include "demand-related" ischemia resulting from mismatch between the decreased supply of well-oxygenated hemoglobin (and blood flow) and the typically high myocardial demand imposed by an often hyperdynamic myocardium, particularly in patients with severe sepsis and septic shock. Demand-related ischemia is common and is frequently encountered in patients with shock and overall poor perfusion from any cause. Insufficient oxygen supply to the myocardium during shock states can cause impaired ventricular contractility and a secondary, superimposed cardiogenic process that further compounds the hemodynamic effects of the pre-existing, primary cause of shock.

Finally, coronary artery vasospasm can cause NSTEMI in critically ill patients. Coronary vasospasm is a rare but recognized complication of administration of high doses of vasopressors. The vasopressors most likely to cause vasospasm are those with unopposed alpha-adrenergic properties [7]. Coronary vasospasm is also a recognized early-complication of coronary bypass surgery [8] and can also be a complication of recreational cocaine use and/or overdose [9].

Treatment of NSTEMI in the ICU should be focused on providing supportive care and treating underlying and potentially causative conditions, while maximizing oxygen delivery to the myocardium and delivering antiplatelet and anticoagulation therapy as soon as possible. In an intubated patient, it is imperative to ensure that the patient is adequately sedated and provided with good analgesia to ensure that excessive work of breathing or ventilator dyssynchrony are minimized, as both processes may increase respiratory muscle work and myocardial oxygen demand. Airway management and mechanical ventilation should be provided to the critically ill patient with NSTEMI and concomitant acute respiratory failure due to pulmonary edema. When treated expeditiously with non-invasive positive pressure ventilation (NIPPV), patients with acute pulmonary edema due to a NSTEMI may avoid the need for intubation and invasive mechanical ventilation. Early NIPPV may potentially even reduce overall mortality in this patient population [10]. Administration of non-invasive continuous positive airway pressure (CPAP) can decrease work of breathing and improve oxygenation, presumably by reducing upper airway resistance [11] and helping to partially recruit fluid-filled and collapsed alveoli. Both non-invasive and invasive positive pressure mechanical ventilation can help decrease left ventricular afterload by raising intrathoracic pressure and effectively reducing transmural pressure across the left ventricle during systole [12]. Non-invasive bi-level positive airway pressure (BiPAP) can help to further reduce patients' work of breathing and similarly improve oxygenation. Of note, some concerns were raised early on by the finding of an increased frequency of myocardial infarction with the use of BiPAP for treatment of pulmonary edema in early observational trials [13], but these concerns have not been substantiated in more recent and larger trials. As such, current guidelines based on contemporary evidence support the use of BiPAP for selected patients with acute pulmonary edema and acute coronary syndrome to minimize the risk of needing endotracheal intubation and invasive mechanical ventilation [14, 15].

In addition to supportive care and treating underlying systemic causes, medical management of a NSTEMI should focus on treatment of the acute myocardial infarction (MI). Aspirin should be given as soon as possible. If no enteral access is available in an intubated patient, an orogastric tube should be placed for administration of aspirin. If there is a contraindication for aspirin administration through the gastric route, rectal aspirin should be given. Without a contraindication to anticoagulation, a patient with a NSTEMI should be systemically anticoagulated with a continuous IV infusion of heparin. Low molecular weight heparin (LMWH) is an alternative consideration for treatment of acute coronary syndrome [16]; however, LMWH should be used with caution in the ICU setting due to its poor reversibility after subcutaneous administration, particularly as critically ill patients are at increased risk for acute bleeding complications.

In addition, treatment of the patient with NSTEMI should include secondary antiplatelet therapy with an ADP receptor antagonist such as clopidogrel. Rate control with beta-blockers should be initiated if clinically possible; however, beta-blockade is often not possible in critically ill patients due to concomitant hypotension and shock. As soon as possible, consultation with a Cardiologist should be obtained to identify the utility of further management options. Specifically, cardiology's early input regarding the risks and benefits of continued medical management versus cardiac catheterization and percutaneous coronary intervention (PCI) is critical, as delayed catheterization may have significant clinical consequences. Glycoprotein IIb/IIIa inhibitors (GPIs) should be initiated when recommended by cardiology, and are typically provided for patients undergoing catheterization.

ST Elevation Myocardial Infarction

Acute STEMI is a true cardiac emergency necessitating rapid evaluation and timely decision making regarding treatment. STEMI is caused by acute plaque rupture and complete occlusion of a coronary artery by formation of an intra-vascular platelet plug. A STEMI presents with sudden onset of severe chest pain or pressure that can be associated with diaphoresis, nausea, and shortness of breath. ECG is diagnostic and will reveal downward concave ST segment elevation in contiguous leads representative of the affected coronary artery territory. Acute ST elevation may be noted on continuous telemetry lead monitoring in the ICU, but the symptoms can be difficult or impossible to detect in an intubated and sedated patient. Acute hemodynamic and/or respiratory decompensation of a previously stable critically ill patient should trigger prompt obtainment of an ECG to ensure that acute myocardial infarction is not the cause of the patient's deterioration. STEMI can have devastating consequences if not treated rapidly, as an untreated STEMI can quickly progress to acute cardiogenic shock with hypotension, acute respiratory failure, and multiorgan failure.

Treatment of a STEMI should initially focus on immediate medical management with anti-platelet therapy with aspirin (PO [per os, or by mouth], PGT [per G-tube] or PR [per rectum]), and anticoagulation with a continuous infusion of unfractionated heparin IV. GPIs may be reasonable in selected patients, and should be initiated in concert with cardiology consultation and recommendations. Best outcomes are achieved with timely restoration of coronary artery patency, coronary artery blood flow, and myocardial perfusion. Clinical options for restoring coronary artery patency include thrombolytic therapy, invasive PCI via cardiac catheterization, or coronary artery bypass grafting (CABG) surgery. PCI is preferred in most patients as it is associated with less adverse outcomes than thrombolytic therapy, specifically a lower prevalence of major bleeding events. Given the significant risks of surgery in critically ill patients, PCI is generally preferred to CABG in most circumstances.

Post-PCI care focuses on continued systemic anticoagulation with the guidance of the cardiology service. Rate control, medical management of potential reperfusion arrhythmias, and vasopressor administration as needed for post-STEMI/post-PCI cardiogenic shock, are all components of post-intervention management. The optimal vasopressor for management of post-STEMI cardiogenic shock is controversial. However, a recent randomized, prospective, head-to-head trial demonstrated that norepinephrine causes fewer adverse events than dopamine in a heterogenous group of critically ill patients with shock [17]. Specifically, norepinerphine caused less tachyarrhythmias than dopamine in all patients, and was associated with decreased mortality in the subgroup of patients with cardiogenic shock [17]. The utility of intra-aortic balloon pump (IABP) counter-pulsation has recently been called into question by a randomized, prospective study that demonstrated that IABP did not confer any mortality benefit over medical management alone in patients with acute myocardial infarction complicated by cardiogenic shock [18].

Cardiac Arrest

Despite aggressive monitoring and care, cardiac arrest and circulatory collapse are still common complications of critical illness. Furthermore, many patients arrive in the ICU after return of spontaneous circulation (ROSC) following an out-of-hospital cardiac arrest. Rapid response teams in the inpatient setting may decrease the rate of cardiac arrest on the general medical and surgical wards and shift the incidence of arrest to the ICU by transferring patients to a higher level of care earlier in their critical illness. There are several underlying causes of cardiac arrest that we review in this section. A large review of registry data from of 51,919 in-hospital cardiac arrests between 1999 and 2005 revealed that the first documented arrhythmia during cardiac arrest was ventricular tachycardia in 3,810 (7 %), ventricular fibrillation in 8,718 (17 %), pulseless electrical activity (PEA) in 19,262 (37 %) and asystole in 20,129 (39 %) of cases [19]. Survival to discharge from the hospital was no different if the initial rhythm at the time of arrest was ventricular tachycardia or ventricular fibrillation (37 %). PEA and asystole were both associated with significantly lower rates of survival to discharge at 12 and 11 %, respectively [18]. Evidence is limited as to what constitutes the best management of in-hospital cardiac arrest, but there are recent data that suggest that post-arrest targeted temperature management (TTM) may confer higher rates of favorable neurologic recovery and survival in patients with PEA and in-hospital cardiac arrest [20, 21], as has already been demonstrated in out-of-hospital arrest due to ventricular fibrillation [22, 23].

For all of the arrhythmogenic causes of cardiac arrest, the key elements of immediate management include performing a primary survey (assessing airway, breathing and circulation), obtaining adequate IV access, providing early defibrillation if clinically indicated, and delivering consistent high-quality chest compressions with minimal interruption.

Ventricular Tachycardia and Ventricular Fibrillation

Ventricular tachycardia (V tach) is a wide complex regular and fast rhythm that is frequently associated with a loss of perfusion to the vital organs, and can result in loss of pulse and cardiac arrest. It is categorized as either V tach with a pulse, or pulseless V tach. Ventricular fibrillation (V fib) results from disorganized electrical activity within the ventricular and is characterized by the lack of discernible QRS complexes on ECG or telemetry monitoring. V tach and V fib most commonly occur as a result of active cardiac ischemia and/or severe electrolyte disturbances, such as hypokalemia or hypomagnesemia. In the ICU, irritation from indwelling vascular access devices, such as central lines or PICC (peripherally inserted central venous catheter) lines inadvertently placed into the ventricle, can also precipitate ventricular ectopy and sustained V tach. V tach and V fib can also be seen in patients with cardiomyopathy or underlying conduction system disturbances from scar tissue involving the ventricular conduction system, the latter resulting from remote myocardial infarction or other inflammatory cardiomyopathies, such as sarcoidosis or viral myocarditis (among other causes).

Treatment of V tach initially hinges on assessing whether or not the patient is hemodynamically stable. For intermittent V tach in a patient who is conscious and hemodynamically stable, administration of an intravenous (IV) beta blocker will often suppress further ectopy. Longer sustained runs of stable V tach are more appropriately managed with IV amiodarone or lidocaine. Amiodarone is generally delivered as a 150 mg IV bolus followed by an infusion, typically at 1 mg/h. Second line agents, such as lidocaine, are less effective than amiodarone and should only be considered if amiodarone is unavailable or contraindicated. Hemodynamically unstable V tach (characterized by patients who are hypotensive or confused, but who have a palpable pulse) is treated similarly to all hemodynamically unstable tachycardias, beginning with immediate *synchronized* cardioversion. If at any point while managing a patient with V tach there is uncertainty regarding the presence or absence of a palpable pulse, it is reasonable to begin cardiopulmonary resuscitation (CPR) and specifically initiate the appropriate pulseless arrest algorithm (e.g., V fib/ pulseless V tach or asystole/PEA).

Pulseless V tach and V fib should both be treated emergently with immediate *defibrillation* (unsynchronized) and initiation of resuscitation based on the American Heart Association Advanced Cardiac Life Support Protocol. Defibrillation is now carried out in a stepwise process to ensure the patient receives uninterrupted chest compressions between each delivered shock prior to assessment of rhythm and evaluation for ROSC. Medical therapy for V fib or pulseless V tach arrest refractory to defibrillation is either a one-time dose of vasopressin 40 units IV or epinephrine 1 mg IV every 3–5 min for the duration of the event.

While animal studies have suggested that vasopressin may lead to improved blood flow to organs and better neurological outcomes after prolonged cardiac arrest [24], the results of vasopressin have been less compelling in human clinical studies. A landmark randomized controlled trial of patients who suffered in-hospital cardiac arrest compared 40 units of vasopressin to 1 mg of epinephrine as initial medical management during cardiac arrest [25]. Patients who did not respond to the first dose of either vasopressin or epinephrine received subsequent doses of epinephrine as a rescue therapy. Of the patients enrolled and randomized, 104 patients received vasopressin and 96 patients were treated with epinephrine. Primary outcomes of survival-to-hospital discharge, survival-to-one-hour, and neurological function were all equivalent between the two groups [25]. A second multicenter, randomized controlled trial compared the use of combined vasopressin plus epinephrine to epinephrine alone for out-of-hospital cardiac arrest [26]. This trial included nearly 3,000 patients and the primary outcome was on survival-to-hospital admission. Secondary outcomes included ROSC, survival-to-hospital discharge, good neurologic recovery, and 1-year survival [26]. This trial again also failed to demonstrate any significant difference between the two medications. Of note, this trial did re-verify the overall poor prognosis associated with out-of-hospital cardiac arrest, with approximately 20 % of patients surviving to hospital admission, 29 % of patients achieving ROSC, and a staggering 2 % of patients surviving to both hospital discharge and to 1 year post-arrest [26].

Lidocaine was previously the agent of choice for medical treatment of refractory V tach and V fib but has since been replaced by amiodarone in the most up-to-date Advanced Cardiac Life Support (ACLS) algorithms. An earlier randomized controlled trial of patients with out-of-hospital cardiac arrest and refractory V tach or V

Table 1.2 Causes of PEA
and asystolic cardiac arrest

Common causes of PEA and asystolic cardiac arrest
Hypovolemia/hypotension
Severe metabolic acidosis
Hyperkalemia/hypokalemia
Hypothermia
Hypoxemia
Thrombosis (acute MI/PE)
Toxins (overdose)
Tension pneumothorax
Tamponade

fib demonstrated a significant increase in survival-to-hospital admission with administration of 300 mg of amiodarone when compared to placebo (44 versus 34 %, $p=0.03$) [27]. Another randomized trial 3 years later demonstrated a statistically significant increase in survival-to-hospital admission in patients with shock-resistant, out-of-hospital V fib patients who received amiodarone versus lidocaine (22.8 versus 12.0 %, $p=0.009$) [28].

Pulseless Electrical Activity

PEA is a common cause of cardiac arrest in the ICU. PEA is characterized by continued electrical activity on telemetry monitoring without effective cardiac output, systemic circulation, or a palpable pulse. In addition to prompt cardiopulmonary resuscitation, the underlying causes of PEA must be considered and directly treated to provide the patient the best chance of surviving an acute PEA arrest. The most common causes of PEA arrest include severe hypovolemia, hypoxia, acidosis, hyperkalemia and hypokalemia, hypothermia, tension pneumothorax, pericardial tamponade, drug ingestion, myocardial infarction, and massive pulmonary embolism (Table 1.2).

The immediate management of a PEA arrest is similar to a V tach/V fib arrest, as clinicians should rapidly perform a primary survey, ensure there is adequate IV access, initiate high-quality chest compressions, and provide fluid resuscitation based on the standard ACLS protocol. Again, the focus of the ACLS algorithm is high-quality, uninterrupted chest compressions. While performing immediate CPR, clinicians should consider potentially treatable causes of the patient's acute decompensation and PEA arrest. Medical therapy for PEA is epinephrine 1 mg IV every 3–5 min for the duration of the resuscitation. Additional medications such as IV calcium, sodium bicarbonate, insulin, and glucose are also frequently provided during resuscitation, particularly when hyperkalemia or severe acidosis is suspected as a potential or probable cause of PEA. Atropine is no longer advised by the American Heart Association as part of the standard medical treatment algorithm for PEA.

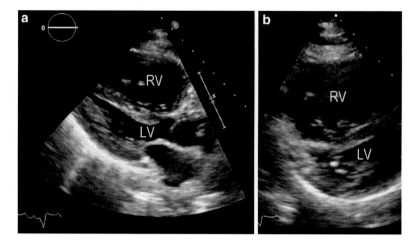

Fig. 1.1 Para-sternal long axis (*panel A* on *left*) and short axis (*panel B* on *right*) views from echocardiogram, demonstrating under-filled left ventricle (LV) and dilated right ventricle (RV) with septal flattening during late systole, leading to asymmetry of left ventricle in cross-section (*panel B*, LV), commonly referred to as the "D-sign", consistent with RV pressure and volume overload, which should raise suspicion for a hemodynamically significant pulmonary embolism

Bedside echocardiogram can be very helpful in evaluating and guiding treatment of patients in PEA arrest. Rapid assessment of cardiac contractility during brief pauses in CPR can allow for differentiation between true PEA (absence of echocardiographic cardiac activity) and "pseudo-PEA", in which electrical conduction and cardiac contractility are coupled but the cardiac output is insufficient to generate adequate perfusion and a palpable pulse.

Bedside ultrasound can also aid in the assessment of potential causes of PEA by rapidly assessing the structure of the heart and lungs. Using bedside echocardiography it is possible, with proper training, to rapidly assess for the presence of pericardial tamponade, pneumothorax, and acute right ventricular pressure and volume overload, which may raise clinical suspicion for massive PE (Fig. 1.1).

With regard to both bedside echocardiography and bedside ultrasound, it is important to emphasize that chest compressions should not be stopped for these evaluations and resumption of chest compressions should not be delayed by these assessments. Rapid and timely use of ultrasound can be helpful in ruling in or ruling out possible causes of PEA, but resuscitative efforts should not be held or delayed simply to perform ultrasonography.

Without the availability of ultrasound, treatment of PEA arrest will typically focus on rapid detection and treatment of acid/base and electrolyte abnormalities using point-of-care testing, restoration of circulating volume, and potentially empiric needle decompression of the chest or pericardiocentesis in the setting of suspected pneumothorax or pericardial tamponade. It is also not uncommon in the critically ill patient to have more than one cause of PEA present. Thus, it is crucial that the clinician continue to work his or her way through the entire list of possible causes when one intervention fails to restore cardiovascular circulation.

Asystole

Asystole is diagnosed by absence of cardiac electrical activity on telemetry monitoring ("flatline"). The common causes for asystole are similar to the causes of PEA. Asystole is commonly preceded by progressive sinus or junctional bradycardia.

Treatment of asystole is focused on airway management, oxygenation, and chest compressions. When an airway cannot be immediately secured, there should be no delay in initiating CPR and delivering high-quality chest compressions. Oxygen should be delivered by face mask while chest compressions are provided at a rate of 100 compressions per minute. Epinephrine should be administered at a dose of 1 mg IV every 3–5 min for the duration of the arrest. Sodium bicarbonate was formerly considered a therapeutic option for the prolonged arrest; however, it has been removed from the most recent algorithms due to a lack of efficacy and concern that it might promote increased intracellular acidosis. The overall survival rate from aystolic cardiac arrest is poor, even in the ICU setting.

Reperfusion Injury/Post-resuscitation Syndrome/ Targeted Temperature Management

Despite aggressive measures and advances in technology, long-term outcomes and survival from cardiac arrest, both in and out of the hospital, remain poor. Care of the post-arrest patient should focus on the restoration of blood flow and oxygen delivery to vital organs and minimization of reperfusion injury. The post resuscitation syndrome is characterized by anoxic brain injury, post-cardiac arrest myocardial dysfunction, systemic ischemia with reperfusion injury, and a subsequent systemic inflammatory response [29]. The degree of post-resuscitation syndrome is based on a number of factors, including the underlying comorbid state of the patient, the underlying cause of the arrest, the duration of no-flow state, and the adequacy of restoration of perfusion.

The pathophysiology of post-cardiac arrest syndrome is not completely understood but appears to involve several cellular pathways. Global ischemia activates the systemic inflammatory response and causes increased production of cytokines, including IL-1, IL-6, IL-8, TNF-α and increased complement activation, arachadonic acid metabolites, expression of leukocyte adhesion molecules, and chemotaxis of neutrophils into the ischemic tissue [30]. Lack of oxygen delivery to cells leads to decreased ATP synthesis, depletion of intracellular ATP stores, and produces a depolarization of the cellular membrane, opening of the voltage-dependent calcium channels, and decreased mitochondrial membrane potential [30]. This results in an influx of calcium into cells which results in cellular damage. Restoration of oxygen delivery to injured cells can accelerate the production of free radical and reactive oxygen species, including superoxide anions, hydrogen peroxide and free radical hydroxyl groups, all of which can lead to further cytotoxic injury [30].

The global systemic inflammatory response also triggers the coagulation cascade, leading to micro-vascular thrombosis, which can potentially lead to added and prolonged ischemia, and ultimately to multi-organ failure and death. Ischemia of the gut can result in breakdown in the epithelial mucosal membrane, which can allow for bacterial translocation into the circulation and subsequent sepsis and multi-organ failure.

Post-cardiac arrest hypotension is a mixed form of cardiogenic and distributive shock [31]. Typically this shock state is characterized by severe and global, but reversible, left ventricular dysfunction, which begins quickly after ROSC and generally resolves within 48–72 h [31]. Management of post-arrest hypotension should be focused on rapid evaluation of left ventricular function with beside echocardiography and initiation of vasopressors and ionotropes to maximize cardiac output and reperfusion. Oxygen should be delivered to a point sufficient to restore cellular oxidative metabolism, but with care to avoid excessive oxygen tension. A large multi-center cohort study of 120 hospitals and 6,326 patients found that post-arrest patients treated with hyperoxia within 24 h of arrest ($PaO_2 > 300$ mmHg) had a significantly higher in-hospital mortality of 63 versus 45 % among patients with more physiologically normal PaO_2 levels [32]. Carbon dioxide levels should be kept within normal range by adjusting of patients' minute ventilation while they are mechanically ventilated. Excessive hyperventilation can lead to decreased $PaCO_2$ and resultant vasoconstriction of the cerebral vasculature with compromise of cerebral perfusion and added threat to favorable neurologic recovery.

Reperfusion injury to the brain is a common occurrence following ROSC. Two landmark studies demonstrated that cooling cardiac arrest survivors, specifically after V tach/V fib arrest, to a temperature of 33–34 degrees Celsius (°C) was associated with decreased mortality and an increase in favorable neurologic recovery [21, 22]. For this reason it has become common practice, and a recommendation by the American Heart Association, to provide TTM immediately following the ROSC in patients who have suffered V fib or V tach cardiac arrest. The application of controlled patient cooling is believed to decrease the harmful effects of reactive oxygen species and cellular calcium influx toxicity, presumably through a reduction in cerebral metabolism and oxidative chemistry. More recent evidence demonstrates that maintaining post-cardiac arrest patients at a temperature of 36 degrees Celsius is non-inferior to 33 degrees, and that avoiding fever with TTM may be the most important intervention to optimize neurologic recovery after ROSC [33].

Evidence to support the use of TTM is strongest for survivors of V tach/V fib cardiac arrest [22, 23], but this practice has been expanded to other causes of cardiac arrest [33]. There is currently no solid evidence available from randomized clinical trials to strongly support the use of TTM for non-shockable rhythms, but the rationale for doing so is the same pathophysiologic processes that occur after V tach and V fib arrest likely occur after PEA and asystolic arrest. The data to support the practice of TTM of non-shockable rhythms include retrospective cohort, non-randomized prospective observational studies, and one large randomized controlled trial and the results are mixed with regard to favorable neurological recovery [21, 34, 35]. A recent meta-analysis of randomized and non-randomized studies appears to support TTM for in-hospital and out-of-hospital arrest due to non-shockable

Table 1.3 Methods to induce cooling via targeted temperature management to achieve therapeutic hypothermia (return of spontaneous circulation is abbreviated as ROSC)

Initiation of therapeutic hypothermia
Determine if patient is appropriate for cooling (comatose [GCS < 8], ROSC < 60 min, hemodynamically stable)
Place ice packs in groin, axilla, and neck
Bolus with 20–30 ml/kg iced saline
Place cooling blankets
Consider medication to manage sedation and prevention of shivering
Anticipate close monitoring and management of serum electrolytes (check levels at least every 4–6 h during initiation and maintenance of therapeutic hypothermia, as well as during rewarming)
Assess and follow coagulation profile

cardiac causes, but the authors acknowledge a substantial risk for bias and poor quality of evidence [20]. As with any clinical intervention, clinicians need to weigh the risks and benefits when deciding whether to initiate TTM for patients who have suffered PEA or asystolic arrest.

Overall, however, TTM should at least be considered for all survivors of cardiac arrest who remain unresponsive or if the GCS remains <8 following ROSC (Table 1.3). There are several important contraindications to the initiation of therapeutic cooling, including severe hemodynamic instability, continued unstable arrhythmias, and the presence of active hemorrhage. Withholding therapeutic cooling should also be considered in patients who have had a prolonged period of compromised perfusion, generally limiting practice to those with less than 60 min before ROSC. The likelihood of favorable neurologic outcome is felt to rapidly diminish beyond this duration of down time.

Rapid induction of cooling can be achieved by applying ice packs in the patient's groin, axilla, and neck, with close attention to the integrity of the skin at least every 15 min after application. In addition to ice packs, rapid cooling can be achieved by administering cold intravenous fluids, typically chilled to 4 °C and administered as a 20–30 ml/kg bolus (Table 1.2). Care should also be taken during cooling to prevent shivering, which can prolong the time to achieve target temperature. Prevention of shivering can often be achieved with opiates, acetaminophen, buspirone, intravenous magnesium, and skin counter-warming measures alone [34]. While most effective in shivering prevention, neuromuscular blocking agents are often reserved as a last resort at some centers, while they are used uniformly at others. It is imperative that goal temperature be achieved as quickly as possible and every effort should be made to achieve goal core temperature of 33 °C within 6 h (ideally 2 h [22]) of ROSC. Core temperature is best monitored with the aid of either a bladder or esophageal probe. Once the goal core temperature has been reached, patients are typically maintained at that temperature for 24 h with the aid of cooling blankets or pads.

TTM is associated with a number of risks. The most common adverse side-effects of cooling include electrolyte abnormalities (particularly hypokalemia and hyperglycemia), hypotension, coagulopathy and bleeding, bradycardia, ventricular arrhythmias, and breakdown in skin integrity due to adherent cooling devices. The majority of these complications can be managed without discontinuation of the hypothermic protocol. Frequent monitoring of electrolytes and aggressive electrolyte repletion during the cooling and maintenance phase is obligatory, and often requires assessment and management of electrolyte concentrations every 4–6 h.

Rewarming is typically executed slowly and cautiously after the target temperature has been maintained for 24 h. Rewarming is done with the aid of a cooling/heating apparatus to achieve a rise in the core temperature by no greater than 0.5 °C/h. During this time, it is important to continue monitoring electrolytes for reverse directional shifts. Once rewarming has been achieved, typically accepted to be a core temperature 36 °C or greater, neurologic function can be thoroughly and legitimately re-assessed.

Pericardial Tamponade

Pericardial tamponade is a life-threatening condition that can quickly lead to obstructive shock. Tamponade is caused by the accumulation of fluid or blood into the pericardial sack, but can at times result from massive mediastinal hemorrhage. It is a common misconception that large amounts of pericardial fluid are necessary to create tamponade physiology. Development of tamponade physiology primarily depends upon the rate at which fluid or blood accumulates in the pericardial space, and the ability of the pericardium to distend and accommodate the fluid. Tamponade and obstructive shock occur due to impaired diastolic filling of the less muscular right ventricle (and atrium) once the pericardial pressure exceeds right atrial pressure. The lack of right-sided diastolic filling leads to a drastic fall in right ventricular stroke volume and compromise of left ventricular preload and, in turn, a collapse in left-sided cardiac output. The physiology of cardiac tamponade is not unlike that of a tension pneumothorax, and immediate attention is needed to differentiate between the two conditions since the immediate and obligatory management of each condition is drastically different.

There are a host of conditions that can lead to pericardial effusion in the ICU setting and increase the risk of tamponade. Some of the most common causes of pericardial effusion seen by the ICU care provider include post-MI pericarditis, peri-infarction ventricular wall rupture, pericardial effusion after cardiac surgery (i.e., "Dressler's Syndrome"), blunt chest trauma, connective tissue disorders, malignancy, uremia, and aortic dissection. Physical exam findings of pericardial effusion and tamponade include increased jugular venous distention, distant or muffled heart sounds, and a narrow pulse pressure. *Pulsus paradoxis* can also be detected by demonstrating a drop in the systolic blood pressure by more than 10 mmHg with inspiration in the non-intubated patient. This phenomenon is sometimes easier to detect by witnessing significant respirophasic variation in the arterial line tracing with invasive blood pressure monitoring (provided the patient is not in A fib). A 12-lead ECG can be helpful in corroborating the suspicion of a significant pericardial effusion (and tamponade) when the tracing demonstrates low voltage or the presence of *electrical alternans*, which is caused by the shifting of the electrical cardiac axis via movement of the heart back and forth within a fluid-filled

Fig. 1.2 Para-sternal long axis view of echocardiogram obtained in a patient with both pleural effusion (pl) and pericardial effusion (pc). The labels "LV" and "RV" represent the left and right ventricle, respectively, and "a" identifies the descending aorta. Note that pericardial fluid (pc) abuts and travels anterior to the descending aorta, while pleural fluid (pl) settles inferior to the descending aorta

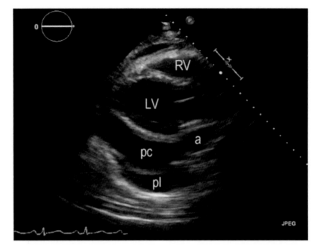

pericardium. One can only rely upon the chest radiograph to demonstrate an enlarging cardiac silhouette when the pericardial fluid has been slowly accumulating, and the pericardium has had sufficient time to distend and accommodate the increasing fluid. The most common method now used in the ICU to diagnose pericardial effusion and tamponade is bedside echocardiography.

Bedside echocardiography can quickly establish the presence of pericardial effusion in either the subcostal view or the parasternal long axis view. A pericardial effusion can easily be seen as a dark anechoic stripe surrounding the myocardium. Close attention is needed to distinguish between pericardial and pleural fluid when fluid is detected. The subcostal view is insufficient to make this determination, and it is recommended that the parasternal long axis view be used to distinguish between fluid tracking anterior to the descending aorta (pericardial fluid) and fluid tracking posterior to the descending aorta (pleural fluid) (Fig. 1.2). Echocardiographic findings concerning for tamponade physiology include inversion or collapse of the right atrium and right ventricle during diastole. This is best done by recording a loop of several cardiac cycles and re-examining systole and diastole at a slower, more controlled rate. Echocardiographic images obtained during tamponade can also reveal a large, fixed and dilated inferior vena cava without respirophasic variation.

Treatment of tamponade involves determining the safest and most immediate method of removing pericardial fluid or blood via pericardiocentesis. For patients in whom the suspicion is high for rapid reaccumulation of fluid, a pericardial drain or window should be considered to prevent recurrence.

Clinical Summary of Recommendations

1. Management of A fib should be based on clinical stability of the patient. Strong consideration should be made for anticoagulation of new onset A fib due to increased risk of in-hospital mortality and stroke, particularly in patients with severe sepsis.

2. Acute coronary syndrome is often difficult to detect in intubated and sedated ICU patients. A low threshold for assessment with ECG and biomarkers should be maintained, especially in rapidly deteriorating patients.
3. Management of cardiac arrest in the ICU setting should always focus on high-quality chest compressions and treatment of correctable causes of cardiovascular instability.
4. Basic bedside ultrasound skills can be of great assistance in evaluating the various causes of shock.
5. Strong consideration for post-cardiac arrest TTM should be given for patients with in-hospital and out-of-hospital cardiac arrest, resulting from both shockable and non-shockable rhythms (when the goals of care are compatible with the practice) in order to provide the best chance for a favorable neurologic recovery.

References

1. Annane D, Sebille V, Duboc D, Le Heuzey JY, Sadoul N, Bouvier E, et al. Incidence and prognosis of sustained arrhythmias in critically ill patients. Am J Resp Crit Care Med. 2008;178(1):20–5.
2. Walkey AJ, Wiener RS, Ghobrial JM, Curtis LH, Benjamin EJ. Incident stroke and mortality associated with new-onset atrial fibrillation in patients hospitalized with severe sepsis. JAMA. 2011;306(20):2248–54.
3. Chapman MJ, Moran JL, O'Fathartaigh MS, Peisach AR, Cunningham DN. Management of atrial tachyarrhythmias in the critically ill: a comparison of intravenous procainamide and amiodarone. Intensive Care Med. 1993;19(1):48–52.
4. Moran JL, Gallagher J, Peake SL, Cunningham DN, Salagaras M, Leppard P. Parenteral magnesium sulfate versus amiodarone in the therapy of atrial tachyarrhythmias: a prospective, randomized study. Crit Care Med. 1995;23(11):1816–24.
5. Balser JR, Martinez EA, Winters BD, Perdue PW, Clarke AW, Huang W, et al. Beta-adrenergic blockade accelerates conversion of postoperative supraventricular tachyarrhythmias. Anesthesiology. 1998;89(5):1052–9.
6. Hanna EB, Glancy DL. ST-segment depression and T-wave inversion: classification, differential diagnosis, and caveats. Cleve Clin J Med. 2011;78(6):404–14.
7. Yasue H, Touyama M, Kato H, Tanaka S, Akiyama F. Prinzmetal's variant form of angina as a manifestation of alpha-adrenergic receptor-mediated coronary artery spasm: documentation by coronary arteriography. Am Heart J. 1976;91(2):148–55.
8. Lockerman ZS, Rose DM, Cunningham Jr JN, Lichstein E. Postoperative ST-segment elevation in coronary artery bypass surgery. Chest. 1986;89(5):647–51.
9. Minor Jr RL, Scott BD, Brown DD, Winniford MD. Cocaine-induced myocardial infarction in patients with normal coronary arteries. Ann Intern Med. 1991;115(10):797–806.
10. Masip J, Roque M, Sanchez B, Fernandez R, Subirana M, Exposito JA. Noninvasive ventilation in acute cardiogenic pulmonary edema: systematic review and meta-analysis. JAMA. 2005;294(24):3124–30.
11. Shepard Jr JW, Pevernagie DA, Stanson AW, Daniels BK, Sheedy PF. Effects of changes in central venous pressure on upper airway size in patients with obstructive sleep apnea. Am J Resp Crit Care Med. 1996;153(1):250–4.
12. Caples SM, Gay PC. Noninvasive positive pressure ventilation in the intensive care unit: a concise review. Crit Care Med. 2005;33(11):2651–8.

13. Mehta S, Jay GD, Woolard RH, Hipona RA, Connolly EM, Cimini DM, et al. Randomized, prospective trial of bilevel versus continuous positive airway pressure in acute pulmonary edema. Crit Care Med. 1997;25(4):620–8.
14. Masip J, Betbese AJ, Paez J, Vecilla F, Canizares R, Padro J, et al. Non-invasive pressure support ventilation versus conventional oxygen therapy in acute cardiogenic pulmonary oedema: a randomised trial. Lancet. 2000;356(9248):2126–32.
15. Nava S, Carbone G, DiBattista N, Bellone A, Baiardi P, Cosentini R, et al. Noninvasive ventilation in cardiogenic pulmonary edema: a multicenter randomized trial. Am J Resp Crit Care Med. 2003;168(12):1432–7.
16. Eikelboom JW, Anand SS, Malmberg K, Weitz JI, Ginsberg JS, Yusuf S. Unfractionated heparing and low-molecular weight heparin in acute coronary syndrome without ST elevation: a meta-analysis. Lancet. 2000;355(9219):1936–42.
17. De Backer D, Biston P, Devriendt J, Madl C, Chochrad D, Aldecoa C, et al. Comparison of dopamine and norepinephrine in the treatment of shock. N Engl J Med. 2010;362(9):779–89.
18. Thiele H, Zeymer U, Neumann FJ, Ferenc M, Olbrich HG, Hausleiter J, et al. Intraaortic balloon support for myocardial infarction with cardiogenic shock. N Engl J Med. 2012;367(14):1287–96.
19. Meaney PA, Nadkarni VM, Kern KB, Indik JH, Halperin HR, Berg RA. Rhythms and outcomes of adult in-hospital cardiac arrest. Crit Care Med. 2010;38(1):101–8.
20. Kim YM, Yim HW, Jeong SH, Klem ML, Callaway CW. Does therapeutic hypothermia benefit adult cardiac arrest patients presenting with non-shockable initial rhythms? A systematic review and meta-analysis of randomized and non-randomized studies. Resuscitation. 2012;83(2):188–96.
21. Lundbye JB, Rai M, Ramu B, Hosseini-Khalili A, Li D, Slim HB, et al. Therapeutic hypothermia is associated with improved neurologic outcome and survival in cardiac arrest survivors of non-shockable rhythms. Resuscitation. 2012;83(2):202–7.
22. Hypothermia after Cardiac Arrest Study Group. Mild therapeutic hypothermia to improve the neurologic outcome after cardiac arrest. N Engl J Med. 2002;346(8):549–56.
23. Bernard SA, Gray TW, Buist MD, Jones BM, Silvester W, Gutteridge G, et al. Treatment of comatose survivors of out-of-hospital cardiac arrest with induced hypothermia. N Engl J Med. 2002;346(8):557–63.
24. Wenzel V, Lindner KH, Baubin MA, Voelckel WG. Vasopressin decreases endogneous catecholamin plasma concentrations during cardiopulmonary resuscitation in pigs. Crit Care Med. 2000;28(4):1096–100.
25. Stiell IG, Hebert PC, Wells GA, Vandemheen KL, Tang AS, Higginson LA, et al. Vasopressin versus epinephrine for inhospital cardiac arrest: a randomised controlled trial. Lancet. 2001;358(9276):105–9.
26. Gueugniaud PY, David JS, Chanzy E, Hubert H, Dubien PY, Mauriaucourt P, et al. Vasopressin and epinephrine vs. epinephrine alone in cardiopulmonary resuscitation. N Engl J Med. 2008;359(1):21–30.
27. Kudenchuk PJ, Cobb LA, Copass MK, Cummins RO, Doherty AM, Fahrenbruch CE, et al. Amiodarone for resuscitation after out-of-hospital cardiac arrest due to ventricular fibrillation. N Engl J Med. 1999;341(12):871–8.
28. Dorian P, Cass D, Schwartz B, Cooper R, Gelaznikas R, Barr A. Amiodarone as compared with lidocaine for shock-resistant ventricular fibrillation. N Engl J Med. 2002;346(12):884–90.
29. Stub D, Bernard S, Duffy SJ, Kaye DM. Post cardiac arrest syndrome: a review of therapeutic strategies. Circulation. 2011;123(13):1428–35.
30. Mongardon N, Dumas F, Ricome S, Grimaldi D, Hissem T, Pene F, et al. Postcardiac arrest syndrome: from immediate resuscitation to long-term outcome. Ann Intensive Care. 2011;1(1):45.
31. Storm C, Nee J, Roser M, Jorres A, Hasper D. Mild hypothermia treatment in patients resuscitated from non-shockable cardiac arrest. Emerg Med J. 2012;29(2):100–3.
32. Kilgannon JH, Jones AE, Shapiro NI, Angelos MG, Milcarek B, Hunter K, et al. Association between arterial hyperoxia following resuscitation from cardiac arrest and in-hospital mortality. JAMA. 2010;303(21):2165–71.

33. Nielsen N, Wetterslev J, Cronberg T, Erlinge D, Gasche Y, Hassager C, et al. Targeted tempera-
    ture management at 33 degrees C versus 36 degrees C after cardiac arrest. N Engl J Med.
    2013;369(23):2197–206.
34. Testori C, Sterz F, Behringer W, Haugk M, Uray T, Zeiner A, et al. Mild therapeutic hypother-
    mia is associated with favourable outcome in patients after cardiac arrest with non-shockable
    rhythms. Resuscitation. 2011;82(9):1162–7.
35. Choi HA, Ko SB, Presciutti M, Fernandez L, Carpenter AM, Lesch C, et al. Prevention of
    shivering during therapeutic temperature modulation: the Columbia anti-shivering protocol.
    Neurocrit Care. 2011;14(3):389–94.

Chapter 2
Renal Complications

Elizabeth J. Lechner and Michael G. Risbano

Abstract Acute kidney injury (AKI) is a common problem in critically ill patients and is associated with adverse clinical outcomes, including increased mortality. Elevation in serum creatinine is the primary diagnostic indicator of AKI. Critically ill patients pose a diagnostic and therapeutic challenge as their clinical circumstances are frequently changing, and alterations in serum creatinine and glomerular filtration rate often lag behind the onset of renal injury. Analysis of urine sediment, osmolality, electrolytes, and renal ultrasound can aid in the diagnosis of AKI and distinguish between prerenal, postrenal and intrinsic causes of renal failure. Some of the most common causes of AKI encountered by intensivists will be discussed here, including ischemic injury, medication-related nephrotoxicity, rhabdomyolysis, acute tubulointerstitial nephritis, and vascular processes. Treatment of AKI depends on the etiology and often includes removal of an injurious medication or exposure. In addition, fluid administration is a major component of therapy in most cases. Renal replacement therapy is available for more severe cases of AKI with critical electrolyte abnormalities, severe acidemia, or massive volume overload refractory to non-invasive medical treatment.

Keywords Acute kidney injury • Acute renal failure • Prerenal, postrenal and acute tubular necrosis • Renal replacement therapy • Acidosis • Fluid management

E.J. Lechner, M.D.
University of Pittsburgh Medical Center, Montefiore Hospital,
3459 Fifth Avenue, NW 628, Pittsburgh, PA 15213, USA
e-mail: lechnerlj@upmc.edu

M.G. Risbano, M.D., M.A., F.C.C.P. (✉)
Division of Pulmonary, Allergy and Critical Care Medicine, University of Pittsburgh
Medical Center, Montefiore Hospital, 3459 Fifth Avenue, NW 628, Pittsburgh,
PA 15213, USA
e-mail: risbanomg@upmc.edu

J.B. Richards and R.D. Stapleton (eds.), *Non-Pulmonary Complications of Critical Care:* 19
A Clinical Guide, Respiratory Medicine, DOI 10.1007/978-1-4939-0873-8_2,
© Springer Science+Business Media New York 2014

Introduction

Contemporary preferred terminology for acute renal failure (ARF) is acute kidney injury (AKI) [1]. AKI is not a disease process in isolation, rather it is a clinical syndrome that occurs rapidly and impairs the kidney's ability to eliminate waste products. Critically ill patients often develop AKI, and AKI is associated with adverse clinical outcomes including increased hospital length of stay and mortality. Even modest increases in serum creatinine (0.3–0.4 mg/dL) advances mortality [2]. Recognizing and diagnosing AKI in critically ill patients is challenging due to dynamic and frequently changing clinical circumstances. In this chapter we review the broad categories of AKI encountered in critically ill patients and discuss how to address contemporary diagnostic strategies and treatment options.

Epidemiology

Due to the variety of definitions associated with AKI, the estimated prevalence of AKI in critically ill patients can greatly vary. AKI affects up to 25 % of intensive care unit (ICU) patients with a reported mortality ranging from 15 to 60 % [3]. AKI requiring renal replacement therapy (RRT) is an independent risk factor for in-hospital mortality, which can be as high as 70 %. AKI is associated with increased health care costs, length of stay, and risk of developing chronic kidney disease. Risk factors for the development of AKI are variable and include advanced age, sepsis, cardiac surgery, diabetes, rhabdomyolysis, pre-existing renal disease, hypovolemia and shock. While kidney injury occurring outside the hospital can usually be attributed to an isolated cause, AKI that evolves during hospitalization, particularly during critical illness, generally has a worse prognosis and may result from multiple renal insults including hypovolemia, surgery, decreased cardiac output, medication effects (anesthetics, diuretics, nephrotoxic drugs), or radiographic contrast agents.

Definition of Acute Kidney Injury

In a broad sense, ARF is defined as a rapid decrease in the glomerular filtration rate (GFR), occurring over a period of minutes to days. As the rate of production of metabolic waste exceeds the rate of renal excretion, serum urea and creatinine concentrations rise [2]. However, the lack of a precise and universally accepted definition for ARF has limited clinical and translational research. Consensus conferences and publications from the Acute Dialysis Quality Initiative (ADQI), American Society of Nephrology (ASN), ARF Advisory group, the International Society of Nephrology (ISN), National Kidney Foundations (NKF), and the Kidney Disease Improving Global Outcomes (KDIGO) groups have worked to identify and correct these knowledge gaps and to develop a universal definition.

Table 2.1 Comparison of RIFLE, AKIN and KDIGO criteria for acute kidney injury

		Serum creatinine criteria	Urine output criteria
RIFLE	Risk	1.5-fold increase in creatinine OR decrease in GFR by 25 %	<0.5 mL/kg/h for 6 h
	Injury	Two-fold increase in creatinine or decrease in GFR by 50 %	<0.5 mL/kg/h for 12 h
	Failure	Three-fold increase in creatinine or decrease in GFR by 75 %	<0.3 mL/kg/h for 24 h or anuria for 12 h
	Loss	Need for renal replacement therapy for more than 4 weeks	
	ESRD	Need for renal replacement therapy for more than 3 months	
AKIN	Stage 1	Increase to ≥0.3 mg/dL or ≥1.5 to <2.0 times baseline)	<0.5 mL/kg/h for 6 h
	Stage 2	Increase to ≥2.0 to <3.0 times baseline	<0.5 mL/kg/h for 12 h
	Stage 3	Increase to ≥3.0 times baseline	<0.3 mL/kg/h for 24 h or anuria for 12 h
KDIGO	Stage 1	Increase to 1.5–1.9 times baseline OR ≥0.3 mg/dL	<0.5 mL/kg/h for 6–12 h
	Stage 2	Increase to 2.0–2.9 times baseline	<0.5 mL/kg/h for ≥12 h
	Stage 3	Increase to 3.0 times baseline OR increase to ≥4.0 mg/dL	<0.3 mL/kg/h for ≥24 h OR anuria for ≥12 h OR initiation of renal replacement therapy

In 2007, a collaborative research focus group between the ASN, ISN, NKF and the European Society of Intensive Care Medicine recommended that the term *acute kidney injury* replace the term *acute renal failure*. This emphasizes that an acute decline in kidney function is often secondary to an injury causing functional or structural changes in the kidneys [4, 5]. The ADQI developed the Risk, Injury, Failure, Loss and End-stage kidney (RIFLE) criteria (Table 2.1) which defines AKI as an increase in serum creatinine by ≥1.5× baseline within 7 (or fewer) days. This RIFLE criterion stratifies patients into three categories of severity: risk, injury, and failure, and defines two outcomes of AKI: need for RRT for >4 weeks (loss) and permanent kidney failure (end-stage renal disease or ESRD) based on serum creatinine, GFR, and urine output. The Acute Kidney Injury Network (AKIN) group subsequently modified the definition of AKI to be an abrupt (within 48 h) increase in serum creatinine concentration of ≥0.3 mg/dL from baseline, a percentage increase in serum creatinine concentration of ≥50 %, or oliguria. The AKIN criteria removed criteria for GFR used by the RIFLE definition and focused on changes in serum creatinine and urine output to define three stages of AKI. Additionally, patients were categorized as having *Failure* if they were initiated on RRT, regardless of serum creatinine or urine output at the time of initiating RRT (Table 2.1). Most recently, the KDIGO guidelines further modified both the RIFLE and AKIN criteria, utilizing changes only in serum creatinine and urine output, and not changes in GFR, for staging. KDIGO maintains the AKIN definition that the absolute increase in serum creatinine of 0.3 mg/dL must occur within 48 h, but the time frame for a 50 % increase in serum creatinine is 7 days, as defined by the RIFLE criteria. When using any of these criteria, patients are classified according to the parameter that classifies them in the most severe stage of injury.

Diagnosis and Assessment of Kidney Injury

History

Obtaining a patient's history is important in determining the etiology of AKI. Many critically ill patients have hypertension, diabetes, vascular disease, chronic glomerulonephritis, and other chronic underlying conditions that can cause chronic kidney disease. Knowledge of the patient's baseline creatinine (if available) is essential, as is knowledge of prior episodes of AKI or prior need for RRT. Confirming the patient's medications and any recent medication changes should be done, as NSAIDS, ACE inhibitors, diuretics and antibiotics may contribute to renal dysfunction. Additionally, recent episodes of hypotension or administration of intravenous contrast should be noted.

Signs and Symptoms

AKI can be asymptomatic in ICU patients, but some patients may complain of nausea, vomiting, anorexia, hiccups, lethargy or gastrointestinal bleeding. Uremic patients may experience asterixis, altered level of consciousness, and/or seizures. Uremic acidosis may cause Kussmaul breathing, and hyperkalemia may cause cardiac arrhythmias.

Assessment of Intravascular Volume

A focused physical exam, with an emphasis on assessing intravascular volume status, is important in evaluating patients with AKI. Decreased skin turgor and mucosal dehydration, tachycardia, orthostatic blood pressure, and/or decreased urine output all indicate an increased likelihood of whole body volume depletion. Reciprocally, lower extremity or sacral edema, elevated jugular venous distention, cardiac rubs/gallops, ascites, pleural effusions and/or pulmonary crackles may indicate volume overload.

Intravascular volume assessment of the ICU patient by the physical exam alone is often not sensitive or specific, and adjunctive studies are often needed to increase the accuracy of clinical volume assessment. Measuring central venous pressure (CVP) either noninvasively or with a central venous catheter has been traditionally utilized as an indicator of volume status and responsiveness to fluid challenge; however, the clinical utility of measuring CVP has recently been challenged [6]. Regardless, use of CVP as a target for intravascular volume assessment and volume responsiveness continues to be widely used in clinical practice.

Laboratory Data

Serum Creatinine

While diagnosing AKI in critically ill patients is complicated by patients' dynamic and frequently changing clinical conditions, serum creatinine remains the primary means of assessing renal function and dysfunction. Age, sex, race, muscle mass, catabolic state and medications, however, can adversely affect renal function and must be considered when interpreting creatinine levels. Formulae for estimating GFR from serum creatinine, such as the Modification of Diet in Renal Disease (MDRD) formula or the Cockcroft and Gault equation, estimate steady-state creatinine clearance. Creatinine is primarily produced by muscle tissue and released into the circulation at a rate of 15–25 mg/kg/day and 10–20 mg/kg/day for middle-aged males and females, respectively. Creatinine excretion primarily depends on glomerular filtration, with very little creatinine secreted into the tubules or reabsorbed into the systemic circulation. Therefore, for the serum creatinine concentration to increase >1 mg/dL, the GFR must decrease by half. As such, serum creatinine concentration is not a particularly reliable measure of renal function in critically ill patients, as patients' renal function may rapidly change with only an associated modest change in creatinine. As changes in serum creatinine often lag behind acute renal injury, creatinine initially underestimates the degree of injury. Thus, other indicators of kidney injury must be utilized in conjunction with creatinine to reliably and accurately detect early AKI. Specifically, urine output, urine sediment, osmolality, electrolytes, and renal ultrasound may increase the precision with which early AKI is detected, as well as assist in identifying possible etiologies (Fig. 2.1). Often, depending upon the clinical scenario, critically ill patients with AKI will have a variety of these diagnostic studies performed simultaneously.

Serum Urea

Urea is a nitrogen-containing breakdown product of protein catabolism primarily excreted by the kidneys. Under normal conditions urea is filtered and 35–50 % is reabsorbed by the renal tubules. At times of decreased renal perfusion, up to 90 % of urea may be reabsorbed. As creatinine is not reabsorbed, urea increases more rapidly with deceased renal blood flow, and particularly with prerenal failure. Prerenal failure is suspected when a blood urea nitrogen to creatinine ratio (BUN:Cr) is increased from the normal ratio of 10:1 to $\geq$20:1. Of note, BUN levels can increase in the absence of renal failure, due to corticosteroid use, upper gastrointestinal (GI) bleeding with metabolism of blood and reabsorption of urea from the GI tract, and increased protein load from overfeeding or starvation (both of which result in increased protein metabolism and urea production).

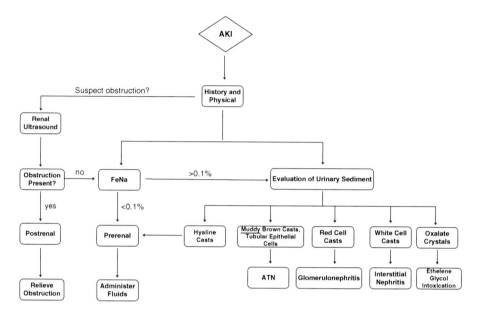

Fig. 2.1 Algorithm for diagnosis and treatment of acute kidney injury. Renal ultrasound may help diagnose obstructive uropathy by identifying hydronephrosis or bladder distension. Fractional excretion of sodium (FeNa) can distinguish between prerenal and intrinsic causes. The intrinsic cause can be identified through examination of the urinary sediment

Other Diagnostic Lab Tests

Other blood tests can be used in conjunction with serum creatinine and urea nitrogen to help determine the etiology of the AKI. Hypercalcemia and hyperuricemia may indicate an underlying malignancy. Elevated creatine kinase may signify rhabdomyolysis. Serum immunoelectrophoresis is abnormal in myeloma. Peripheral eosinophilia is suggestive of allergic interstitial nephritis. An osmolal gap (difference between measured and calculated osmolalities) suggests ethylene glycol or other non-ethanol alcohol toxicity [5].

Urine Output

Acute oliguria is defined as less than 400 mL of urine output per day, and may be the earliest sign of impaired renal function. Unfortunately, oliguria is an insensitive indicator of impending renal failure, as the absence of oliguria does not preclude nonoliguric renal failure.

Urine Sediment

Examination of the urinary sediment is helpful in distinguishing between the various causes of renal failure. In prerenal failure, hyaline and fine granular casts are usually present. In intrinsic renal failure due to acute tubular necrosis (ATN), muddy brown granular casts and tubular epithelial cells can predominate. White-cell casts and eosinophils may represent interstitial nephritis, and red-cell casts are typical in glomerulonephritis [5]. Heme-positive urine in the absence of erythrocytes suggests myoglobinuria or hemoglobinuria, and supports the diagnosis of rhabdomyolysis or transfusion reaction. The presence of oxalate crystals in the urine suggests ethylene glycol intoxication [5].

Urine Electrolytes and Osmolality

Urine osmolality, urine sodium concentration, fractional excretion of sodium (FE_{Na}), and the ratio of urine to plasma creatinine can differentiate between the causes of AKI. FE_{Na} distinguishes between prerenal azotemia and ATN:

$$FE_{Na} = \frac{\text{Urine Na (mEq/L)}}{\text{Urine Cr (mg/dL)}} \times \frac{\text{Serum Cr (mg/dL)}}{\text{Serum Na (mEq/L)}} \times 100$$

One of the earliest signs of tubular damage is decreased ability to concentrate the urine. ATN is characterized by a urine osmolality of less than 350 mOsm/kg, U_{Na} concentration greater than 40 mmol/L, and FE_{Na} greater than 1.0 % [6]. Prerenal azotemia is associated with a urine osmolality greater than 500 mOsm/kg, a U_{Na} concentration less than 20 mmol/L, and a FE_{Na} of less than 1.0 %. The accuracy of these indices is decreased with volume resuscitation, dopamine, mannitol, and diuretics. Therefore, urine specimens used to determine urine osmolality, U_{Na} (urinary concentration of sodium) and FE_{Na} should be collected before any such therapies are initiated. If a patient has recently received diuretics, the fractional excretion of urea (FE_{Ur}) can be used instead of the FE_{Na}.

$$FE_{Ur} = \frac{\text{Urine Ur (mg/dL)}}{\text{Urine Cr (mg/dL)}} \times \frac{\text{Serum Cr (mg/dL)}}{\text{Serum Ur (mg/dL)}} \times 100$$

Normal values of FE_{Ur} are 50–65 %, and a FE_{Ur} of <35 % indicates renal hypoperfusion. Note that the FE_{Ur} cannot distinguish between prerenal failure and ATN. Furthermore, the FE_{Ur} may be less accurate in patients experiencing osmotic diuresis.

Imaging Studies

Renal ultrasound (US) is often the first line imaging technique for critically ill patients with AKI. Renal US can accurately measure kidney size and detect hydronephrosis without the use of intravenous (IV) contrast. Small kidneys (evidence of chronic kidney disease) and horseshoe or unilateral kidney (evidence of congenital abnormalities) can assist in contextualizing a patient with AKI. Although evaluation of renal perfusion can be assessed by Doppler can determine renal viability by presence or absence of flow, the measurements are not quantitative. Obtaining accurate US images in ICU patients can be technically difficult and may require an experienced operator. In obstructive renal failure, computed tomography (CT) imaging can evaluate the level and site of obstruction. The decision to administer IV contrast for vascular assessment is often made on an individual patient basis.

Biomarkers

As serum creatinine is a slow and sometimes insensitive marker of kidney injury, several novel biomarkers for AKI are under investigation, though they are not yet available for routine use. Cystatin-C, a cysteine–proteinase inhibitor, is a small protein produced by nucleated cells that is freely filtered across the glomerulus, and therefore reflects GFR. Cystatin-C levels rise earlier than creatinine in critically ill patients with AKI. Cystatin-C levels are independent of muscle mass, allowing for more accurate estimation of GFR than serum creatinine [7]. Neutrophil gelatinase (NGAL), a 25-kDa protein, is up-regulated rapidly after AKI and can be measured in the urine or serum using enzyme-linked immunosorbent assay (ELISA) or fluorescence immunoassay. It has shown particular promise as a marker of AKI in patients with liver failure, with recent studies demonstrating that urinary NGAL can detect AKI in cirrhotic patients and can distinguish hepatorenal syndrome (HRS) from other causes of renal injury [7].

Causes of AKI

Some of the most common causes of AKI in critically ill patients are listed in Table 2.2. The causes are usually classified into one of three categories: prerenal, postrenal, or intrinsic.

Prerenal

Prerenal failure occurs due to decreased circulating blood volume, due to hypovolemia or a relative decrease in effective blood volume due to sepsis, hepatic failure, anaphylaxis, or vasodilatory drugs. Hemorrhage, gastrointestinal fluid loss

Table 2.2 Common causes of prerenal, intrinsic, and postrenal AKI in the ICU

Prerenal	Intrinsic	Postrenal
Sepsis	Acute tubular necrosis	Prostatic hypertrophy
Hypovolemia	Drugs	Prostate or cervical tumors
Hemorrhage	Toxins	Ureteral or urethral stones
GI fluid loss	Microcapillary occlusion	Neurogenic bladder
Surgery	Glomerular occlusion	Ureteral obstruction
Burns	Rhabdomyolysis	(i.e., from RP
Anaphylaxis	Hemolysis (HUS/TTP)	lymphadenopathy)
Hepatic failure	Tumor lysis syndrome	Intra-abdominal hypertension
Vasodilatory drugs	Vascular	
Renal-artery or renal-vein occlusion	Glomerulonephritis	
	Acute interstitial nephritis	
	Intra-abdominal hypertension	

(diarrhea, vomiting, or nasogastric suction), renal losses (diuretics or glycosuria), trauma, surgery, and burns are other common etiologies of prerenal failure in critically ill patients. The renal structure and microstructure remain preserved early in prerenal failure. A reduction in the GFR coupled with an increased stimulus for salt and water reabsorption leads to high urine-to-plasma creatinine ratio. Urine sodium concentration is typically low. Elderly patients are particularly susceptible to prerenal azotemia due to a predisposition to hypovolemia and high prevalence of renal-artery atherosclerotic disease. Concomitant exposure to certain medications including angiotensin converting enzyme (ACE) inhibitors, diuretics, nonsteroidal anti-inflammatory drugs (NSAIDs), tacrolimus, and cyclosporine can also precipitate prerenal azotemia. Prerenal AKI is usually fully reversible if the underlying cause is rapidly identified and treated [5].

Postrenal

Postrenal AKI, caused by obstruction of the urinary outflow tract, leads to hydronephrosis and enlargement of the renal pelvic cavity, with minimal distention of the renal papilla and few microscopic changes. It usually occurs due to ureteral or bladder-outlet obstruction from external compression with mass effect, tumor, or intrarenal obstruction due to crystals or renal calculi. Prostatic hypertrophy, prostate or cervical cancers, or retroperitoneal disorders are the most common causes. Neurogenic bladder can also result in functional obstruction. Renal ultrasound can be used to visualize obstructive uropathy and hydronephrosis and make the diagnosis. Like prerenal AKI, the potential for full recovery is good if the etiology of postrenal failure is determined and the obstruction is relieved quickly. The potential for recovery is inversely related to the duration of the obstruction.

Table 2.3 Nephrotoxic medications and mechanism of injury

Drugs that may cause acute renal failure in the ICU and possible mechanisms of injury
Radiocontrast agents (mechanism unknown)
Aminoglycosides (direct cellular toxicity from tubular cell accumulation)
Amphotericin (direct tubular cell toxicity)
Nonsteroidal anti-inflammatory drugs (prostaglandin blockade with afferent arteriolar vasoconstriction)
Angiotensin-converting enzyme inhibitors (efferent arteriolar vasodilatation)
Angiotensin receptor blockers (efferent arteriolar vasodilatation)
β-Lactam antibiotics (interstitial nephropathy)
Cisplatin (tubular cell toxicity)
Cyclosporin A (afferent arteriolar vasoconstriction and interstitial nephropathy)
FK-506 (tacrolimus) (afferent arteriolar vasoconstriction and interstitial nephropathy)

Reprinted with permission from Bellomo R. Acute renal failure. Semin Respir Crit Care Med. 2011 Oct;32(5):639–50

Intrinsic

Intrinsic AKI is due to parenchymal injury of the blood vessels, glomeruli, tubules, or interstitium, and most commonly occurs after periods of prolonged or severe ischemia or exposure to nephrotoxins [2]. Damage to the tubular epithelium leads to sloughing of cellular debris and formation of casts which can occlude the tubular lumen. Prerenal AKI can lead to ATN if the renal perfusion is severe and the duration is long enough to cause tubular cell death. Congestive heart failure, cirrhosis and HRS, medications, sepsis, and renal vascular diseases such as renal artery thrombosis, renal artery stenosis, vasculitides, malignant hypertension, and hemolytic uremic syndrome are common causes [5].

Drugs and toxins can cause intrinsic renal failure by direct damage to the renal tubular cells, reduction in renal perfusion, rhabdomyolysis, drug precipitation causing intratubular obstruction, or allergic interstitial nephritis. Antimicrobials, radiocontrast agents, and chemotherapeutic agents are common causes of drug-induced AKI (Table 2.3).

Specific Etiologies of AKI

Ischemic Injury

When renal perfusion pressure drops, autoregulation maintains normal blood flow and GFR. Prostaglandins mediate a drop in afferent glomerular arteriolar resistance and sustain glomerular capillary pressure. An increase in efferent glomerular arteriolar resistance mediated by angiotensin II also supports glomerular capillary pressure. However, when renal perfusion pressure drops below the autoregulatory range, endogenous vasoconstrictors increase afferent arteriolar resistance, which reduces glomerular capillary pressure and GFR, resulting in functional prerenal pathophysiology. Initially, the postglomerular capillary bed perfusing the renal tubules has diminished blood flow and pressures, but the tubules remain intact. Increasing severity and duration of ischemia, however, causes structural tubular damage and further renal dysfunction. Impaired sodium reabsorption by injured tubular epithelial cells increases sodium concentration in the tubular lumen and leads to polymerization of the Tamm–Horsfall protein, which contributes to cast formation [2].

Depletion of ATP leads to a number of critical alterations in metabolism. Cytoskeletal disruption leads to sloughing of cells from the brush-border membrane and obstruction of downstream tubules. Proteases and phospholipases are activated and cause oxidant injury to tubular cells and endothelial cells of the peritubular capillaries. Oxidant injury together with an increase in production of vasoconstrictors such as endothelin leads to vasoconstriction, congestion, hypoperfusion, and expression of adhesion molecules, which initiates leukocyte infiltration causing obstruction of the microcirculation and release of proinflammatory and chemotactic cytokines, reactive oxygen species, and proteolytic enzymes which damage tubular cells [2].

Elderly patients or those with atherosclerosis, hypertension, or pre-existing chronic renal failure are particularly susceptible to acute ischemic injury. While ischemic AKI classically occurs after an acute drop in systolic blood pressure below 90 mmHg during shock, normotensive ischemic ARF can also occur, involving milder degrees of low-perfusion states, in patients with increased susceptibility.

Contrast-Induced Nephropathy

Contrast-induced nephropathy (CIN) is acute deterioration of renal function after intravenous radiocontrast administration. Generally there is an increase in serum creatinine concentration more than 0.5 mg/dL or 25 % above baseline within 48 h of contrast administration [8]. The exact mechanism behind CIN is not clear. Though the incidence of CIN is low in the general population, critically ill patients are at increased risk due to multiple coexisting renal insults including hypotension, concomitant administration of nephrotoxic medications, sepsis, diabetes, cirrhosis, nephritic syndrome, and congestive heart failure.

There is no specific treatment for CIN once it develops, so prevention is a major focus. Ascorbic acid, fenoldopam, atrial natriuretic peptides, calcium channel blockers, prostaglandin E1, and endothelin receptor antagonist have been studied as preventative medications, but none have demonstrated an absolute benefit [9]. N-acetylcysteine (NAC) has also been proposed as a preventive therapy against CIN, but results across multiple studies remain inconsistent [10]. Contemporary management therefore centers upon intravenous fluid loading and using iso-osmolar contrast agents to minimize the risk of CIN [11]. Some studies have shown that sodium bicarbonate may confer more protection against CIN as compared to saline [12, 13]. The Renal Insufficiency Following Contrast Media Administration (REMEDIAL) study compared 326 at-risk patients with chronic kidney disease receiving intravenous contrast, and demonstrated that sodium bicarbonate and NAC infusions prevented CIN compared to normal saline and NAC [12]. Additionally, the Reno-Protective Effect of Hydration with Sodium Bicarbonate Plus N-Acetylsteine in Patients Undergoing Emergency Percutaneous Coronary Intervention (RENO) study evaluated 111 patients undergoing emergency percutaneous coronary intervention and demonstrated that rapid infusion of sodium bicarbonate plus NAC before contrast injection was both safe and effective in preventing CIN [13]. Follow-up studies, however, have reported conflicting results, [14, 15], and a meta-analysis concluded that patient heterogeneity may significantly influence the benefit of sodium bicarbonate [16]. In high-risk patients with chronic renal failure, hemofiltration has been reported to prevent CIN, though the clinical applicability of this is limited [17].

Nephrotoxic Drugs

Many drugs commonly administered in the ICU have nephrotoxic potential. Direct nephrotoxicity can lead to prerenal AKI, intrinsic AKI, or tubular obstruction. Renal syndromes such as renal tubular acidosis, Fanconi-like syndrome, and nephrogenic diabetes insipidus may also occur. Indirect nephrotoxicity occurs when agents damage non-renal tissues and produce breakdown products that cause renal failure (drug-induced hemolytic anemia or rhabdomyolysis), or when they interfere with the metabolism of other nephrotoxic medications. Though many medications may cause renal damage, anti-infective agents are some of the most commonly administered agents with nephrotoxic potential. Risk factors for development of AKI induced by antimicrobials include duration of therapy, excessive drug serum levels, pre-existing impaired kidney function, renal hypoperfusion, sepsis, and concurrent use of other nephrotoxic medications. The most successful strategy to prevent antimicrobial-induced kidney insufficiency is to decrease a patient's exposure to these agents, including limiting use based on pathogen susceptibility and limiting treatment duration to recommended treatment courses for the specific infection. For renally cleared agents, dosing should be adjusted according to creatinine clearance, acknowledging this may only be a rough estimate of GFR in critically ill patients. Monitoring medication serum concentrations may also help prevent dose-related renal toxicity. Of note, serum creatinine levels can increase with use of trimethoprim-sulfamethoxazole as this medication competes with creatinine for tubular secretion, not due to an actual decrease in GFR.

Vancomycin

Vancomycin is a key antibiotic for treating Gram-positive bacteria, particularly methicillin-resistant *Staphylococcus aureus* (MRSA). Vancomycin is primarily eliminated by renal excretion through glomerular filtration as well as active tubular secretion. The exact mechanism of vancomycin-induced nephrotoxicity is not well understood, but is thought to involve proximal renal tubular cell necrosis, oxidative stress, and mitochondrial damage [18].

Elevated vancomycin trough levels are a significant predictor of nephrotoxicity. A retrospective analysis of patients with MRSA pneumonia treated with vancomycin demonstrated that patients with higher vancomycin trough levels (levels ≥15 µg/mL) and prolonged treatment duration (courses ≥14 days) were more likely to develop renal toxicity, defined as a 0.5 mg/dL or greater than 50 % increase in baseline serum creatinine [19]. However, as the temporal relationship between elevated trough concentrations and development of nephrotoxicity was unclear, it is difficult to discern whether elevated trough levels represent a cause or effect of the accompanying renal failure. The concomitant use of vancomycin and aminoglycosides also significantly increases the risk of renal toxicity even more than when receiving any one therapy alone [18].

Patients typically recover from vancomycin-induced nephrotoxicity if the antibiotic is discontinued or dosage is appropriately adjusted [18].

Aminoglycosides

Aminoglycosides cover both Gram-negative bacilli and Gram-positive cocci, and despite years of use, bacterial resistance to aminoglycosides has not significantly increased. The most common complication of aminoglycoside administration is nephrotoxicity, estimated to occur in 10–20 % of patients receiving aminoglycosides [20]. Risk factors for development of aminoglycoside nephrotoxicity include increased age, diabetes, cirrhosis, chronic kidney disease, metabolic disturbances, concomitant use of other potentially nephrotoxic drugs (furosemide, ACE inhibitor, NSAIDs, vancomycin, colistin, cephalosporins, piperacillin, clindamycin, or iodinated contrast media), prolonged duration of therapy, or high concentrations of the drug.

Aminoglycosides are primarily cleared through the kidneys. They are filtered by the glomerulus, after which they reach the proximal tubule epithelial cells and bind to the brush-border membrane. Accumulation of aminoglycosides in endosomes and lysosomes results in cellular apoptosis and necrosis and decreased GFR [20].

Nephrotoxicity due to aminoglycosides generally occurs during treatment or a few days after discontinuation of treatment, with a mean delay of 9 days between first administration of the drug and resultant nephrotoxicity. However, increases in plasma creatinine associated with aminoglycoside toxicity have been reported to occur as late as 21 days after initiation of therapy. Recovery of renal function usually occurs after discontinuation of the drug without the need for RRT.

Standard (multiple-daily) and once-daily dosing regimens are equivalent with regard to bacteriologic cure, although once-daily dosing reduces mortality and incidence of nephrotoxicity [20]. The convenience of once-daily dosing and cost-reduction are additional benefits.

Nephrotoxic anti-infective agents should be used with caution, especially in patients with additional risk factors for kidney injury. However, in some cases prompt treatment of life-threatening infections must take precedence over the potential for nephrotoxicity. Guidelines recommend monitoring of drug levels when possible to ensure appropriate dosing, and limiting the duration of treatment to the minimum time needed to treat the infection [21].

Nonsteroidal Anti-Inflammatory Drugs

NSAIDs cause AKI by inhibiting prostaglandins. Prostaglandins are produced from cell membrane lipid precursors through enzymatic activity of cyclooxygenases. Prostaglandins are vasodilators, and are particularly important for maintaining renal perfusion in conditions of prolonged vasoconstriction such as chronic kidney disease, volume depletion, effective arterial volume depletion (heart failure, nephrotic syndrome, and cirrhosis), prolonged use of vasoactive medications such as norepinephrine or vasopressin, or severe hypercalcemia with renal arteriolar vasoconstriction. NSAIDs inhibit cyclooxygenase, leading to a reduction in prostaglandin synthesis, which can result in reversible renal ischemia, decreased glomerular filtration and AKI [22].

Increase in plasma creatinine concentration can occur at any time during NSAID use but usually occurs during the first 3–7 days of therapy. Urinalysis generally does not demonstrate hematuria or proteinuria. Hyaline casts or renal tubular epithelial cell casts may be seen.

NSAID-induced AKI can be minimized by limiting or avoiding NSAID use in high-risk patients. In addition, NSAIDs should be avoided in patients requiring iodinated contrast or other nephrotoxic medications. NSAID-induced AKI is treated by discontinuing the offending agent. Volume resuscitation may also benefit patients with coexisting volume depletion. Renal recovery may occur quickly; however, time to recovery is affected by the presence of underlying chronic kidney disease or concomitant renal insults. Further evaluation, including possible renal biopsy, should be considered if recovery does not occur within 3–7 days.

Acute Interstitial Nephritis

Acute interstitial nephritis (AIN) is an allergic reaction caused by a variety of drugs, including penicillins, cephalosporins, ciprofloxacin, rifampin, sulfonamides, cimetidine, allopurinol, and NSAIDs. AIN can also be due to infectious (Legionnaire's disease, cytomegalovirus, and Hantavirus), autoimmune (lupus), alloimmune (renal transplant rejection), and infiltrative (sarcoidosis, leukemia, and lymphoma) processes. AIN is associated with a classic triad of fever, rash, and eosinophilia. Urinalysis may show leukocyturia with eosinophils, leukocyte casts, and low-grade proteinuria. Tubular dysfunction occurs in the majority of patients with AIN, with interstitial infiltrates composed of lymphocytes, macrophages, eosinophils, and plasma cells. The diagnosis is usually made based on clinical history and supported by laboratory findings, and can be confirmed by renal biopsy. AIN is usually reversible after discontinuing the offending agent or treating the underlying disease. Corticosteroids administered early (within 7 days of diagnosis) can improve the recovery of renal function [23].

Glomerulonephritis/Vasculitis

Acute glomerulonephritis and vasculitis often results in transfer to the ICU for management of associated renal or respiratory failure. Renal failure due to glomerulonephritis and vasculitis includes: postinfectious glomerulonephritis, rickettsial infection, bacterial endocarditis, Goodpasture's syndrome, systemic lupus erythematosis, granulomatosis with polyangiitis, and Henoch–Schönlein purpura. Diagnosis is based on clinical presentation. Urinalysis typically shows nephritic sediment with red cells as well as white and red cell casts. Additional laboratory studies include antinuclear antibody, anti-GBM antibodies, serum complement levels (C3, C4), anti-neutrophil cytoplasmic antibodies, and antistreptolysin antibodies. Renal biopsy is typically recommended to obtain the correct diagnosis and guide management.

Rhabdomyolysis

AKI is a complication of rhabdomyolysis, and represents 7–10 % of all cases of AKI in the USA. The outcome of rhabdomyolysis is worse when complicated by AKI, with a reported mortality of 59 % among critically ill patients with the coexisting conditions [24]. The exact mechanism by which rhabdomyolysis impairs glomerular filtration is unclear, but intrarenal vasoconstriction, direct and ischemic tubule injury, and tubular obstruction all likely play a role [24]. Myoglobin is concentrated in the renal tubules and precipitates in the tubules with the Tamm–Horsfall protein. This process is enhanced by volume depletion, renal vasoconstriction, and acidosis. Though there is no defined threshold value of serum creatine kinase above which the risk of AKI is certain, AKI is unlikely when initial creatine kinase levels are less than 15,000–20,000 U/L.

Patients with AKI due to rhabdomyolysis usually experience volume depletion due to sequestration of water in injured muscles. The mainstay of treatment is early, aggressive volume repletion, with some patients requiring up to 10 L of fluid per day [24]. The type of fluid used for repletion remains controversial. The use of sodium bicarbonate to alkalinize the urine has been considered to have potential benefit, but studies have not been definitive [24]. Large volumes of normal saline may be required to resuscitate a patient with rhabdomyolysis. This can result in the development of a hyperchloremic metabolic acidosis. Therefore changing IV fluids to either sodium bicarbonate or lactated ringers may be a reasonable option. As an osmotic agent, there is hypothetical benefit for mannitol in rhabdomyolysis as it increases urinary flow and mobilizes fluid from injured muscles; however, studies have not shown benefit from its use [24]. Loop diuretics have also been studied but have also not shown any clear benefit.

Electrolyte abnormalities can occur as a result of the release of cellular components during rhabdomyolysis, particularly hyperkalemia, hyperphosphatemia, hyperuricemia, high anion-gap metabolic acidosis, and hypermagnesemia, and further complicate and exacerbate accompanying AKI. In cases of severe AKI with refractory hyperkalemia, acidosis, or volume overload, RRT may be necessary. Conventional hemodialysis does not remove myoglobin effectively due to its molecular size. Continuous venovenous hemofiltration or hemodiafiltration may have some efficacy in removing myoglobin, but larger studies are needed to assess the effect on outcomes.

Vascular Causes of ARF

Vascular diseases are an important yet often overlooked cause of AKI. Vascular processes can be divided into small-vessel and large-vessel diseases.

Small-Vessel Disease

Atherosclerosis with embolization of atherosclerotic plaques to the kidneys is an increasingly common cause of small vessel disease in the elderly population. Scleroderma can lead to fibrosis and narrowing of the small arteries in the kidneys. Although uncommon, scleroderma renal crisis is the sudden onset of oliguric renal failure, hypertension, and grade 3 or 4 hypertensive retinopathy in patients with scleroderma. Malignant hypertension can lead to acute renal vascular damage with fibrinoid necrosis and intimal thickening of the small arteries and arterioles. Clinical signs may include oliguria, proteinuria, hematuria, thrombocytopenia, and microangiopathic hemolytic anemia. The most common cause of malignant hypertension is underlying renal disease, though essential hypertension and medication noncompliance are also frequently responsible. Other less common causes of malignant hypertension that should be considered, particularly in difficult to treat cases, include renal artery stenosis, primary aldosteronism, and pheochromocytoma [25].

Other rare causes of small vessel renovascular disease include hemolytic-uremic syndrome (HUS), thrombotic thrombocytopenic purpura (TTP), and acute cortical necrosis.

Large-Vessel Disease

Renal artery stenosis (RAS) is usually caused by atherosclerosis of the main renal arteries; fibromuscular hyperplasia is a rare cause of RAS. RAS leads to decreased perfusion pressure and release of renin by the kidneys, which leads to hypertension. Over time, the kidneys decrease in size and become atrophic, glomerular filtration decreases, and oliguria/anuria ensues. Serum renin levels, radionuclide scans after administration of captopril, Doppler studies, or renal arteriography may be useful for confirming a suspected diagnosis of RAS. Renal infarction, caused by acute embolism or thrombosis, most commonly occurs in older patients with coronary disease or atrial fibrillation [25].

Hepatorenal Syndrome

Hepatic and renal failure commonly coincide in critically ill patients, frequently due to drug intoxication and/or infections. Prerenal azotemia associated with advanced cirrhosis is common phenomena, and prerenal azotemia refractory to volume resuscitation is termed HRS. In HRS, splanchnic vasodilation leads to decreased effective arterial circulating volume and compensatory activation of the renin-angiotensin and sympathetic systems to maintain blood pressure. Catecholamine and angiotensin production increases, causing intrarenal vasoconstriction [7], resulting in a prerenal state with low urine sodium (<10 mEq/L) and low FE_{Ur} (<20 %), and a bland urine sediment.

HRS is associated with a very high mortality. Etiologies of HRS include GI hemorrhage, spontaneous bacterial peritonitis and excessive diuretic use. When a cirrhotic patient demonstrates signs of prerenal failure, aggressive fluid resuscitation with crystalloid or albumin is indicated to attempt to reverse the process. Extravascular volume overload may limit resuscitation efforts; however, in hypoalbuminemic patients with prohibitive pleural effusions or ascites, thoracentesis or paracentesis with concomitant IV albumin replacement may be indicated.

Pharmacologic management of HRS includes α-agonists, norepinephrine, vasopressin analogs, and combination therapies, which may improve or reverse HRS in a minority of patients. Pentoxifylline may decrease the incidence of AKI in patients with acute alcoholic hepatitis. Intravenous albumin significantly reduces the incidence of AKI and mortality in cirrhotic patients with spontaneous bacterial peritonitis, and decreases the incidence of AKI after large-volume paracentesis. RRT can be a bridge to transplantation in patients with HRS and liver failure, but does not significantly change outcomes in the absence of liver transplantation [7].

Complications of Renal Failure

Bleeding

Increased risk of bleeding has long been recognized as a complication of renal injury; however, the pathophysiology remains poorly understood. Prolonged bleeding from puncture sites, subdural hematomas, and bleeding from mucous membranes including nasal, gastrointestinal, and genitourinary sites are the most common manifestations [26]. Although platelet counts and coagulation factors are often normal in patients with AKI, platelet adhesiveness is reduced [27]. Prolonged bleeding time is a useful clinical laboratory test for assessment of bleeding risk [26]. Anticoagulation during hemodialysis can transiently worsen bleeding risk. However, RRT can improve the bleeding defect. Other medical therapies such as administration of cryoprecipitate, desmopressin, and estrogens can also improve bleeding due to AKI and uremia. Platelet transfusion is generally ineffective because transfused platelets will behave like the patient's own uremic platelets. Red blood cell transfusion in anemic patients can correct prolonged bleeding time. Erythropoietin can improve anemia associated with renal insufficiency and reduce the need for repeated transfusions, but it acts slowly and may not be useful in the acute setting [26].

Cardiovascular/Infectious/Neurologic Complications

Cardiovascular complications such as congestive heart failure, pulmonary edema, and hypertension may occur as a result of salt and water retention. Arrhythmias have been reported to occur in 10–30 % of patients. Infections are a leading cause of morbidity and mortality in patients with AKI, primarily respiratory or urinary tract infections. Neurologic problems may also be seen and include confusion, ataxia, somnolence, and seizures [5].

Nephrogenic Systemic Fibrosis

Administration of IV gadolinium in the setting of kidney injury is associated with increased risk of nephrogenic systemic fibrosis (NSF). NSF has been described in chronic renal failure with or without dependence on hemodialysis, in AKI, and in renal transplant patients. The precise extent of renal failure that is associated with NSF is not clear, though a GFR <30 mL/min/1.73 m^2 increases risk. High doses of IV gadolinium have been implicated as a cause, as gadolinium has been found within the tissue of patients with NSF. In patients with renal dysfunction, hemodialysis can remove approximately 93 % of infused gadolinium [28]. The American College of Radiology recommends that use of gadolinium contrast in patients with a GFR <30 mL/min/1.73 m^2 be reserved for absolutely essential cases and notes that no single gadolinium contrast in renal dysfunction can be safely administered [29]. If gadolinium must be given to a patient on hemodialysis, several sessions of hemodialysis performed after administration of gadolinium may decrease the risk of developing NSF [29].

Treatment

Treatment of AKI in the ICU is complicated as AKI is usually due to multifactorial etiologies, and is not necessarily due to a single process or insult.

Fluid Management in the Critically Ill

The mainstay of treatment for renal hypoperfusion due to hypovolemia from septic shock is goal-directed fluid resuscitation to rapidly and aggressively restore end-organ perfusion. Rivers' seminal paper on goal-directed fluid therapy targeted CVP (8–12 mmHg) or pulmonary capillary wedge pressure, mixed venous saturations (>70 %) and improved cardiac output as physiological endpoints [30]. This algorithm for volume resuscitation requires rapid administration of fluids or blood within a 6-h window. In a post-hoc analysis of the Vasopressin in Septic Shock Trial, patients in the highest quartile of CVP (>12 mmHg) had lowest survival at both 12 h and 4 days, and those with CVP <8 mmHg had better survival. Current sepsis guidelines recommend maintaining mean arterial pressure (MAP) greater than or equal to 65 mmHg with crystalloid, colloids or vasopressors [31]. It is unknown whether this is adequate to prevent renal failure. The Fluids and Catheters Treatment Trial (FACTT) suggested that in patients with acute lung injury, conservative fluid management may not be detrimental to kidney function. Specifically there was no significant difference in need for RRT between patients in the conservative versus liberal fluid strategy groups, although creatinine concentration was slightly higher in the conservative-strategy group [32]. Given these considerations, once appropriate resuscitation is achieved it is reasonable to transition to either maintaining euvolemia or even actively removing fluid [31].

Crystalloids Versus Colloids

Crystalloids and colloids are the two main types of fluids used for resuscitation, and there has been long-standing debate regarding the superiority and safety of one versus the other. Crystalloid solutions are inexpensive and readily available. Colloid solutions can be synthetic (hydroxyethyl starches) or natural (albumin). Due to their larger molecular weight, colloids remain in the bloodstream longer than crystalloids. However, colloids confer no survival advantage as compared to crystalloids [33, 34]. In addition, some hyperosmotic colloids have been associated with development of renal failure [35].

Hydroxyethyl starch is a synthetic colloid derived from partially hydrolyzed and variably hydroxyethylated plant starch. A systematic review of 38 randomized controlled trials comparing hydroxyethyl starch to crystalloids, albumin, or gelatin for acute fluid resuscitation in critically ill patients found that hydroxyethyl starch was associated with increased mortality, increased AKI, and increased need for RRT after exclusion of seven trials for scientific misconduct [36]. The Saline versus Albumin Fluid Evaluation (SAFE) Study randomized and evaluated 6,997 patients admitted to the ICU to receive either 4 % albumin or normal saline for fluid resuscitation. Although patients in the normal saline infusion arm initially received more IV fluids, blood products, had a positive fluid balance, and had higher CVPs, there was no difference in 28-day mortality or need for RRT between groups [37].

Despite the increased cost associated with use of albumin, the Surviving Sepsis Guidelines advocate using crystalloid or albumin for volume resuscitation in patients with sepsis with hypovolemic shock [31]. They recommend against the use of hydroxyethyl starch [31].

Vasopressors

In patients with persistent hypotension despite adequate fluid resuscitation, vaso-pressors should be used to increase MAP and/or cardiac output to optimize organ perfusion. The impact of vasopressors can be inferred from observed increases in urine output and creatinine clearance, and decreases in serum creatinine levels. However, there are no data to support the use of one vasopressor over another for improving renal function [21]. Though the Vasopressin and Septic Shock Trial (VASST) did suggest that vasopressin could reduce progression to severe AKI com-pared with norepinephrine in a small subgroup of patients with less severe septic shock, this study is not generalizable to a large population [37]. Dopamine stimu-lates renal dopamine receptor-1 and can increase renal blood flow and diuresis. Though initially thought to have a protective effect against kidney injury, this has not been proven in human studies and dopamine's use for this purpose is not recom-mended by consensus guidelines [21].

Nutrition

Adequate nutrition should be ensured, as malnutrition is associated with increased morbidity and mortality in patients with AKI. Critically ill patients have accelerated protein breakdown and increased caloric needs, and daily caloric intake of 25–30 kcal/kg of body weight may be required [2, 5]. Intake of potassium and phosphate is typi-cally restricted for patients with renal dysfunction because of impaired renal excre-tion. Hypokalemia and hypophosphatemia due to cellular uptake or external losses can occur, and patients should be monitored for need of careful supplementation.

Renal Replacement Therapy

Acute dialysis-dependent renal failure portends a poor prognosis and is associated with in-hospital mortality of 60–70 %. Indications for RRT include electrolyte abnormalities (elevated potassium or phosphate), acidemia, or volume overload refractory to medical management. The need for RRT can occur with or without a significantly elevated serum creatinine concentration. Encephalopathy, pericarditis, and coagulopathy are late complications of AKI requiring RRT.

Optimal timing of initiation of RRT is controversial. Though it is reasonable to conclude that early initiation of RRT may be beneficial in order to avoid dangerous metabolic, fluid, and electrolyte derangements of uremia, there are no outcomes data to support this sentiment [38]. In fact, some have argued to withhold RRT until definite indications are present to minimize risks of complications associated with catheter placement, hemodynamic instability and cardiac arrhythmias during dialysis, or delayed renal recovery [2].

Types of RRT

Types of renal replacement for AKI include peritoneal dialysis, intermittent hemodialysis, and continuous renal replacement therapy (CRRT). Acute peritoneal dialysis is infrequently used in developed countries and will not be discussed in this chapter.

Intermittent hemodialysis is performed using venovenous access for a few hours a day at variable intervals. Sustained, low efficiency dialysis (SLED) or extended daily dialysis are forms of intermittent hemodialysis in which the duration of dialysis is extended to 6–12 h to allow for more gradual removal of solutes and fluid. CRRT is performed continuously (24 h per day) through either arteriovenous or venovenous vascular access using much slower blood flow rates and achieving slower solute clearance per unit of time compared to intermittent hemodialysis. Continuous venovenous hemofiltration, continuous venovenous hemodialysis, and continuous venovenous hemodiafiltration are the most common sub-modalities of CRRT. CRRT requires continuous anticoagulation, thus increasing risk of bleeding. Additionally, continuous exposure to an extracorporeal circuit can result in nutritional depletion, subtherapeutic antibiotic levels, or infection.

A systematic review of randomized controlled trials and prospective cohort studies found intermittent hemodialysis and CRRT lead to similar clinical outcomes in patients with AKI [38]. A recent randomized trial of intermittent hemodialysis versus CRRT demonstrated that even sicker patients could be safely treated with intermittent hemodialysis. Thus, given the significantly higher cost of CRRT, intermittent hemodialysis may be preferable in patients with AKI requiring RRT. However, in patients with severe hemodynamic instability, CRRT is still preferred.

Anticoagulation with unfractionated heparin is recommended to maintain activated partial thromboplastin time between 1 and 1.4 times the upper limit of normal. In patients with high risk of bleeding, regional citrate anticoagulation can be administered.

Acid–Base Regulation by the Kidneys

The systemic acid–base balance is maintained when the renal net acid excretion equals the body's net endogenous acid production. Under normal conditions, the 80–85 % of filtered bicarbonate (HCO_3^-) is reabsorbed through the proximal convoluted tubules (PCT), where carbonic anhydrase II (CA II) splits cytosolic H_2CO_3 into H^+ and HCO_3^-. Bicarbonate then exits the cell through the basolateral

Table 2.4 Causes of metabolic acidosis

High anion gap metabolic acidosis	Normal (hyperchloremic) anion gap metabolic acidosis
Acute kidney injury	Administration of normal saline
Chronic kidney disease	Chronic kidney disease
Diabetic ketoacidosis[a]	Adrenal insufficiency
Alcoholic ketoacidosis	Hyporeninemic hypoaldosteronism
Lactic acidosis	Proximal renal tubular acidosis
Salicylate intoxication	Distal renal tubular acidosis
Toxic alcohol intoxication	Diarrhea
(methanol, ethylene glycol,	Intestinal, pancreatic, or biliary fistulae
diethylene glycol, propylene glycol)	Pseudoaldosteronism
Pyroglutamic acidosis	Drugs (spironolactone, prostaglandin inhibitors,
Fasting ketoacidosis	triamterene, amiloride, trimethoprim, pentamidine)
Toluene intoxication[a]	Ureterosigmoidostomy, ureteroileostomy
	Diabetic ketoacidosis[a]
	Toluene intoxication[a]

[a]Can have a high or normal anion gap

Na^+/HCO_3^- co-transporter. Carbonic anhydrase IV (CA IV), which is located in the lumen of the tubule, promotes dissociation of luminal H_2CO_3 into CO_2 and H_2O to prevent buildup of a proton gradient. The major determinants of HCO_3^- reabsorption include luminal HCO_3^- concentration, luminal pH, luminal flow rate, peritubular partial pressure of CO_2 (pCO_2), and luminal and peritubular concentrations of angiotensin II. HCO_3^- that is not reabsorbed in the PCT gets reabsorbed by the thick ascending limb of the loop of Henle via the NHE_3 Na^+/H^+ exchanger and an electrogenic H^+-ATPase. Some HCO_3^- is also reabsorbed in the collecting duct via an H^+-ATPase. With normal renal function, very little HCO_3^- is excreted in the urine and the urine pH is usually below 6.0 [39].

Metabolic Acidosis

Metabolic acidosis is common in critically ill patients, characterized by a primary reduction in the serum HCO_3^- concentration, resulting in a decrease in the arterial partial pressure of carbon dioxide (P_aCO_2) and a decrease in blood pH. Metabolic acidosis occurs when the body's normal mechanisms of acid–base homeostasis are overwhelmed by an increased acid production or bicarbonate loss (Table 2.4).

In response to acidosis, increase in H^+ and HCO_3^- transport along the nephron, increased ammoniagenesis, and increased availability of urinary buffers such as phosphate leads to reduction (or elimination) of HCO_3^- from the urine, and increased NH_4 excretion. Endothelin-1, produced by endothelial cells and proximal tubule cells in response to acidosis, stimulates renal H^+ and HCO_3^- transport. Cortisol is secreted by the adrenal cortex in response to acidosis and stimulates renal H^+ and HCO_3^- transport in the proximal tubule. Parathyroid hormone acts on the proximal tubule to inhibit phosphate reabsorption, which acts as a urinary buffer [39].

Metabolic acidosis triggers a secondary ventilatory response to decrease P_aCO_2. The expected P_aCO_2 for the serum HCO_3^- concentration can be calculated using Winter's formula ($P_aCO_2 = 1.5[HCO_3^-] + 8 \pm 2$). A measured P_aCO_2 different than the value calculated using Winter's formula indicates the presence of a coexisting primary respiratory alkalosis or acidosis [39].

The serum anion gap ($[Na^+] - ([Cl^-] + [HCO_3^-])$) may be useful in determining the etiology of a metabolic acidosis. Normal anion gap is 6–12 mmol/L. Low serum albumin reduces the calculated anion gap by ~2.3 mmol/L for every 1.0 g/dL decrease in serum albumin concentration. When the change in HCO_3^- concentration exceeds the change in anion gap, it can be inferred that a coexisting hyperchloremic acidosis is present. Conversely, if the change in HCO_3^- concentration is lower than the change in anion gap, a coexisting metabolic alkalosis is present [39].

Acute metabolic acidoses are treated by addressing the underlying disorder. Administration of sodium bicarbonate has not been shown to be clinically beneficial. However, sodium bicarbonate should be considered in patients with ketoacidosis and serum pH below 7.1 or hemodynamic instability. Bicarbonate may also be considered in severe lactic acidosis with significant acidemia and/or hemodynamic instability. Increasing minute ventilation in mechanically ventilated patients to reduce the P_aCO_2 or dialysis may also be appropriate in some cases [39].

Summary of Key Points

- Acute kidney injury (AKI) has largely replaced the term acute renal failure.
- Serum creatinine concentration remains the primary measurement for the diagnosis of AKI.
- The causes of AKI can be classified into prerenal, postrenal, and intrinsic. Urinary sediment and urine electrolytes can be used to differentiate between the various causes.
- The mainstay of therapy is fluid resuscitation with crystalloid solutions. There is no survival benefit of colloids over crystalloids.
- Intermittent hemodialysis and CRRT result in similar clinical outcomes; however, patients with severe hemodynamic instability may still require CRRT.
- The kidneys are important for maintaining normal acid–base balance.

References

1. Bellomo R, Ronco C, Kellum JA, Mehta RL, Palevsky P. Acute renal failure – definition, outcome measures, animal models, fluid therapy and information technology needs: the second international consensus conference of the acute dialysis quality initiative (ADQI) group. Crit Care. 2004;8:R204–12.
2. Abuelo JG. Normotensive ischemic acute renal failure. N Engl J Med. 2007;357:797–805.
3. Uchino S, Kellum JA, Bellomo R, Doig GS, Morimatsu H, Morgera S, et al. Acute renal failure in critically ill patients: a multinational, multicenter study. JAMA. 2005;294:813–8.

4. Mehta RL, Kellum JA, Shah SV, Molitoris BA, Ronco C, Warnock DG, et al. Acute kidney injury network: report of an initiative to improve outcomes in acute kidney injury. Crit Care. 2007;11:R31.
5. Thadhani R, Pascual M, Bonventre JV. Acute renal failure. N Engl J Med. 1996;334: 1448–60.
6. Marik PE, Cavallazzi R. Does the central venous pressure predict fluid responsiveness? An updated meta-analysis and a plea for some common sense. Crit Care Med. 2013;41:1774–81.
7. Verna EC, Wagener G. Renal interactions in liver dysfunction and failure. Curr Opin Crit Care. 2013;19:133–41.
8. Tepel M, Aspelin P, Lameire N. Contrast-induced nephropathy: a clinical and evidence-based approach. Circulation. 2006;113:1799–806.
9. Stone GW, McCullough PA, Tumlin JA, Lepor NE, Madyoon H, Murray P, et al. Fenoldopam mesylate for the prevention of contrast-induced nephropathy: a randomized controlled trial. JAMA. 2003;290:2284–91.
10. McCullough PA. Radiocontrast-induced acute kidney injury. Nephron Physiol. 2008;109: p61–72.
11. Adolph E, Holdt-Lehmann B, Chatterjee T, Paschka S, Prott A, Schneider H, et al. Renal insufficiency following radiocontrast exposure trial (REINFORCE): a randomized comparison of sodium bicarbonate versus sodium chloride hydration for the prevention of contrast-induced nephropathy. Coron Artery Dis. 2008;19:413–9.
12. Briguori C, Airoldi F, D'Andrea D, Bonizzoni E, Morici N, Focaccio A, et al. Renal insufficiency following contrast media administration trial (REMEDIAL): a randomized comparison of 3 preventive strategies. Circulation. 2007;115:1211–7.
13. Recio-Mayoral A, Chaparro M, Prado B, Cozar R, Mendez I, Banerjee D, et al. The renoprotective effect of hydration with sodium bicarbonate plus n-acetylcysteine in patients undergoing emergency percutaneous coronary intervention: the RENO study. J Am Coll Cardiol. 2007;49:1283–8.
14. Maioli M, Toso A, Leoncini M, Gallopin M, Tedeschi D, Micheletti C, et al. Sodium bicarbonate versus saline for the prevention of contrast-induced nephropathy in patients with renal dysfunction undergoing coronary angiography or intervention. J Am Coll Cardiol. 2008;52: 599–604.
15. Brar SS, Shen AY, Jorgensen MB, Kotlewski A, Aharonian VJ, Desai N, et al. Sodium bicarbonate vs sodium chloride for the prevention of contrast medium-induced nephropathy in patients undergoing coronary angiography: a randomized trial. JAMA. 2008;300:1038–46.
16. Hogan SE, L'Allier P, Chetcuti S, Grossman PM, Nallamothu BK, Duvernoy C, et al. Current role of sodium bicarbonate-based preprocedural hydration for the prevention of contrast-induced acute kidney injury: a meta-analysis. Am Heart J. 2008;156:414–21.
17. Klarenbach SW, Pannu N, Tonelli MA, Manns BJ. Cost-effectiveness of hemofiltration to prevent contrast nephropathy in patients with chronic kidney disease. Crit Care Med. 2006;34: 1044–51.
18. Elyasi S, Khalili H, Dashti-Khavidaki S, Mohammadpour A. Vancomycin-induced nephrotoxicity: mechanism, incidence, risk factors and special populations. A literature review. Eur J Clin Pharmacol. 2012;68:1243–55.
19. Jeffres MN, Isakow W, Doherty JA, Micek ST, Kollef MH. A retrospective analysis of possible renal toxicity associated with vancomycin in patients with health care-associated methicillin-resistant staphylococcus aureus pneumonia. Clin Ther. 2007;29:1107–15.
20. Boyer A, Gruson D, Bouchet S, Clouzeau B, Hoang-Nam B, Vargas F, et al. Aminoglycosides in septic shock: an overview, with specific consideration given to their nephrotoxic risk. Drug Saf. 2013;36:217–30.
21. Brochard L, Abroug F, Brenner M, Broccard AF, Danner RL, Ferrer M, et al. An official ATS/ERS/ESICM/SCCM/SRLF statement: prevention and management of acute renal failure in the ICU patient: an international consensus conference in intensive care medicine. Am J Resp Crit Care Med. 2010;181:1128–55.

22. Whelton A. Nephrotoxicity of nonsteroidal anti-inflammatory drugs: physiologic foundations and clinical implications. Am J Med. 1999;106:13S–24.
23. Praga M, Gonzalez E. Acute interstitial nephritis. Kidney Int. 2010;77:956–61.
24. Bosch X, Poch E, Grau JM. Rhabdomyolysis and acute kidney injury. N Engl J Med. 2009;361:62–72.
25. Abuelo JG. Diagnosing vascular causes of renal failure. Ann Intern Med. 1995;123:601–14.
26. Weigert AL, Schafer AI. Uremic bleeding: pathogenesis and therapy. Am J Med Sci. 1998;316:94–104.
27. Eknoyan G, Wacksman SJ, Glueck HI, Will JJ. Platelet function in renal failure. N Engl J Med. 1969;280:677–81.
28. Saitoh T, Hayasaka K, Tanaka Y, Kuno T, Nagura Y. Dialyzability of gadodiamide in hemodialysis patients. Radiat Med. 2006;24:445–51.
29. Kanal E, Barkovich AJ, Bell C, Borgstede JP, Bradley Jr WG, Froelich JW, et al. Acr guidance document for safe mr practices: 2007. AJR Am J Roentgenol. 2007;188:1447–74.
30. Rivers E, Nguyen B, Havstad S, Ressler J, Muzzin A, Knoblich B, et al. Early goal-directed therapy in the treatment of severe sepsis and septic shock. N Engl J Med. 2001;345:1368–77.
31. Dellinger RP, Levy MM, Rhodes A, Annane D, Gerlach H, Opal SM, et al. Surviving sepsis campaign: international guidelines for management of severe sepsis and septic shock: 2012. Crit Care Med. 2013;41:580–637.
32. Wiedemann HP, Wheeler AP, Bernard GR, Thompson BT, Hayden D, deBoisblanc B, et al. Comparison of two fluid-management strategies in acute lung injury. N Engl J Med. 2006;354:2564–75.
33. Finfer S, Bellomo R, Boyce N, French J, Myburgh J, Norton R. A comparison of albumin and saline for fluid resuscitation in the intensive care unit. N Engl J Med. 2004;350:2247–56.
34. Roberts I, Alderson P, Bunn F, Chinnock P, Ker K, Schierhout G. Colloids versus crystalloids for fluid resuscitation in critically ill patients. Cochrane Database Syst Rev. 2004;18, CD000567.
35. Schortgen F, Girou E, Deye N, Brochard L. The risk associated with hyperoncotic colloids in patients with shock. Intensive Care Med. 2008;34:2157–68.
36. Zarychanski R, Abou-Setta AM, Turgeon AF, Houston BL, McIntyre L, Marshall JC, et al. Association of hydroxyethyl starch administration with mortality and acute kidney injury in critically ill patients requiring volume resuscitation: a systematic review and meta-analysis. JAMA. 2013;309:678–88.
37. Russell JA, Walley KR, Singer J, Gordon AC, Hebert PC, Cooper DJ, et al. Vasopressin versus norepinephrine infusion in patients with septic shock. N Engl J Med. 2008;358:877–87.
38. Pannu N, Klarenbach S, Wiebe N, Manns B, Tonelli M. Renal replacement therapy in patients with acute renal failure: a systematic review. JAMA. 2008;299:793–805.
39. Kraut JA, Madias NE. Metabolic acidosis: pathophysiology, diagnosis and management. Nat Rev Nephrol. 2010;6:274–85.

Chapter 3
Neurologic Complications

John P. Kress

Abstract Neurological complications are common in intensive care unit (ICU) survivors. As survival from severe critical illness has become more commonplace, patients and care providers are faced with the reality of recovery from both physical and psychological dysfunction. Suspension of physical and mental activity is a reality for many ICU patients. In such a state of suspended animation, physical and neurocognitive function deteriorate quickly. Recent data suggest that minimization of ICU sedation and maintaining activity through programs of early mobilization can improve both physical and neurocognitive functional status. ICU delirium is a common problem with both short- and long-term consequences. Future research is needed to better understand which strategies best prevent ICU delirium.

Keywords Respiratory failure • Physical therapy • Occupational therapy • Mobilization • Mechanical ventilation • ICU-acquired weakness • Muscle atrophy • Critical care • Neuropathy • Sedation

Introduction

Over the last few decades, outcomes in critically ill patients have improved dramatically. The reasons for this include, but are not limited to, a better understanding of pathophysiologies common to intensive care unit (ICU) patients, technological improvements in the treatment of various states of organ dysfunction, and evidence-based clinical investigations in the ICU. Increased survival of critically ill patients, coupled with increasing severity of patients' pre-hospital health and chronic

J.P. Kress, M.D. (✉)
Department of Medicine, Section of Pulmonary and Critical Care, University of Chicago,
5841 South Maryland, MC 6026, Chicago, IL 60637, USA
e-mail: jkress@medicine.bsd.uchicago.edu

J.B. Richards and R.D. Stapleton (eds.), *Non-Pulmonary Complications of Critical Care:*   45
A Clinical Guide, Respiratory Medicine, DOI 10.1007/978-1-4939-0873-8_3,

diseases, has resulted in extreme degrees of both physical and mental neurological dysfunction in many ICU survivors. Rehabilitation for such patients can be very long and frustrating, particularly in survivors of acute respiratory distress syndrome (ARDS), sepsis, and/or the systemic inflammatory response syndrome (SIRS).

Bed rest during intensive care is routine in most settings and has been the standard of care since ICUs have been in existence. This practice subjects patients to a circumstance that can be referred to as a state of "suspended animation," which affects both mind and body. The harmfulness of bed rest was described quite eloquently by authors such as Asher as early as the 1940s [1]. In modern ICUs, advances in life support allow practitioners to maintain homeostasis of "vital" organ systems (e.g., cardiac, pulmonary, and renal) despite extreme acuity of illness; however, patients receiving intensive critical care support are often deeply sedated, and homeostasis of the nervous and musculoskeletal systems is often lost. Heavy use of potent sedative and analgesic drugs causes patients to remain immobilized for extended time periods. That intensive critical care support and high doses of sedatives result in the loss of neuromuscular homeostasis could be rationalized as the "cost" of life support during acute illness. However, recent evidence suggests that heavy sedation is unnecessary, even harmful to patients, and this has begun to lead to a change in patient care strategies. Relatedly, there is increasing awareness that along with decreasing sedative dosing, prolonged bed rest need not be the default strategy in ICU care anymore.

In conjunction with the move away from deep sedation in ICU patients, literature describing long-term problems that ICU survivors face has become increasingly recognized. A landmark study in 2003 by Margaret Herridge and colleagues described the outcomes of survivors of the ARDS 1 year following hospital discharge. Patients were interviewed and evaluated for both physical and mental functional problems. In this group of 109 young patients (median age of 45 years), 100 % noted loss of muscle bulk, proximal muscle weakness, and fatigue. Fifty percent of the patients were unemployed 1 year after discharge [2]. Even at 5 years post discharge, the 64 remaining patients from the original cohort still had physical limitations, with 6-min walk tests and physical component scores on the Short Form-36 Health Survey (SF-36) lower than normal subjects [3] (Fig. 3.1). By 5 years post discharge, most of the 64 survivors had returned to work, suggesting that adaptation to physical handicaps was a common coping mechanism.

ICU-Acquired Weakness

While it may seem self-evident that the prolonged physical immobilization that is so common in critically ill and mechanically ventilated ICU patients leads to neuromuscular weakness, the science supporting this concept is actually quite limited. This is despite the fact that immobilization is a well-known phenomenon associated with neuromuscular dysfunction in other settings, such as orthopedic injury with casting and space travel. As an example, in 1995, a report by Griffiths and colleagues evaluated the effects of continuous passive motion of one leg in ICU patients

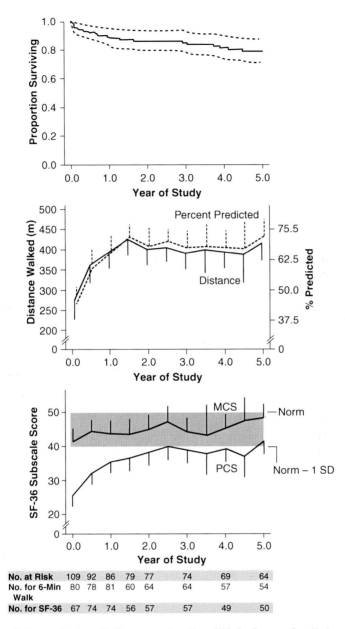

Fig. 3.1 Survival rates, 6-min walk distance, and quality of life for 5 years after discharge from the intensive care unit. Exact survival times were used for these analyses. In the *top graph*, the *solid line* is the Kaplan–Meier survival curve from 0 to 5 years; *dashed lines* represent the 95 % confidence interval. The *middle graph* shows the distance walked in 6 min in meters (*solid line*) and the percent of the predicted distance (*dashed line*). The *bottom graph* shows the physical-component score (PCS) and the mental-component score (MCS) on the Medical Outcomes Study 36-Item Short-Form Health Survey (SF-36); scores range from 0 to 100, with higher scores indicating better health status. *Vertical bars* in the *middle and bottom graphs* represent half 95 % confidence intervals. Reprinted from with permission Herridge MS, Tansey CM, Matté A, et al. Functional disability 5 years after acute respiratory distress syndrome. N Engl J Med. 2011;364(14):1293–304

subjected to neuromuscular blockade during respiratory failure [4]; the patients' contralateral leg served as a control. Muscle fiber atrophy was prevented, and muscle DNA to protein ratios (an established index of wasting), and muscle protein content were reduced less profoundly in the leg receiving passive range of motion. The authors concluded that in critically ill patients, an intervention as simple as passive muscle stretching could preserve the architecture of muscle fibers. Apart from this report, there had been little research on the effects of immobility in the ICU until very recently (see below). Now, with increasing numbers of debilitated ICU survivors, the syndrome of *ICU-acquired weakness* has received increasing attention in the critical care community.

ICU-acquired weakness is a major neurologic complication seen in many critically ill patients. It is a syndrome with many different causative pathophysiologic mechanisms. In 1984, Charles Bolton and colleagues first described a neuropathic change in critically ill patients characterized by histopathological evidence of primary axonal degeneration without demyelination. Motor nerves were affected more profoundly than sensory nerves [5]. The investigators described this phenomenon as *critical illness polyneuropathy*. In critical illness polyneuropathy, nerve electrophysiological studies demonstrate that while nerve conduction velocity is preserved, the amplitudes of compound muscle and sensory nerve action potentials are reduced. Symmetrical muscle weakness is a common clinical finding, and it is typically most notable in proximal muscle groups (e.g., hips and shoulders). It is important to note that critical illness polyneuropathy can affect respiratory muscles, and therefore can lead to problems with weaning from mechanical ventilation. Accordingly, some experts recommend that patients who fail weaning trials be evaluated for the presence of critical illness polyneuropathy. While there are no interventions currently available to treat critical illness polyneuropathy, testing for and diagnosing this syndrome may provide important prognostic information for patients and families.

In critical illness myopathy there is histopathologic evidence of selective loss of myosin thick filaments and even muscle necrosis. Patients with critical illness myopathies have reduced amplitude and increased duration of compound muscle action potential on electrophysiological studies.

A distinguishing clinical feature of critical illness myopathy, when compared to neuropathy, is the preservation of sensory function. However, this clinical distinction can be obscured by the effects of sedative medications, acute ICU delirium, or other clinical processes that impair patients' ability to report the presence or absence of intact sensory function. With regard to prognosis, critical illness myopathy tends to recover more fully than neuropathy. Critical illness myopathy is a primary myopathy, rather than a secondary myopathy that occurs as a result of neuromuscular uncoupling. Secondary myopathies result from direct nerve injury or prolonged neuromuscular blockade (typically in conjunction with corticosteroid use).

Weakness in critically ill patients is often due to both neuropathy and myopathy. Therefore, the term "ICU-acquired weakness" is used to describe any patient who has clinically evident weakness with no plausible etiology other than critical illness. This all-encompassing term acknowledges that ICU-acquired weakness is a syndrome, rather than a specific, discrete disease process. The differential diagnosis of weakness in ICU patients is broad, and includes catabolic muscle-wasting states, metabolic

Table 3.1 Risk factors for developing ICU-acquired weakness

Risk factors for ICU-acquired weakness
Sepsis
Systemic inflammatory response syndrome (SIRS)
Multi-organ system failure
Hyperglycemia
Immobilization
Corticosteroids
Neuromuscular blocking agents

Table 3.2 Medical Research Council Scale (MRC)

Medical research council scale
Muscle groups (right and left) assessed in the measurement of the MRC
• Abduction of the arm
• Flexion of the forearm
• Extension of the wrist
• Flexion of the leg
• Extension of the knee
• Dorsal flexion of the foot
MRC scale for each of the above muscle groups
0 = No visible contraction
1 = Visible contraction without movement of the limb (not existent for hip flexion)
2 = Movement of the limb but not against gravity
3 = Movement against gravity over (almost) the full range
4 = Movement against gravity and resistance
5 = Normal
Perfect score is 60, and ICU-acquired weakness is defined by MRC score <48

derangements such as hyperglycemia, prolonged immobility, joint contractures and drug toxicities. Table 3.1 lists common risk factors for ICU-acquired weakness.

ICU-acquired weakness is diagnosed most commonly using the Medical Research Council (MRC) scale, with the strengths of various muscle groups in the upper and lower extremities graded on a scale of 0–5 (a combined score of less than 48 defines ICU-acquired weakness, see Table 3.2). Although this tool has limitations with regard to specificity (e.g., ICU delirium or pain, which may result in lower scores despite normal neuromuscular function), it remains the most widely utilized clinical means of diagnosing ICU-acquired weakness.

Strategies to Reduce Neurological Complications in Critical Illness

In the last few years, early mobilization of ICU patients has been reported as a way of combating ICU-acquired weakness. The specific approach to mobilization of ICU patients varies from study to study; however, the core of a successful early mobilization strategy is a team of physical and occupational therapists working with critically ill patients in the ICU. Therapists work to get patients out of bed sooner than has been traditionally done for critically ill patients. The motivation for early mobilization of critically ill patients is the awareness that neuromuscular deconditioning during critical illness is rapid and potentially permanent. Accordingly, even intubated and mechanically ventilated patients are eligible for early mobilization.

Mobilization Protocols

Mobilization protocols with physical and occupational therapists do require that patients are awake and able to follow instructions. As noted above, contemporary awareness that minimizing or even avoiding sedative and analgesic drug use allows patients to be more alert and more interactive with their surroundings, providing an opportunity for early mobilization. This demonstrates that achieving successful early mobilization is truly a multidisciplinary effort involving nurses, respiratory therapists, physicians, and physical and occupational therapy teams.

One of the earliest reports of mobilization in ICU patients was a descriptive study by Bailey and colleagues in 2007, in which her group described a novel strategy of mobilizing mechanically ventilated patients in their ICU [6]. The patients received minimal sedation, so that the mobilization team (which consisted of a nurse, physical therapist, respiratory therapist, and a critical care technician) could begin physical therapy and mobilization as soon the patients were responsive to verbal stimulation. Clinical parameters for initiating early mobilization included: (1) ventilator settings of $FiO_2 \leq 0.6$ and $PEEP \leq 10$ cm H_2O, (2) absence of orthostatic hypotension, (3) patients did not require continuous catecholamine infusions.

The mobilization team used a sequential approach, in which exertional activities progressed according to a patient's level of tolerance. The typical activity sequence started with sitting on the edge of the bed, then progressed to sitting in a chair after bed transfer, and ultimately progressed to assisted ambulation. Such a progressive approach is standard practice for physical and occupational therapists in other settings, and it naturally translates to the ICU. In this study, more than 40 % of activities, including ambulation, occurred in patients who were intubated and mechanically ventilated. Adverse events were very rare, and included five falls, five notable changes in blood pressure, three severe decreases in oxygen saturation, and one medical device removal. Obviously, all of these events also occasionally occur in sedentary ICU patients, so indicating that the low rate of adverse events in this study does not preclude performing early mobilization the benefits of early mobilization almost certainly outweigh the risks, when performed by a trained multidisciplinary team.

The effect of reduced sedation and its impact on mobility can be inferred from an interesting study by DeJonghe and colleagues [7]. These investigators described a tool known as Adaptation to the Intensive Care Environment (ATICE) instrument, which assesses Consciousness (with Awakeness and Consciousness subdomains) and Tolerance (with Calmness, Ventilatory Synchrony and Face Relaxation subdomains). This study was a "before-after" trial, in which the "after" intervention consisted of a sedation algorithm driven by bedside nursing staff. Reduced doses of sedation when nurses followed the algorithm resulted in reduced time to awakening, reduced time requiring mechanical ventilation, and reduced ICU length of stay. The occurrence of pressure sores was halved. It is reasonable to presume that decreased sedative dosing resulting in patients being more awake and requiring fewer days of mechanical ventilation led to this important result.

Mobilization in Mechanically Ventilated Patients

A prospective trial of early mobilization in mechanically ventilated medical ICU patients was published by Morris and colleagues in 2008. The primary outcome of the trial was the frequency with which mobility could occur in the ICU. Daily sedative interruption was performed to permit patients to be awake and able to follow instructions. Once patients were awake, a progressive sequential approach to mobility similar to that described by Bailey and colleagues was followed (Fig. 3.2). A total of 330 patients were enrolled in a non-randomized block allocation manner. Eighty percent of patients in the group assigned to mobilization had at least one physical therapy session versus 47 % in the usual care group. There were no adverse events reported in the trial. Patients who were mobilized were out of bed 5 days sooner than control patients, and they had a 2 day reduction in hospital length of stay. At 1 year of follow up, the intervention group had a significantly lower chance of death or hospital readmission [8].

Bedside Ergometry

A Belgian group, led by Burtin and colleagues, subsequently performed a randomized controlled trial of early exercise using a bedside bicycle ergometer attached to the foot of the patient's bed. Both medical and surgical critically ill patients were enrolled [9]. Patients in this trial had relatively long stays in the ICU, as the bicycle ergometer was generally initiated approximately two weeks after admission to the ICU. The feet of each subject were strapped to the bicycle pedals, so that cycling could be passive if the patient was unable to follow instructions, or active in alert patients. The study targeted improvements in neurological function, specifically strength and functional parameters. This simple intervention substantially reduced neurological complications. At hospital discharge, patients in the intervention group had significantly better quadriceps strength, 6-min walk distance, and SF-36 physical function scores. Cycling sessions were well tolerated in this group of critically ill patients. There were a total of 425 cycling sessions in the study, with no serious adverse events. Mild adverse events were rare, and cycling sessions had to be stopped only 4 % of the time for oxygen desaturation and unexpected blood pressure changes.

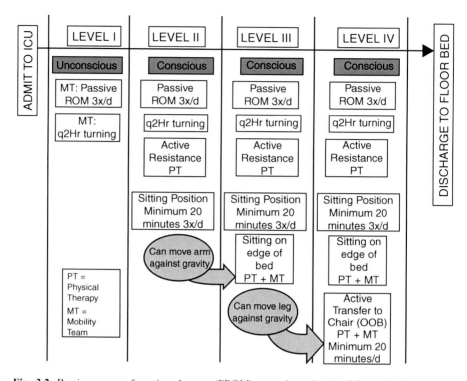

Fig. 3.2 Passive range of motion therapy (PROM) started on day 1 of Protocol (level I). As patients demonstrated consciousness and increased strength (see *circles* with *arrows* above), they were moved to the next level. Physical therapy (PT) would be first attempted at level II. The protocolized intervention ceased when patient was transferred to a floor bed, after which time patients within both "Protocol" and "Usual Care" groups received usual care mobility therapy (MT) as dictated by the floor physician teams (out of bed [OOB]). Reprinted with permission from Morris PE, Goad A, Thompson C, et al. Early intensive care unit mobility therapy in the treatment of acute respiratory failure. Crit Care Med. 2008;36(8):2238–43

Multi-Disciplinary Approach to Early Mobilization

Also in 2009, Schweickert and colleagues published a prospective randomized blinded trial of very early physical and occupational therapy from the initiation of mechanical ventilation [10]. This work was novel for several reasons. First, it was the first randomized and blinded study evaluating early mobilization in mechanically ventilated ICU patients. Second, mobilization began almost immediately—most patients began mobilization within one and a half days following endotracheal intubation, limited only by the inability of investigators to obtain informed consent. This study demonstrates the feasibility of very early mobilization in selected critically ill and mechanically ventilated patients.

Other studies have demonstrated clearly that neuromuscular weakness occurs very rapidly in mechanically ventilated patients. For example, Levine and colleagues demonstrated diaphragmatic atrophy after less than one day of full ventilatory

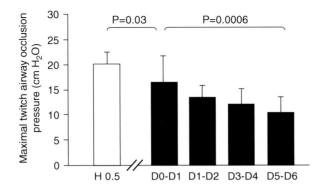

Fig. 3.3 Electron microscopy image of diaphragm in patient receiving long-term mechanical ventilation showing disorganized sarcomere structure. Reprinted with permission of the American Thoracic Society. Copyright © 2014 American Thoracic Society. Jaber S, Petrof BJ, Jung B, et al. Rapidly progressive diaphragmatic weakness and injury during mechanical ventilation in humans. Am J Respir Crit Care Med. 2011;183(3):364–71. Official Journal of the American Thoracic Society

support [11]. Jaber and colleagues also noted diaphragm injury with resultant diaphragm weakness 1 day after initiating mechanical ventilation (Fig. 3.3) [12].

Given the rapidity with which neuromuscular weakness and deconditioning occur in this patient population, the aim of Schweickert and colleagues' study of very early mobilization was to prevent neurological complications before they happened. Patients from medical ICUs undergoing mechanical ventilation for less than 72 h who were functionally independent prior to admission to the ICU were enrolled. The intervention group followed a progressive physical and occupational therapy regimen focused on mobilization and maintenance of the ability to perform functional tasks (i.e., activities of daily living [ADLs]). There were no differences in any other aspect of medical care between the two groups, as evidence-based standardized care was provided to all patients. Specifically, all patients underwent daily sedative interruptions, daily spontaneous breathing trials, early enteral nutrition, and tight glucose control.

Once they were awake, a physical and occupational therapy team worked with patients in the intervention group in a progressive, step-wise manner. The mobilization team led patients through sequential activities such as sitting at the edge to the bed, engaging in simulated activities of daily living, transfer training, and assisted ambulation. Control patients also received physical and occupational therapy, but this was done later in their hospital course and was initiated by the primary clinical team rather than being reflexively initiated for all patients. A separate group of therapists who were blinded to patient randomization assignments performed evaluations of functional outcomes. The primary endpoint of this trial focused on avoiding neurological complications so that patients would maintain independent functional status at the time of hospital discharge. Functional independence was defined *a priori* as the ability to perform ADLs (bathing, dressing, eating, grooming, transfer from bed to chair, toileting) and the ability to walk independently.

The intervention group that underwent early mobilization was active even while intubated and mechanically ventilated. While being mechanically ventilated, bed mobility occurred 76 % of the time (a median of 1.7 days after intubation); standing occurred 33 % of the time (median 3.2 days after intubation); chair sitting occurred 33 % of the time (median 3.1 days after intubation); and ambulation occurred 15 % of the time (median 3.8 days after intubation; median ambulation distance 15 ft). The early mobilization group had reduced neurological dysfunction, as evidenced by a 1.7 fold increase functional independence at hospital discharge (59 vs. 35 %; $p = 0.02$). There were no differences in the amount of sedative medications administered to patients in the intervention versus the control groups. Despite this, the duration of mechanical ventilation was reduced (3.4 versus 6.1 days; $p = 0.02$). The number of days of ICU delirium was reduced by 50 % in the intervention group (2.0 versus 4.0 days, $p = 0.03$). The early mobilization patients had better maximal walking distances (33.4 versus 0 m, $p = 0.004$) and were able to perform more ADLs at hospital discharge (6 versus 4, $p = 0.06$). More patients in the early mobilization group were discharged home (43 versus 24 %; $p = 0.06$). Despite the fact that virtually all patients screened for inclusion in the intervention group were considered candidates for mobilization, adverse events were rare. Even high-risk patients mobilized without adverse events. High-risk patients included those with acute lung injury (58 % of all mobilization sessions), morbid obesity (41 % of all mobilization sessions), shock requiring vasoactive infusions (17 % of all mobilization sessions), and patients requiring renal replacement therapy (9 % of all mobilization sessions).

In 2010, Needham and colleagues [13] designed a quality improvement project focused on reducing sedation and delirium and increasing mobilization in ICU patients. Using a multidisciplinary team, including full time physical and occupational therapists, routine mobilization replaced a previous routine of bed rest and deep sedation. The group reported less sedative and opiate use and reduced ICU delirium. In conjunction with these findings, critically ill patients underwent more intensive rehabilitation and were able to achieve a higher level of functional mobility. These improved neurological outcomes translated into reduced length of stay, as ICU length of stay decreased by an average of 2.1 days and hospital length of stay decreased by 3.1 days.

Electrical Muscle Stimulation

Electrical muscle stimulation (EMS) is a strategy that has been studied as a means of reducing neuromuscular deconditioning in critically ill patients. Routsi and colleagues reported improved MRC scores and a reduced incidence of ICU-acquired neuromyopathy in patients randomized to EMS on the vastus lateralis, vastus medialis and peroneous longus muscles of both lower extremities [14]. Critical illness polyneuromyopathy (defined as MRC score < 48) was diagnosed in 12.5 % of patients in the EMS group as compared to 39.3 % in the control group (OR = 0.22; CI: 0.05–0.92, $p = 0.04$). The raw median MRC score was higher in the EMS group as compared to the control group [58 (33–60) versus 52 (2–60) respectively, median (range), $p = 0.04$]. This study is very interesting as preliminary evidence of a novel approach to prevent ICU-acquired weakness. Two major limitations of this trial are the lack of blinding of the MRC scores, which have an inherent subjectivity, and the very large dropout of patients originally enrolled in the trial. One hundred and forty patients were originally enrolled, but only 52 were evaluated for critical illness polyneuromyopathy. If future studies can confirm these preliminary findings, ECM could become a beneficial strategy for many patients.

Neurocognitive Complications of Critical Illness: Delirium and Post Traumatic Stress Disorder (PTSD)

In addition to physical manifestations of neurological complications, derangements in mental function are also very common in critically ill patients. ICU delirium has received a tremendous amount of attention over the last decade. ICU delirium is defined as an acute state of confusion characterized by fluctuating mental status, inattention, and either altered level of consciousness or disorganized thinking [15].

Delirium

A sentinel study by Ely and colleagues in 2004 reported that a high percentage of ICU patients suffer from delirium. In this trial, ICU delirium was independently associated with increased mortality at 6 months, increased hospital length of stay, fewer days alive without mechanical ventilation, and markedly increased likelihood of cognitive impairment at hospital discharge. The Confusion Assessment Method for the ICU (CAM-ICU) and the Intensive Care Delirium Screening Checklist are both well-validated delirium screening tools, and the recent Clinical Practice Guidelines for the Management of Pain, Agitation, and Delirium in Adult Patients in the Intensive Care Unit recommend use of one of these tools for all ICU patients [16]. Most ICU patients experience hypoactive delirium, which practitioners may not notice without using a delirium assessment tool to diagnose an acute confusional state.

There are several important risk factors for ICU delirium. Risk factors include pre-existing chronic conditions (e.g., hypertension, alcoholism), as well as consequences of the patient's acute critical illness (e.g., sepsis, congestive heart failure). As such, risk factors may be difficult or impossible to modify. However, there are aspects of critical care that can be modified to reduce the risk of patients developing acute delirium. Specific examples of such modifiable aspects of critical care include medications (especially sedatives and analgesics), immobilization, and sleep deprivation.

It is important to remember that delirium is a syndrome rather than a specific disease. Accordingly, there are many proposed pathophysiological mechanisms of delirium, including neurotransmitter derangements, hypoxia, hypoperfusion, inflammation, and/or drug effects. Though the data regarding biomarkers and neuroimaging are still preliminary and these tools are not yet a standard component of contemporary clinical care, such modalities have potential as tools for diagnosing and tracking delirium in critically ill patients. As a specific example, Ely and colleagues identified the apolipoprotein E4 allele as a strong independent predictor of delirium duration [17]. The same group of investigators demonstrated preliminary utility of neuroimaging, by demonstrating that reduced brain volumes and disrupted white matter integrity were both related to delirium duration [18, 19]. Such findings are intriguing, though mechanistically, the pathogenic and clinical implications of these results remain to be fully understood. Therefore, these tools are not yet ready for clinical use in the management of patients with ICU delirium.

Treating Delirium

Pharmacological Agents

Though haloperidol is often used to treat delirium in ICU patients, there is no convincing evidence that this therapy definitively results in improved clinical outcomes. In 2002, the Society of Critical Care Medicine's (SCCM) recommendations for the treatment of delirium recommended considering haloperidol. However, given the lack of compelling clinical evidence, the updated 2013 SCCM Clinical Practice Guidelines for the Management of Pain, Agitation, and Delirium in Adult Patients in the Intensive Care Unit stated: "there is no published evidence that treatment with haloperidol reduces the duration of delirium in adult ICU patients; the guidelines did note that atypical antipsychotics may reduce the duration of delirium in adult ICU patients, though this received a C recommendation (i.e., "low/very low") [16].

Alpha-2 agonists are another class of medications with the potential to address ICU delirium. Clonidine has been used for many years to treat hypertension and acute withdrawal from alcohol, cocaine, and heroin. It is available in Europe and South American in a parenteral formulation, whereas in the United States it is only available for enteral or transdermal use. Dexmedetomidine is also an alpha-2 agonist, and is much more potent as compared to clonidine. Dexmedetomidine has both sedative and analgesic properties. Patients receiving dexmedetomidine are able to interact reliably with their caregivers, yet remain tranquil. Several trials comparing dexmedetomidine to other conventional sedatives (e.g., benzodiazepines and propofol) have been performed. In 2007, the Maximizing Efficacy of Targeted Sedation and Reducing Neurological Dysfunction (MENDS) trial compared dexmedetomidine to lorazepamin in ICU patients requiring continuous sedation for greater than 24 h. Acute brain dysfunction (i.e., delirium or coma) was reduced in the patients receiving dexmedetomidine as compared to lorazepam [20].

In 2009, the Safety and Efficacy of Dexmedetomidine Compared with Midazolam (SEDCOM) trial was published [21]. SEDCOM was a much larger study than the MENDS trial, as 375 patients were enrolled. Dexmedetomidine and midazolam were equally effective with regard to achieving sedation goals. In addition, patients randomized to receive dexmedetomidine had a reduced prevalence of delirium as compared to patients randomized to receive midazolam. It is impossible to determine whether this was due to a high "deliriogenic" propensity of midazolam or some protective effect of dexmedetomidine. Most recently, Jakob and colleagues reported the results of two separate randomized controlled trials [22]. One compared dexmedetomidine to midazolam, while the other compared dexmedetomidine to propofol. In both trials, patients receiving dexmedetomidine were more arousable, better able to communicate pain, and more able to cooperate with nursing care. Delirium, however, was not directly measured in these trials.

Long-Term Cognitive and Psychological Maladjustment

The duration of ICU delirium has been reported as a predictor of long-term cognitive impairment by numerous investigators. Furthermore, duration of ICU delirium is a predictor of subsequent mortality. Post traumatic stress disorder (PTSD) occurs in approximately 10 % of ICU survivors [23]. Variables that are associated with PTSD after discharge from the ICU include delirium [24], recall of delusional memories [25], prolonged sedation, and physical restraint with no sedation. In a recent review, Hipp and Ely relay the perspective of and advice from an ICU physician after she herself suffered from ICU delirium. Given her experience as both an ICU patient as well as an ICU doctor, her insights into the experience of being critically ill and delirious is quite provocative and important for intensive care physicians and care teams to bear in mind. The summary of her recommendations are: (1) Get the patient out of bed; (2) Do not restrain patients either physically or with medications unless absolutely necessary; (3) Do not deny patients their experience; treat them as adults, not children; (4) Be patient, even when patients are agitated and "misbehave"; (5) Be aware of the long-term consequences of delirium, such as hallucinations and PTSD; (6) Surround the patient with familiarity (e.g., family and loved ones) [26].

Summary of Recommendations and Conclusion

Neurological complications are common in critically ill patients. ICU survivors recovering from respiratory failure requiring mechanical ventilation often have neuromuscular weakness and functional impairment. It is clear that surviving acute critical illness is often followed by a phase of long and often incomplete neuromuscular and neurocognitive recovery. Maintaining animation of patients with regard to both physical and mental function is critical to optimizing outcomes and reducing ICU-related neurological complications. A multidisciplinary care plan for critically ill patients is essential to optimize neurological outcomes. The ABCDE approach (Awakening and Breathing Coordination, Delirium Monitoring, Early Mobility, and Exercise) [27], as reported by others and outlined in this chapter, appears to be the best way to reduce such complications. In conclusion, to minimize neuromuscular and neurocognitive complications of critical illness, pertinent strategies are summarized in Table 3.3.

Table 3.3 Summary of recommendations to minimize neurological complications

Minimize sedative administration: use a validated sedation strategy such as a nursing algorithm or daily sedative interruption

Engage patients in *early mobilization* strategies

Bicycle ergometry is a safe and simple means of reducing ICU-acquired weakness

Electrical muscle stimulation may be useful for reducing ICU-acquired weakness, but further research is needed

Antipsychotics should be used sparingly for treating ICU delirium given limited evidence regarding clinical outcomes

Early mobilization reduces ICU delirium

Dexmedetomidine is associated with reduced delirium when compared to benzodiazepines, but not propofol

Post-traumatic stress disorder can be reduced by *daily sedative interruption* and *enhancing factual rather than delusion memories*

References

1. Asher RA. The dangers of going to bed. Br Med J. 1947;2(4536):967.
2. Herridge MS, Cheung AM, Tansey CM, Matte-Martyn A, Diaz-Granados N, Al-Saidi F, et al. One-year outcomes in survivors of the acute respiratory distress syndrome. N Engl J Med. 2003;348(8):683–93.
3. Herridge MS, Tansey CM, Matte A, Tomlinson G, Diaz-Granados N, Cooper A, et al. Functional disability 5 years after acute respiratory distress syndrome. N Engl J Med. 2011;364(14):1293–304.
4. Griffiths RD, Palmer TE, Helliwell T, MacLennan P, MacMillan RR. Effect of passive stretching on the wasting of muscle in the critically ill. Nutrition. 1995;11(5):428–32.
5. Bolton CF, Gilbert JJ, Hahn AF, Sibbald WJ. Polyneuropathy in critically ill patients. J Neurol Neurosurg Psychiatry. 1984;47(11):1223–31.
6. Bailey P, Thomsen GE, Spuhler VJ, Blair R, Jewkes J, Bezdjian L, et al. Early activity is feasible and safe in respiratory failure patients. Crit Care Med. 2007;35(1):139–45.
7. De Jonghe B, Bastuji-Garin S, Fangio P, Lacherade JC, Jabot J, Appere-De-Vecchi C, et al. Sedation algorithm in critically ill patients without acute brain injury. Crit Care Med. 2005;33(1):120–7.
8. Morris PE, Griffin L, Berry M, Thompson C, Hite RD, Winkelman C, et al. Receiving early mobility during an intensive care unit admission is a predictor of improved outcomes in acute respiratory failure. Am J Med Sci. 2011;341(5):373–7.
9. Burtin C, Clerckx B, Robbeets C, Ferdinande P, Langer D, Troosters T, et al. Early exercise in critically ill patients enhances short-term functional recovery. Crit Care Med. 2009;37(9):2499–505.
10. Schweickert WD, Pohlman MC, Pohlman AS, Nigos C, Pawlik AJ, Esbrook CL, et al. Early physical and occupational therapy in mechanically ventilated, critically ill patients: a randomised controlled trial. Lancet. 2009;373(9678):1874–82.
11. Levine S, Nguyen T, Taylor N, Friscia ME, Budak MT, Rothenberg P, et al. Rapid disuse atrophy of diaphragm fibers in mechanically ventilated humans. N Engl J Med. 2008;358(13):1327–35.
12. Jaber S, Petrof BJ, Jung B, Chanques G, Berthet JP, Rabuel C, et al. Rapidly progressive diaphragmatic weakness and injury during mechanical ventilation in humans. Am J Respir Crit Care Med. 2011;183(3):364–71.
13. Needham DM, Korupolu R, Zanni JM, Pradhan P, Colantuoni E, Palmer JB, et al. Early physical medicine and rehabilitation for patients with acute respiratory failure: a quality improvement project. Arch Phys Med Rehabil. 2010;91(4):536–42.

14. Routsi C, Gerovasili V, Vasileiadis I, Karatzanos E, Pitsolis T, Tripodaki E, et al. Electrical muscle stimulation prevents critical illness polyneuromyopathy: a randomized parallel intervention trial. Crit Care (London). 2010;14(2):R74.

15. Ely EW, Shintani A, Truman B, Speroff T, Gordon SM, Harrell Jr FE, et al. Delirium as a predictor of mortality in mechanically ventilated patients in the intensive care unit. JAMA. 2004;291(14):1753–62.

16. Barr J, Fraser GL, Puntillo K, Ely EW, Gelinas C, Dasta JF, et al. Clinical practice guidelines for the management of pain, agitation, and delirium in adult patients in the intensive care unit. Crit Care Med. 2013;41(1):278–80.

17. Ely EW, Girard TD, Shintani AK, Jackson JC, Gordon SM, Thomason JW, et al. Apolipoprotein E4 polymorphism as a genetic predisposition to delirium in critically ill patients. Crit Care Med. 2007;35(1):112–7.

18. Morandi A, Rogers BP, Gunther ML, Merkle K, Pandharipande P, Girard TD, et al. The relationship between delirium duration, white matter integrity, and cognitive impairment in intensive care unit survivors as determined by diffusion tensor imaging: the VISIONS prospective cohort magnetic resonance imaging study*. Crit Care Med. 2012;40(7):2182–9.

19. Gunther ML, Morandi A, Krauskopf E, Pandharipande P, Girard TD, Jackson JC, et al. The association between brain volumes, delirium duration, and cognitive outcomes in intensive care unit survivors: the VISIONS cohort magnetic resonance imaging study*. Crit Care Med. 2012;40(7):2022–32.

20. Pandharipande PP, Pun BT, Herr DL, Maze M, Girard TD, Miller RR, et al. Effect of sedation with dexmedetomidine vs lorazepam on acute brain dysfunction in mechanically ventilated patients: the MENDS randomized controlled trial. JAMA. 2007;298(22):2644–53.

21. Riker RR, Shehabi Y, Bokesch PM, Ceraso D, Wisemandle W, Koura F, et al. Dexmedetomidine vs midazolam for sedation of critically ill patients: a randomized trial. JAMA. 2009;301(5):489–99.

22. Jakob SM, Ruokonen E, Grounds RM, Sarapohja T, Garratt C, Pocock SJ, et al. Dexmedetomidine vs midazolam or propofol for sedation during prolonged mechanical ventilation: two randomized controlled trials. JAMA. 2012;307(11):1151–60.

23. Jones C, Backman C, Capuzzo M, Flaatten H, Rylander C, Griffiths RD. Precipitants of posttraumatic stress disorder following intensive care: a hypothesis generating study of diversity in care. Intensive Care Med. 2007;33(6):978–85.

24. Jackson JC, Hart RP, Gordon SM, Hopkins RO, Girard TD, Ely EW. Post-traumatic stress disorder and post-traumatic stress symptoms following critical illness in medical intensive care unit patients: assessing the magnitude of the problem. Crit Care (London, England). 2007;11(1):R27.

25. Jones C, Griffiths RD, Humphris G, Skirrow PM. Memory, delusions, and the development of acute posttraumatic stress disorder-related symptoms after intensive care. Crit Care Med. 2001;29(3):573–80.

26. Hipp DM, Ely EW. Pharmacological and nonpharmacological management of delirium in critically ill patients. Neurotherapeutics: J Am Soc Exp Neurotherapeutics. 2012;9(1):158–75.

27. Morandi A, Brummel NE, Ely EW. Sedation, delirium and mechanical ventilation: the 'ABCDE' approach. Curr Opin Crit Care. 2011;17(1):43–9.

Chapter 4
Hematologic Complications

Ralitza Martin, Annette Esper, and Greg S. Martin

Abstract Critically ill patients are at high risk of developing various hematologic complications that may be present on admission or occur during their stay in the Intensive Care Unit (ICU). Often times the etiology of specific hematologic abnormalities is unclear and the diagnosis may be challenging due to the complexity of critically ill patients. This chapter will focus on diagnosis and management of the most commonly encountered hematologic problems in the critically ill such as anemia, neutropenia, thrombocytopenia, coagulopathy and thrombotic complications, with specific focus on diagnosis and management of these conditions.

Keywords Hematologic • Complications • ICU • Anemia • Erythrocytosis • Thrombocytopenia • Thrombocytosis • Neutropenia • Leukocytosis • Coagulopathy • HIT • DIC • TTP • HELLP • DVT • PE • Transfusion

Anemia in the ICU

Anemia is a very common problem in critically ill patients, with nearly two-thirds of patients in the Intensive Care Unit (ICU) have a hemoglobin <12 g/dl, and almost all develop anemia at some point during their stay [1]. Although there remains considerable controversy regarding the optimal hemoglobin levels in the ICU, careful

R. Martin, M.D. (✉) • G.S. Martin, M.D., M.Sc.
Division of Pulmonary, Allergy and Critical Care, Emory University School of Medicine,
49 Jesse Hill Jr. Drive, Pulmonary, Atlanta, GA 30303, USA
e-mail: ralitza.martin@emory.edu; greg.martin@emory.edu

A. Esper, M.D., M.Sc.
Division of Pulmonary, Allergy and Critical Care Medicine, Grady Memorial Hospital,
Emory University, 49 Jesse Hill Jr. Drive, FOB, Pulmonary, Atlanta, GA 30303, USA
e-mail: aesper@emory.edu

J.B. Richards and R.D. Stapleton (eds.), *Non-Pulmonary Complications of Critical Care:*
A Clinical Guide, Respiratory Medicine, DOI 10.1007/978-1-4939-0873-8_4,
© Springer Science+Business Media New York 2014

management can improve morbidity and mortality [2]. In this section we will briefly review the physiology, etiologies and effects of anemia and potential treatment strategies.

Red Blood Cell Function

Red blood cells (RBCs) are the main transporting vessel for oxygen and carbon dioxide, have potent antioxidant capacity, enhance hemostasis by directing platelets to the vessel wall, and actively participate in vasoregulation. These functions may be compromised by critical illness. The regular life span of RBCs is approximately 120 days which means that there must be constant production of new cells. This process requires crucial factors such as iron, zinc, folate, and vitamin B12 as well as the influence of several hormones including erythropoietin (EPO), thyroxin, androgens, cortisol, and catecholamines. With aging, properties of the RBC change, including oxygen binding affinity, ability to deform during microvascular transit, and structural morphology which marks it for destruction by the spleen and reticuloendothelial system (RES) [1]. Due to inflammation, nutritional deficiencies, renal failure, and decreased EPO levels, these changes occur even sooner and shorten the life span of RBCs in critical illness.

Etiology of Anemia in Critical Illness

There are three major causes of anemia in the ICU: blood loss, increased RBC destruction and decreased RBC production (see Table 4.1).

Blood Loss

The average daily loss of 40–70 ml of blood in the ICU from diagnostic phlebotomy exceeds the normal physiologic replacement rate of 15–20 ml/day and can lead to higher transfusion requirements. The volume of blood loss is higher for patients with more organ dysfunction and who have intravascular lines in place which facilitate easy access for phlebotomy [3]. The amount of blood loss due to surgery can be very significant but varies depending on the type of procedure—ranging from 3 units during total hip arthroplasty to 6 units during bilateral total knee arthroplasty [2]. Physiologic stress, especially in those with head trauma and who are mechanically ventilated, can lead to stress ulceration and acute bleeding. In one prospective study, 10 % of all patients admitted to the ICU developed bleeding [3]. The gastrointestinal (GI) tract is the most common site, accounting for up to 30 % of all significant bleeding in the ICU. Pro-inflammatory cytokines, coagulopathy, renal failure, and malnutrition can exacerbate acute bleeding [2,3].

Table 4.1 Etiologies of anemia

Anemia due to blood loss/sequestration
- Active hemorrhage
  - Rapid—GI bleed, trauma, hematoma
  - Slow—ulcer, gastritis
- Phlebotomy
- Surgical procedure
- Dilutional (intravenous fluids, pregnancy)

Anemia due to decreased red blood cell production
- Bone marrow suppression (inflammation, infection, drugs, alcohol)
- Bone marrow infiltration (tumor, infection)
- Bone marrow disorder (myeloproliferative disorders, leukemia, myelodysplastic syndrome)
- Nutritional deficiency (vitamin B12, folic acid)
- Low levels of stimulating hormones (EPO in chronic renal failure, TSH in hypothyroidism)

Anemia due to red blood cell destruction
- *Hemolysis*
  - Extravascular
    - Intrinsic: sickle cell, G6PD deficiency, spherocytosis, thalassemia
    - Extrinsic: liver disease, autoimmune conditions
  - Intravascular
    - Infusion of hypotonic solutions
    - Transfusion reaction
    - Systemic infections
    - Trauma from valves/intravascular devices
    - Drug effect

Decreased Production

Anemia in the ICU can also be attributed to decreased production of RBCs which can be caused by many factors, including reduced concentrations of EPO, blunted response to EPO, toxic effects of medications, nutritional deficiencies of essential substrates (iron, vitamin B12, folate), bone marrow fibrosis, or tumor infiltration of the bone marrow. Unlike healthy individuals where decreased hemoglobin levels and hypoxia trigger almost immediate production and release of EPO, this response is blunted in the critically ill patient. This blunted response can be explained by the high prevalence of renal failure in this population. In addition, inflammatory cytokines (e.g., interleukin-1, transforming growth factor (TGF)-β, and tumor necrosis factor (TNF)-α) inhibit EPO gene transcription in renal juxtaglomerular cells and the response to EPO in the bone marrow, suppress iron release from storage sites, and increase iron sequestration.

Toxic effects of medications on the bone marrow should also be considered in the evaluation of anemia. In addition to chemotherapeutic agents, known for their myelosuppressive effects, many other medications commonly used in the ICU can decrease bone marrow activity, including antibiotics, corticosteroids, histamine-2 blockers, and others [2,3].

Increased RBC Destruction

In critical illness there is increased RBC destruction due to several reasons, including decreased RBC deformability and reduced life span. Hemolysis can also contribute to anemia. Hemolysis can be *intrinsic*, i.e., the cells are destroyed due to a defect in the RBCs themselves. Some of these defects are inherited (e.g., thalassemia, sickle cell disease, glucose-6-phosphate dehydrogenase (G-6-PD) deficiency) or defects may be acquired as in autoimmune diseases, malaria, hepatitis, and disseminated intravascular coagulation (DIC). In *extrinsic* hemolysis normal RBCs are produced but are destroyed iatrogenically. Examples include infusion of hypotonic solutions, mechanical valves, intra-aortic balloon pumps, as well as toxic effects of commonly used medications such as antibiotics, sulfa drugs, and acetaminophen [2].

Evaluation

Anemia has several physiologic effects on the body including a decrease in intravascular volume and viscosity leading to increased cardiac output, heart rate, stroke volume, and oxygen extraction.

It is important to recognize that anemia is associated with increased morbidity and mortality in the ICU [1]. It can be particularly problematic in patients with ischemic heart disease or cerebrovascular disease. Many studies have shown an association between anemia and adverse outcomes in congestive heart failure (CHF), acute myocardial infarction and chronic kidney disease [4]. It can contribute to failure to liberate from mechanical ventilation, demand ischemia, and death. While anemia may be associated with poorer outcomes in ICU patients, it is crucial to note that aggressive correction of anemia through liberal blood transfusions and erythropoietic agents has also been shown to be harmful [4].

Hemoglobin level is the most useful laboratory measurement for diagnosing and monitoring anemia, with normal values between 12 and 16 g/dl for women and 13 and 19 g/dl for men. The hematocrit (HCT) is a rough estimate and is approximately three times the hemoglobin value. Low hemoglobin and haptoglobin, along with an elevated lactate dehydrogenase (LDH) and elevated serum indirect bilirubin, indicate a hemolytic process and a Coombs test can help distinguish the cause of a hemolytic anemia. The reticulocyte count can indicate whether the marrow response is adequate. Review of the peripheral blood smear can offer additional information regarding potential causes of anemia, including assessing for evidence of RBC destruction (e.g., schistocytes) and characterizing RBC morphology (e.g., determining RBC size and chromicity).

To evaluate for iron deficiency, anemia serum iron, serum ferritin and transferring saturation are used as markers to assess total body iron stores. *Serum iron* is not a particularly reliable test because it is altered by a variety of conditions including infection, inflammation, neoplasm, and liver disease. Its sensitivity and specificity are 78 and 35 %, respectively, and thus it should not be used alone in determining the etiology of anemia. Serum ferritin is an acute phase reactant, is increased with chronic inflammation, and can also be affected by acute inflammation, infection, and malnutrition. Although a low ferritin level is highly suggestive of iron deficiency (sensitivity and specificity are 71 and 69 %, respectively), an iron-deficient patient can have a high ferritin level. The normal range for ferritin is between 100 and 800 ng/ml. Although cut-off values for iron supplementation in the ICU have not been established, some authors suggest using ferritin <100 ng/ml as an indication to begin iron therapy. *Transferrin saturation* provides information about the amount of iron available for erythropoiesis. The National Kidney Foundation recommends values of 20–50 %. Transferrin saturation of <20 % indicates diminished iron availability and depending on the clinical setting, the need for iron supplementation. However, in critically ill patients with low transferrin saturation and high ferritin levels, this can indicate functional iron deficiency [2].

Management

The first step in managing anemia is to determine its etiology and type. Once the etiology is confirmed the best approach is to eliminate the risk factors (e.g., ensure stress ulcer prophylaxis, discontinue offending medications, minimize blood draws, identify source of bleeding) and decide on the need for intervention.

Transfusion

Blood transfusion is the most commonly used treatment for anemia in the ICU. More than one-third of all ICU patients receive transfusion, with the frequency increasing to 70 % when the ICU stay exceeds 1 week. There remains much controversy regarding the best transfusion practice. The primary goal of transfusion in volume-replete, non-hemorrhagic patients is to improve tissue oxygen delivery. This goal needs to be weighed against multiple potential problems associated with giving allogenic blood such as transfusion reactions, transfusion-related infections, transfusion-related acute lung injury (TRALI), transfusion-associated circulatory overload (TACO), and transfusion-related immunomodulation (TRIM).

While modern blood banking has decreased the risk of transfusion-transmitted viral or bacterial infections, the risk of transfusion reaction, TRALI, TACO, and TRIM remain and can contribute to morbidity and health care costs. Two studies in general ICU patients, the Anemia and Blood Transfusion in the Critically Ill (ABC trial) in 2002 [5] and CRIT (Anemia and Blood Transfusion in the Critically Ill—Current Clinical Practice in the United States) in 2004 [6]), found blood transfusions to be an independent predictor of death, and a randomized trial in 1999 found that critically ill patients who were transfused at a higher hemoglobin threshold of 10 g/dl had poorer outcomes than those transfused at a lower threshold of 7 g/dl [4].

Storage

Some of the complications of transfusions could potentially be explained by the changes that occur during packed red blood cell (PRBC) storage. The Food and Drug Administration (FDA) limits the maximum duration of storage to 42 days to ensure adequate cellular integrity. The mean storage time of PRBCs transfused in US ICUs is 16–21 days. Detrimental changes to PRBCs occurring during preservation and storage include decreased concentration of adenosine triphosphate (ATP) and 2,3-diphosphoglycerate (DPG), as well as accumulation of pro-inflammatory cytokines, with the hypothesized effects of these changes being potent nitric oxide scavenging, vasoconstriction, loss of normal RBC-mediated vasoregulation, and immunosuppression. Studies investigating the association between length of PRBC storage duration and mortality have not been conclusive; however, there are two ongoing trials addressing this matter (Age of Blood Evaluation—ABLE [7], and Red Cell Storage Duration—RECESS [8]).

Leukoreduction

The practice of leukoreduction has the hypothetical benefit of reducing transmission of viruses, febrile non-hemolytic transfusion reactions, human leukocyte antigen (HLA) alloimmunization, nosocomial infections, and death. Currently the majority of PRBC transfusions in the US are leukocyte reduced. Although there have been studies that have shown reduced morbidity and mortality after universal leukocyte reduction, randomized trials have failed to find benefit.

Transfusion Thresholds

Data suggest that hemoglobin levels of 7–9 g/dl in the non-bleeding ICU patient are generally well tolerated. One should also consider that blood is a very costly and scarce resource. The hallmark trial that helped establish the current guidelines for transfusion threshold is the TRICC trial (Transfusion Requirements in Critical Care) [4]. In this trial the authors found no difference in mortality at 30 days between a restrictive approach (transfusion for hemoglobin <7 g/dl) versus a liberal approach (hemoglobin <10 g/dl) in critically ill non-bleeding patients. Interestingly, one recently published trial also demonstrated that a restrictive approach is not only safe in patients with active GI bleeding, but it also significantly reduced morbidity and mortality [9].

There remains controversy regarding transfusion in specific groups of patients such as those with ischemic heart disease or active GI bleeding, who have failed liberation from mechanical ventilation, and receiving early resuscitation for septic shock. More research is necessary to understand the optimal approach to transfusion practices in these patients.

Blood Substitutes

There are two categories of blood substitutes/oxygen carrying agents: hemoglobin solutions and perfluorocarbons. These agents have high affinity for oxygen and although conceptually promising, they are yet to be proven as a safe alternative to blood and remain investigational [2].

Erythropoietin

Erythropoietin (EPO) is an endogenous hormone produced by the kidney that promotes production of RBCs in the bone marrow. Critically ill patients have decreased circulating concentrations of EPO, as well as a blunted response to it, which initially increased interest in determining whether administration of exogenous EPO could improve outcomes. Several trials have since demonstrated that in the environment of restrictive transfusion, EPO therapy does not improve survival and may increase thrombotic complications. One potential explanation for this lack of efficacy may be due to the significant lag time between administering EPO and its onset of action. It is important to note that when EPO therapy is considered, it should always be given concomitantly with iron supplementation to ensure maximum benefit. Neither epoetin alfa nor darbepoetin alfa (the latter having an increased half-life and bioactivity) are approved for the treatment of anemia of critical illness.

Iron Supplementation

As already mentioned, iron supplementation is required when considering erythropoietic agents. Although animal studies have suggested that iron promotes infections, this has not been proven in clinical studies. While oral iron has poor absorption and can interact with other drugs, intravenous (IV) iron supplementation can provide rapid repletion of systemic iron stores. The previously reported rare complication of anaphylactic reaction with IV iron dextran has not been observed in other preparations such as iron gluconate and iron sucrose.

Minimization of Blood Loss

Small-volume phlebotomy tubes, point-of-care testing, non-invasive testing (such as CO_2 monitors and pulse oximeters), and reinfusion of discarded samples from indwelling lines are all strategies that can minimize blood loss through phlebotomy. In addition, reducing the number of laboratory studies in ICU patients can be done safely without compromising care and the need for labs. This strategy has been termed "learning not to know."

Summary

In conclusion, anemia is a very common condition in the ICU and is associated with poor outcomes and higher healthcare resource utilization. In addition to tailoring guidelines and recommendations on safest therapeutic interventions to the needs of each patient with regard to management of anemia, it will likely be beneficial for ICU protocols on blood conservation techniques to be developed.

Erythrocytosis/Polycythemia

While erythrocytosis is a relatively uncommon finding in the ICU setting, it can be seen in various diseases and can be associated with thrombotic or hemorrhagic complications. The term erythrocytosis is often used interchangeably with the term polycythemia, and is suspected when the serum HCT is >48 % in women and >52 % in men, and the serum hemoglobin (hemoglobin) concentration is >16.5 g/dl and >18.5 g/dl in women and men, respectively. Since both measurements represent concentration relative to volume, polycythemia can be classified as relative or absolute. *Relative* polycythemia can occur when the plasma volume is reduced as a result of intravascular volume depletion (diarrhea, vomiting, massive capillary leak) which causes hemoconcentration. *Absolute* polycythemia is accompanied by an increase in RBC mass and can be further divided into primary and secondary polycythemias [10] (see Table 4.2).

Table 4.2 Etiologies of erythrocytosis

Relative
–   Intravascular volume depletion

Absolute
–   *Primary*
   •   Polycythemia vera (PV), primary congenital and familial polycythemia
–   *Secondary*
   •   Conditions associated with chronic hypoxemia:
       Congenital heart disorders
       COPD
       Obstructive sleep apnea (OSA)/obesity hypoventilation syndrome (OHS)
       Tobacco use
       High altitude
   •   Drugs
       Androgens
       Corticosteroids
   •   Other
       Post renal transplant, renal cell carcinoma, polycystic kidney disease

Etiology of Erythrocytosis

The *primary polycythemias* include polycythemia vera (PV) and primary familial and congenital polycythemia (PFCP). PV is associated with the Janus kinase 2 (JAK2) mutation and low or normal EPO levels. Thrombosis is very frequently noted, with two-thirds of thrombotic episodes occurring either at presentation or before diagnosis of PV. Arterial thrombotic events are more common than venous events in patients with PV, with transient ischemic attacks, ischemic strokes, and myocardial infarctions being the most common thrombotic complications. Patients with PV who undergo surgical procedures are also at a higher risk of post-operative thrombotic complications.

Secondary polycythemia is associated with hypoxemia due to cyanotic heart and/ or pulmonary disease. EPO production is triggered when PaO_2 is sustained at <67 mmHg. Chronic obstructive pulmonary disease (COPD), obstructive sleep apnea (OSA), obesity hypoventilation syndrome (OHS), high altitude, tobacco use, and carbon monoxide poisoning are common conditions that have been linked to secondary polycythemia. Other less common conditions associated with secondary polycythemia are post-renal transplant erythrocytosis (found in up to 15 % of renal allograft recipients), renal cell carcinoma, polycystic kidney disease, hepatocellular carcinoma, and pheochromocytoma. Polycythemia may also be secondary to drugs such as corticosteroids or androgens [10].

Evaluation

The first step in establishing the cause of erythrocytosis is ruling out secondary causes which can often be determined by careful history and physical examination. Measuring the EPO level can also be helpful, with increased levels consistent with a hypoxic state and low levels being virtually diagnostic for PV. The diagnosis of PV can also be confirmed by molecular testing for JAK2 mutation.

Management

As mentioned, patients with erythrocytosis, and specifically those with PV, are at a much higher risk of thrombotic complications which are often noted on presentation. While the goal of treatment in the ICU is to manage the complications of PV, the long-term goal after resolution of a patient's critical illness is to reduce the risk by reducing the HCT to 42 % in women and 45 % in men. This is achieved by daily low-dose aspirin, phlebotomy and in patients who are high risk (age >60, prior thrombotic events) myelosuppressive therapy with pegylated interferon or hydroxyurea may be indicated [10].

Neutropenia in the ICU

Since neutrophils play a key role in the innate immune defense against microbes, neutropenia is a predisposing risk factor for infections. Neutropenia is defined as an absolute neutrophil count (ANC) of less than 1,500 cells/µL. We differentiate mild (ANC 1,000–1,500 cells/µL), moderate (500–1,000 cells/µL) and severe (ANC <500 cells/µL) neutropenia. Agranulocytosis is specifically defined as <200 cells/µL [11]. This stratification aids in predicting infection risk, as in general patients with chronic (lasting >3 months) severe neutropenia are at risk for major pyogenic infections [12]. There are many different causes of neutropenia including congenital, infectious, autoimmune, nutritional deficiencies, malignancy or drug-related. Because the underlying cause of neutropenia may also be associated with an increased risk of infection, it must also be considered when evaluating the patient. For example, patients with neutropenia due to leukemia have a much higher infection risk than those with ethnic neutropenia or chronic idiopathic neutropenia. The most frequent sites of infection in neutropenic patients are skin, oral mucosa and lungs. Importantly, the paucity of neutrophils results in a blunted immune response and decreased frequency or severity of the typical signs and symptoms of an infection.

Etiology of Neutropenia

The major causes of neutropenia in the ICU are infection, malignancy, and medications. However, when patients are diagnosed with neutropenia the clinician should also include other potential causes ethnic neutropenia (more prevalent in the African American population, considered to be benign), congenital neutropenia, immune-mediated neutropenia (seen in patients with systemic autoimmune disorders such as systemic lupus erythematosus (SLE), rheumatoid arthritis (RA), and hypothyroidism), and idiopathic neutropenia (Table 4.3).

Medication-induced neutropenia (not due to chemotherapeutics) is relatively rare but should be considered in every patient with neutropenia. The incidence increases with age, likely because older individuals are exposed to more drugs. Many medications have been implicated, with the most common culprit drugs including lactam antibiotics, cotrimoxazole, anti-thyroid medications, ticlopidine, neuroleptics, antiepileptics, rituximab, and non-steroidal anti-inflammatory medications (NSAIDs). The onset of neutropenia is highly variable depending on the drug and can range from days to weeks after initiation. There are two mechanisms involved: repeated exposure causing myelosuppression, or intermittent exposure leading to immune-mediated antibody production. The latter is most commonly due to β-lactam antibiotics and anti-thyroid medications. A bone marrow biopsy can elucidate the expected duration of neutropenia—if precursors are present but there are no mature cells, recovery can take 5–7 days. If no neutrophil precursors are present, recovery can take up to 14 days. With regard to treatment, the offending medication should be discontinued. There is no clear role for giving granulocyte colony

Table 4.3 Etiologies of neutropenia

Ethnic variations
– African American

Congenital
– Cyclic neutropenia
– Severe congenital neutropenia
– Shwachman–Diamond syndrome

Acquired
– Immune-related (RA, SLE, hyperthyroidism)
– Infectious
  • Sepsis
  • Viral: HIV, HSV, EBV, CMV, Parvovirus B19, Hepatitis A/B/C, measles, rubella
  • Bacterial
  • Parasitic: Malaria, leishmaniasis, babesiosis
– Malignancy (Leukemias, myelodysplastic syndrome)
– Hypersplenism
– Nutritional deficiencies (Vitamin B12, folic acid, copper)
– Medications
  • **Antibiotics** (β-lactam, macrolides, trimethoprim–sulfamethoxazole, sulfanoamides, cephalosporins)
  • **NSAIDS**
  • **Cardiac** (procainamide, quinidine, ACE-inhibitors, digoxin)
  • **Antithyroid** (propylthiouracil, methimazole)
  • **Anticonvulsants** (valproic acid, phenytoin)
  • **Antipsychotics** (clozapine, chlorpromazine)
  • **Antineoplastic agents**

---

stimulating factor (G-CSF) in the setting of neutropenia induced by medications other than chemotherapeutics, but empirically administering broad spectrum antibiotics while awaiting count recovery is warranted if infection is suspected.

Infections

Human Immunodeficiency Virus

One of the major infections associated with neutropenia is human immunodeficiency virus (HIV). Neutropenia is usually caused directly, or by concurrent infections (e.g., bacterial, cytomegalovirus (CMV), mycobacterium avium, histoplasmosis) and medications. Medications commonly associated with neutropenia in patients with HIV include anti-retrovirals (specifically zidovudine), trimethoprim/sulfamethoxazole, and ganciclovir. Factors associated with neutropenia are low CD4 count (<200 cells/μL) and high viral load (>100,000 copies/ml).

Other Infections

In addition to HIV, other viruses have been implicated as causes of neutropenia. Human herpes virus 6 and measles are potential causes of neutropenia in children, and CMV primarily affects immuno-compromised patients, but occasionally causes neutropenia in immunocompetent patients. Sepsis caused by any bacteria can induce neutropenia by consumption of neutrophils in the setting of overwhelming infection. Zoonoses (tularemia, brucellosis) and parasites should be considered in the appropriate clinical setting.

Malignancy

In addition to neutropenia caused by chemotherapeutic medications for treatment of hematologic and solid cancers, certain hematologic malignancies can directly cause neutropenia. Specifically, the acute leukemias and myelodysplastic syndrome (MDS), which is characterized by ineffective hematopoiesis, are frequently associated with neutropenia. Diagnosis of these hematologic malignancies is confirmed with a bone marrow biopsy.

Evaluation

A thorough physical exam and history could reveal the etiology for neutropenia, with specific emphasis on ethnicity, the presence of congenital disorders, underlying malignancy, infectious exposures, and new medications. Review of systems and physical exam should include an assessment for the presence of fever, chills, lymphadenopathy, easy bruising, and recurrent infections. Initial labs should include a complete blood count (CBC) with a differential count and peripheral smear examining for neutrophil abnormalities such as Dohle bodies (infection), immature neutrophil precursors (infection, myelodysplasia), hypoplastic changes (myelodysplasia), and hyperlobulation (nutritional deficiencies). Additional labs could include a reticulocyte count, LDH, erythrocyte sedimentation rate (ESR), rheumatoid factor, antinuclear antibody (ANA), thyroid stimulating hormone (TSH), HIV, vitamin B12, and potentially folate levels. Bone marrow biopsy should be considered in cases where there is a high suspicion for a malignancy to assess for either a primary hematologic malignancy or an infiltrating metastatic solid tumor. In the appropriate clinical scenario, the presence of antibodies against Borrelia burgdorferi should be tested. Granulocyte agglutination test or granulocyte immunofluorescence test for anti-granulocyte antibodies should be assessed in cases where an autoimmune disorder as a cause of neutropenia is suspected [11,12].

Management

Treatment should target the underlying process causing neutropenia. Nutritional deficiencies should be corrected and offending drugs discontinued. In addition, if infection is present, colony stimulating factors (CSFs) may be indicated.

Treatment Guidelines for Infection in Neutropenic Patients with Cancer

Neutropenic fever in the setting of an underlying malignancy is not an uncommon scenario in critical care medicine. In 2010 the Infectious Disease Society of America issued updated guidelines for treatment of patients with neutropenia induced by chemotherapy [13]. Fever is often the only sign of an underlying infection and requires prompt treatment. A scoring system was developed to assess the risk of serious complications in febrile neutropenia. The Multinational Association for Supportive Care in Cancer (MASCC) scoring system considers age, severity of symptoms, prior infections, and type of malignancy in calculating a score that can guide therapy (oral versus intravenous and outpatient versus inpatient antibiotics). Lab tests should include a CBC, serum creatinine, transaminases, and at least 2 blood cultures (with one drawn from each port of central venous catheters [if present] as well as an additional peripheral culture). Other specimens should be obtained for culture as clinically indicated (urine, sputum, cerebrospinal fluid, and other microbiologic cultures). A chest radiograph should also be obtained if respiratory symptoms are present. The following is a brief summary of recommendations regarding care of critically ill patients with malignancy and neutropenic fever.

Choosing Antibiotic Therapy

In critically ill patients with impending or existing organ dysfunction, rapid delivery of empiric antibiotics is crucial. Monotherapy with an anti-pseudomonal β-lactam agent such as cefepime, a carbapenem, or piperacillin-tazobactam is recommended. Other agents may be added to the initial regimen if clinically indicated—vancomycin or linezolid for methicillin-resistant Staphylococcus aureus (MRSA), linezolid or daptomycin for vancomycin-resistant enterococcus (VRE), carbapenem for extended-spectrum β-lactamase (ESBL) producing bacteria. Most patients with penicillin allergy can tolerate cephalosporins, but in patients with a history of immune-mediated hypersensitivity reaction characterized by hives or bronchospasm, the use of aztreonam plus vancomycin to avoid β-lactams or carbapenems is recommended. Afebrile neutropenic patients who have new signs and symptoms of an infection should be evaluated and treated as high-risk patients. A patient receiving a fluoroquinolone as a prophylactic antibiotic should not receive a fluoroquinolone as empiric therapy of an acute infection.

Changing the Antibiotic Regimen

Modification of the initial antibiotic regimen should be guided by clinical and microbiologic data. Infections should be treated with the appropriate antibiotics for the site of the primary infection, and guided by the susceptibilities of any isolated organism.

If vancomycin or other coverage for gram-positive organisms was started, it may be stopped if after 2 days there is no evidence of gram-positive infection.

Patients who remain hemodynamically unstable after receiving their first doses of standard agents should have their regimen broadened to cover resistant gram-negative, gram-positive, anaerobes and fungi.

Duration of Treatment

The duration of treatment is guided by the site of infection and organism involved but should continue at least for the duration of neutropenia (until ANC > 500 cells/ μL).

If no source of infection is identified, guidelines advise to continue empiric therapy until bone marrow recovery. Patients who remain neutropenic beyond completion of the appropriate antibiotic therapy can resume oral fluoroquinolone therapy until marrow recovery.

Empiric Anti-Fungal Coverage

Empiric antifungal therapy should be initiated and clinical investigation for invasive fungal infections should be pursued if there is persistent or recurrent fever after 4–7 days of antibiotics, as well as for patients whose neutropenia is expected to last >7 days.

Viral Treatment

Influenza virus infections should be treated with neuraminidase inhibitors if the strain is susceptible. In the setting of influenza outbreak patients with flu-like symptoms should be treated empirically. Antiviral treatment for herpes simplex virus (HSV) or varicella-zoster virus (VZV) is only indicated if there is clinical or laboratory evidence of active viral disease.

Respiratory virus testing (including assays for influenza, parainfluenza, adenovirus, respiratory syncytial virus (RSV), and human metapneumovirus) and chest X-ray are indicated in patients presenting with upper respiratory symptoms.

Role of Hematopoietic Growth Factors (G-CSF or GM-CSF)

Colony stimulating factors (CSFs) are not routinely recommended for afebrile patients with neutropenia. However, administration of CSFs should be considered in patients at high risk of infection-associated complications or poor clinical outcomes. These high-risk patients include those with expected prolonged (>10 day) or profound (<100 cells/μL) neutropenia, age >65 years of age, pneumonia, hypotension, multisystem organ failure, sepsis, invasive fungal infection, or being hospitalized at the time of the development of fever. As many patients with neutropenic fever cared for in an ICU have sepsis or organ failure, CSF administration may sometimes be warranted.

Catheter-Related Infections

A culture drawn from a central venous or arterial line that is positive up to 120 min faster than a culture drawn from a peripheral venipuncture is a sign of a central line associated blood stream infection (CLABSI). Removal of the catheter is essential for any patient with a suspected or confirmed CLABSI who has sepsis, hemodynamic instability, evidence of endocarditis, persistent bacteremia for more than 72 h despite antibiotics, or evidence of tunnel or pocket infection. In the ICU, patients often demonstrate some degree of hemodynamic instability, so catheter removal is common. Of note, catheter exchange over a wire should not be performed and if central access is needed, a new central venous catheter should be placed at a new insertion site.

Prolonged treatment (4–6 weeks) is recommended for a complicated CLABSI as defined by the presence of deep tissue infection, endocarditis, septic thrombosis or persistent bacteremia and fungemia occurring >72 h after catheter removal in a patient who has received the appropriate antimicrobial therapy.

Environmental Precautions

Standard barrier precautions should be followed, and infection-specific isolation should be used with patients with certain signs or symptoms (e.g., when meningitis is suspected). No fresh or dried plants should be allowed in rooms of neutropenic patients.

Summary

Neutropenia in the ICU can be a common problem, usually caused by infection, malignancy or medications. Treatment targets the underlying pathogenic cause and in the setting of neutropenic fever prompt administration of antibiotics is critical.

Leukocytosis

Leukocytosis is defined as an absolute increase of the white blood count, usually greater than 11,000/μL. The term includes all granulocytes but it often refers to the elevation of the ANC (neutrophilia). Isolated elevation of the lymphocyte, eosinophil or monocyte count is usually much rarer and can help direct the differential diagnosis.

Leukocytosis is very commonly encountered in daily clinical practice. There are numerous causes of leukocytosis including normal physiologic response to infection, inflammation, and/or malignancy. In the ICU the cause of leukocytosis is usually an acute event such as infection, physiologic response to stress, medications (e.g., steroids), or an acute malignancy [14].

Table 4.4 Etiologies of leukocytosis

Primary hematologic disorder
- Leukemia
- Myeloproliferative disorders (PV, ET)
- Congenital neutrophilia

Secondary
– Normal physiologic response
– Infection
– Chronic inflammation
– Stress
– Cigarette smoking
– Drug-induced
  - Corticosteroids
  - Lithium
  - β-Agonists
  - Colony stimulating factors (G-CSF)
– Non-hematologic malignancy
– Marrow stimulation (hemolytic anemia, immune thrombocytopenia, recovery from marrow suppression)

Etiology of Leukocytosis

When the white blood cell (WBC) count is elevated, the usual differential diagnosis includes a primary hematologic disorder (such as leukemia or myeloproliferative disorder) and a secondary response to a challenge (e.g., inflammation or infection). Leukocytosis may be caused by increased WBC production, mobilization from storage, or half-life; decreased migration to peripheral tissues; or a combination of these processes. The clinician should consider the duration, the nature of the cells involved, and other clinical findings to explain the increase in WBC count. *Left shift* refers to an increased percentage of immature granulocytes (bands) in the peripheral blood usually indicating an infectious process. *Leukemoid reaction* represents an exaggerated response which can be malignant or benign in etiology, and the WBC usually exceeds 50,000/μL. *Hyperleukocytosis* refers to a WBC greater than 100,000/μL and is seen almost exclusively in leukemias and myeloproliferative disorders. The excess number of cells can cause sludging in the small vessels of the brain, kidney, and lungs and is an oncologic emergency since impaired blood flow can lead to ischemia [10].

Leukocytosis is generally a manifestation of an underlying disease process and the treatment is almost always focused on that disorder (see Table 4.4).

Evaluation

A careful history and physical exam, CBC with differential, and review of the peripheral smear can offer clues to the etiology of the leukocytosis. Occasionally, bone marrow biopsy and/or cytogenetic and molecular testing along with expert consultation are required [14].

Primary Causes

Hematologic Malignancies

An elevated WBC is often the primary clinical finding leading to the diagnosis of leukemia or myeloproliferative disorder.

Symptoms can be very non-specific and can include fever, fatigue and bruising, but patients can also face life-threatening complications such as disseminated intravascular coagulopathy, leukostasis, and severe infections. A CBC and a peripheral smear (which can have varying amounts of blast cells, from none to more than 100,000/μL) will offer a clue to the diagnosis, but often bone marrow biopsy and cytogenetic or chromosome analysis will be needed for definitive confirmation. Statistically, acute myelogenous leukemia (AML) is the most common type of acute leukemia in adults, followed by acute lymphoblastic leukemia (ALL). An important subset of AML is acute promyelo-cytic leukemia (APL) which often presents with bleeding due to DIC which can lead to fatal pulmonary or cerebral hemorrhage, and requires prompt treatment.

Treatment of newly diagnosed acute leukemia in the ICU is often focused on supportive care and managing complications such as infection. Patients with hyper-leukocytosis and symptoms of leukostasis may need immediate cytoreduction to avoid further complications. This usually will require expert advice and is coordi-nated with induction chemotherapy, cytoreduction agents (such as hydroxyurea), and in some cases leukopheresis. Treatment of tumor lysis syndrome may also be required if urgent cytoreduction is needed.

Chronic lymphocytic leukemia (CLL) and *chronic myelogenous leukemia* (CML) are most often established conditions upon admission and are only rarely first diag-nosed in the ICU. Patients tend to present with less severe symptoms and usually do not require urgent aggressive treatment.

Leukocytosis can be seen also in essential thrombocythemia (ET). Most patients with ET are asymptomatic but some can face an acute thrombotic or hemorrhagic event due to a high number of dysfunctional platelets.

There are additional benign hematologic disorders associated with leukocytosis, but these are mostly inherited conditions, are relatively rare, and beyond the scope of this review.

Secondary Causes of Leukocytosis

In general, secondary causes of leukocytosis can be grouped into infectious and non-infectious categories.

Infectious Causes

Bacterial infections usually cause moderate elevation of the WBC (11,000–30,000/μL) with predominance of neutrophils and bands. While certain infections such as Clostridium difficile or tuberculosis can present with a leukemoid reaction

(WBC > 50,000/μL), it is important to note that some infections can present with leukopenia. Viral infections usually do not cause neutrophilia, but leukocytosis due to lymphocytosis can be observed in the early phase of viral infection.

Monocytosis can be seen in either bacterial or viral infection. Eosinophilia is most commonly caused by drug hypersensitivity and allergic reactions but is also an important response to parasite infection.

Non-infectious Causes

Leukocytosis can be caused by a variety of conditions including chronic inflammatory states secondary to autoimmune and inflammatory bowel disorders, medications, and splenectomy. Almost any malignancy can cause leukocytosis by non-specifically stimulating the bone marrow.

Medications commonly associated with leukocytosis are corticosteroids, lithium, β-agonists and CSFs. Corticosteroids can cause increased demargination and lithium stimulates endogenous CSF production. CSFs are commonly used in patients undergoing chemotherapy and in stem cell transplant patients to stimulate WBC into the peripheral circulation.

Marrow recovery (from chemotherapy), or stimulation of the marrow through other processes (hemolytic anemia or idiopathic thrombocytopenic purpura) can cause leukocytosis as well.

Summary

Leukocytosis is a very common finding in the ICU and can indicate an acute or a chronic process. Most frequently it represents an appropriate physiologic response to an infectious or inflammatory stimulus and less commonly is a manifestation of a primary bone marrow disorder such as leukemia, lymphoma or myeloproliferative neoplasm. Defining the cause requires a careful history, physical examination and review of the peripheral blood smear. Additional testing such as bone marrow biopsy and molecular and cytogenetic analysis may be required. Treatment is usually directed toward the underlying cause.

Thrombocytopenia in the ICU

Thrombocytopenia is generally defined as platelet count of <150,000/μL or a decrease greater than 30–50 % from a patient's prior platelet count. Thrombocytopenia is a very common occurrence in the ICU, with studies reporting prevalence upon admission of 8–67 %. Furthermore, patients may develop thrombocytopenia during their ICU stay with an incidence ranging from 13 to 44 % [15]. Thrombocytopenia may impact both the treatment of critically ill patients (such as the risk of providing deep vein thrombosis [DVT] prophylaxis or performing invasive procedures) and their prognosis. Several studies have indicated that the development of thrombocytopenia is associated with increased length of stay and morbidity, and is an independent predictor of death. These associations have been noted in both pediatric and adult populations, as well as medical and surgical patients. Thrombocytopenia seems to be an especially strong mortality predictor in patients with sepsis. Not surprisingly, patients who develop thrombocytopenia have higher severity of illness scores and patients whose platelet counts do not recover or remain persistently low have a higher mortality. Although one of the most feared complications of severe thrombocytopenia is major bleeding, the cause of excess mortality in thrombocytopenic patients does not seem to be related to uncontrolled bleeding but rather to the process causing the severe thrombocytopenia [16]. Spontaneous bleeding is rarely seen unless platelet count is <10,000/μL.

Etiology of Thrombocytopenia

Risk factors for developing thrombocytopenia in the ICU include high illness severity, organ dysfunction, sepsis, renal failure, trauma, and intravascular catheters/devices. In general, the etiology of thrombocytopenia is multifactorial and is due to some combination of the following mechanisms: increased destruction or consumption, decreased production, dilution and sequestration [17] (see Table 4.5). Most commonly in the ICU the underlying causes of thrombocytopenia are sepsis, DIC, massive transfusion and drugs.

Spurious thrombocytopenia (or also pseudothrombocytopenia) can be seen when platelets clump in collection tubes due to ethylenediaminetetraacetic acid (EDTA)-antibodies or insufficient anticoagulant. This occurs more frequently in patients with sepsis and autoimmune, neoplastic, or liver disease [17]. Platelets clump together and thus are not recognized by automated counter devices. If pseudothrombocytopenia is suspected, the clinician should always examine the peripheral smear to identify clumped platelets and re-draw a sample in a heparin or citrate containing collection tube.

Increased platelet destruction is the most common mechanism for thrombocytopenia in critically ill patients, and may be further divided into immune-mediated and non-immune-mediated.

Non-immune causes of thrombocytopenia include diffuse intravascular coagulopathy (DIC) secondary to sepsis, trauma, malignancy, thrombotic thrombocytopenic purpura/hemolytic uremic syndrome (TTP/HUS), HELLP syndrome (hemolysis, elevated liver enzymes and low platelets—see "Disorders of the hemostatic system" below), and physical destruction (cardiopulmonary bypass, intravascular devices or catheters, artificial valves).

Immune-mediated mechanisms can be primary (idiopathic/immune thrombocytopenic purpura—ITP) or secondary to drugs, autoimmune disease, infection (such as CMV, HIV, Epstein-Barr virus or EBV, parvovirus), and alloimmunization following transfusion or transplantation. ITP is caused by antibodies directed at specific antigens on the platelet surface. Treatment frequently involves steroids,

Table 4.5 Etiologies of thrombocytopenia

Spurious
- EDTA-dependent agglutinins
- Insufficient anticoagulation of collected blood samples

Increased platelet destruction
- *Immune-mediated*
  - Drugs
    Antibiotics
    Heparins
    H2 blockers
    NSAIDS
    Diuretics
    Glycoprotein IIb/IIIa inhibitors
    Antiarrhythmics
    Antiepileptics
  - Autoimmune disorders (SLE)
  - ITP
  - Infection (EBV, CMV, HIV, H. pylori)
  - Alloimmunization (post transfusion, post transplant)
- *Non-immune-mediated*
  - DIC
  - TTP
  - HELLP
  - Mechanical destruction (valves, catheters, cardio-pulmonary bypass)

Decreased platelet production
- Bone marrow suppression secondary to:
  - Drugs or toxins (chemotherapy, alcohol, radiation therapy)
  - Viral infections
  - Nutritional deficiencies (Vit B12, folic acid)
- Liver disease (decreased production of thrombopoietin)

Dilutional or distributional
- Massive transfusion
- Splenic sequestration

intravenous immunoglobulin (IVIG) or IV anti-Rhd antibody [Rh_o(D) Immune Globulin] [16]. Drug-induced thrombocytopenia develops in about 25 % of ICU patients [16]. A number of drugs have been implicated as causes (Table 4.5). This diagnosis requires a high degree of suspicion since there are no clear identifiers, it can occur days after medication exposure, and there may be multiple other possible causes for thrombocytopenia. The mechanism of destruction is through formation of anti-platelet antibodies that bind platelets in the presence of sensitizing drugs or direct drug-platelet interaction resulting in immune destruction. In most cases thrombocytopenia can be reversed if the offending agent is stopped. Heparin is probably the most common non-chemotherapeutic medication drug associated with thrombocytopenia (see heparin-induced thrombocytopenia [HIT] in "Disorders of the hemostatic system").

Dilutional thrombocytopenia and soluble factor deficiencies occur after massive blood product administration. There is no clear blood product transfusion threshold that predicts this event but replacement of the entire blood volume within 24 h or

half within 3–4 h can precipitate dilutional thrombocytopenia [17]. Dilutional coagulopathy is often complicated with large amounts of (acidic) intravenous fluids,
DIC, hypothermia, and hypoperfusion.

Splenomegaly (secondary to portal hypertension or other causes) can cause
thrombocytopenia by pooling and splenic sequestration of platelets, but thrombocytopenia in these patients is also often multifactorial. For example, thrombocytopenia
in patients with cirrhosis may be due to both splenomegaly from portal hypertension
and decreased platelet production (caused by lack of hepatic production of
thrombopoietin).

Decreased Platelet Production

Thrombocytopenia can often be the first sign of bone marrow suppression since
platelets have the shortest life span of all cell lines, especially if consumption/
destruction is increased. In addition to chemotherapeutic agents, there are myriad
additional causes of bone marrow suppression, including non-chemotherapy drugs,
viruses, toxins (e.g., alcohol and radiation therapy), malignant invasion of bone
marrow, and nutritional deficiencies. In the ICU, sepsis and drug-induced decreased
production are very common causes of thrombocytopenia. Many commonly used
medications have been implicated such as vancomycin, penicillins, cephalosporins,
histamine-2 blockers, and anticonvulsants (valproic acid and phenytoin). Once further exposure is avoided the platelet count may recover within 5–7 days, but generally not before 48 h [16].

Evaluation

One of the first steps in evaluating a critically ill patient with thrombocytopenia is
to rule out a laboratory error (e.g., spurious thrombocytopenia). In general, a rapid
decline (within 1–2 days) indicates an immune process (drug or non-drug-related)
and a slow but steady decline is more suggestive of drug-induced thrombocytopenia
resulting from marrow suppression [16]. Consumptive coagulopathy can present
acutely or more slowly, depending on the severity of the process.

Management

Since thrombocytopenia in the ICU is almost universally secondary to another process, the general recommendation is to treat the underlying process and/or remove
the offending agent (in case of drug-induced thrombocytopenia). For treatment of
HIT, TTP/HUS and HELLP, see the respective sections later in this chapter.

As with any other blood product, the risks and benefits of administering platelets
should be considered prior to transfusion. Platelet transfusions are generally not indicated in a non-bleeding patient unless counts fall below 10,000/μL where the risk for

spontaneous bleed is higher. Expert opinion recommends 50,000/µL as a threshold for transfusion in patients undergoing invasive procedures. Platelet transfusion is relatively contraindicated in TTP and HIT because transfusion in these circumstances can fuel thrombosis and potentially have catastrophic consequences. In patients with ITP, immunoglobulin infusions may enhance the response to platelet transfusion in addition to being primarily therapeutic. With advancements of technology, 6–10 units of leukocyte-reduced platelets can be collected from a single donor in one pheresis setting, which can avoid pooling from multiple donors and decrease the incidence of alloimmunization and refractoriness to platelet transfusion. HLA-matched platelet transfusions are used in patients with alloimmunization. As a rule, after transfusing 6–10 units of platelets, the measured platelet count should rise by 17,000–31,000/ µL.

Special treatment consideration should be given to critically ill patients who have platelet dysfunction. One should remember that despite normal counts, platelet activity may be impaired by medications, environment (such as in renal failure) and intrinsic platelet defects (although rare). Medications often implicated in platelet dysfunction are aspirin, clopidogrel, and glycoprotein IIb/IIIa inhibitors such as abciximab, tirofiban, and eptifibatide. It is also important to note that in a bleeding patient who has been exposed to these medications, discontinuation of the drug may not be sufficient to quickly return platelet function to normal and platelet transfusion may be necessary [17].

Despite normal platelet counts, patients with end-stage renal disease (ESRD) often have inadequate platelet function. Biologic mechanisms for this dysfunction are multifactorial and may be explained by uremia causing dysfunctional von Willebrand factor (vWF) thus leading to impaired platelet aggregation. Treatment of bleeding in a patient with ESRD may require dialysis to remove uremic toxins, desmopressin to release vWF from endothelial storage sites, and transfusion of platelets in cases of severe thrombocytopenia or severe bleeding with platelet dysfunction [17].

Thrombocytosis in the ICU

Thrombocytosis, defined in most cases as platelet count >500,000/µL, can be a common finding in the ICU. While the prevalence of thrombocytosis upon admission to the ICU is relatively low (<2 %), prevalence upon discharge is approximately 10 % [18]. It is important to distinguish between primary and secondary (reactive) thrombocytosis since the management and prognosis are quite different.

Etiology

Primary thrombocytosis is due to a clonal/myeloproliferative disorder such as essential thrombocythemia (ET), polycythemia vera (PV), or CML. It is important to note that thrombocytosis does not occur exclusively in ET and can occur in other myeloproliferative disorders, especially PV. These diseases are a risk factor for thrombotic complications, particularly in the elderly, who can face acute myocardial infarction, cerebrovascular accident (CVA), venous thromboembolism (VTE), or a bleeding complication. It is generally felt that reactive thrombocytosis does not increase the risk for thrombotic complications; however, prior research has found that reactive thrombocytosis in the recovery phase of critical illness increased both the risk of VTE after discharge as well as mortality. There is also evidence that splenectomized patients with no evidence of myeloproliferative disorder are at a higher risk for thrombotic events, especially portal, mesenteric and splenic vein thrombosis, if they have persistent thrombocytosis after splenectomy [18].

Secondary (*reactive*) *thrombocytosis* occurs in the absence of a myeloproliferative disorder and is by far the most common cause of thrombocytosis in critically ill patients (>85 % of cases) [19]. Common causes include sepsis, trauma, surgery, splenectomy, chronic inflammation, malignancy, bleeding, and iron deficiency. Reactive thrombocytosis is primarily driven by increased levels of thrombopoietin, catecholamines, interleukin-6, and other cytokines. In most cases there are obvious clinical symptoms of an underlying systemic disease but further investigation may occasionally be required.

Evaluation

Certain laboratory studies can point toward an etiology of thrombocytosis. For example, elevated serum markers of inflammation (ESR, C-reactive protein [CRP]) may suggest a chronic inflammatory condition. Iron studies may be helpful as iron deficiency has been linked to reactive thrombocytosis. Peripheral blood smear may also be useful as platelets are usually of normal size in reactive thrombocytosis, but giant platelets may be seen in essential thrombocythemia (ET). However, none of these tests fully differentiate between reactive and primary thrombocytosis because patients with clonal abnormalities may also have iron deficiency or chronic inflammation. Testing for the JAK2 mutation may be definitive as JAK2 mutations are present in virtually all cases of polycythemia vera (PV) and up to 70 % of cases of ET [20]. If no etiology for thrombocytosis can be identified and the test for JAK2 is negative, then CML should be ruled out by testing for the BCR–ABL oncogene and, as clinically indicated, a bone marrow biopsy.

Management

As mentioned above, thrombocytosis in critically ill patients is most commonly reactive in nature and does not require specific targeted treatment. However, if a patient presents with thrombocytosis *and* a thrombotic event such as acute myocardial infarction (MI), CVA, pulmonary embolism (PE), or peripheral thrombosis, further investigation and consultation with a specialist is warranted. In a symptomatic patient with an already established or suspected clonal disorder, the treatment for thrombocytosis includes aspirin, cytoreduction (using hydroxyurea or anagrelide), interferon gamma, and possibly platelet pheresis [19].

Interestingly, patients with chronic myeloproliferative disorders (ET, PV, CML) with extremely high platelet counts (>1,000,000/μL) are more prone to bleeding episodes as opposed to thrombotic events, likely secondary to increased clearance of vWF via platelet-dependent interactions. Reduction of platelet counts effectively decreases the bleeding tendency [20].

Disorders of the Hemostatic System

Thrombotic Complications in the ICU (Venous Thromboembolism)

Venous thromboembolism (VTE) continues to be a major diagnosis on hospitalization admission. The prevention, diagnosis, and management of DVT and pulmonary embolism (PE) in the critical care setting remains challenging, often because the use of pharmacologic prophylaxis is problematic due to active bleeding or perceived risk of bleeding. Clinical prediction rules, diagnostic algorithms, and laboratory studies such as D-dimer testing are very useful in evaluating outpatients, but are often not applicable in critically ill or have not been validated in the ICU population. As a result, diagnosis and treatment of VTE in critically ill patients remains challenging.

Evidence suggests that critically ill patients should receive prophylaxis against VTE unless contraindicated. In cases where pharmacologic prophylaxis is contraindicated, patients should be placed on mechanical prophylaxis with graduated compression stockings, intermittent pneumatic compression, or both. Although data are not robust, combination prophylaxis (mechanical and pharmacological) is recommended in very high-risk patients such as those with recent major surgery, malignancy, hip fracture, stroke or spinal cord injury, as well as patients who are more than 40 years old with a history of prior VTE. The American College of Chest Physicians (ACCP) recommends against routine use of IVC filters as primary prophylaxis [21].

Despite the increasing awareness of and implementation of DVT prophylaxis measures, the incidence of VTE in the critically ill is still estimated to be between 5 and 25 %. In addition to inherited thrombophilic conditions, patients can have one or more of the following risk factors: age, surgery, trauma, malignancy, prolonged immobilization, stroke/paralysis, CHF, COPD, prior DVT or PE, and indwelling vascular device [22]. There is compelling evidence that obesity is also a risk factor for VTE. Other conditions that have been associated with higher risk of VTE include hormonal agents (replacement therapy in post-menopausal women, tamoxifen, and oral contraceptives), pregnancy, antiphosholipid antibody syndrome (and other inherited or acquired thrombogenic conditions), nephrotic syndrome, and inflammatory bowel disease.

Thromboprophylaxis appears to substantially reduce the risk of VTE (by 60–70 %); however, it is important to note that it does not eliminate the risk entirely [22]. Therefore, if there is a high clinical suspicion for VTE, the use of prophylaxis should not impede pursuing a definitive diagnosis [22].

Clinical Presentation of VTE

Clinical signs of symptomatic DVT depend on the degree of venous obstruction and related inflammation, and can include pain, erythema, and swelling of the involved extremity. However, clinical features alone are not sufficient for diagnosis and objective testing can frequently reveal that DVT is not the cause of these signs and symptoms. Reciprocally, screening studies in high-risk populations have shown a high prevalence of lower extremity thrombi that are not evident clinically. As such, the clinical presentation is neither sensitive nor specific for diagnosis of DVT in the critically ill.

The clinical effects of PE depend on the degree of obstruction, the pre-existing cardiopulmonary reserve, and the physiologic consequences of both hypoxic and humorally mediated vasoconstriction. Symptoms associated with PE can include chest pain, dyspnea, cough, hemoptysis, and circulatory shock. Less than half of patients with PE have clinical evidence of DVT (edema, erythema, tenderness) at the time of PE diagnosis.

The diagnosis of VTE in the critically ill is especially challenging as the accuracy of symptoms, laboratory results, and imaging findings suggestive or diagnostic of VTE can be affected by concomitant critical illnesses. Furthermore, PE does not always present as a dramatic event and can be symptomatically subtle in some patients. Given these considerations, it is not surprising that autopsy data from ICU patients suggest that PE is very often undiagnosed [22].

Diagnosis of DVT

One of the most widely used clinical prediction tools for diagnosing DVT is the Wells score. First described in 1995, this scoring system assigns patients points for different risk factors, placing them into low, moderate and high-risk categories. While this scoring system has been well validated in outpatients and in the Emergency Department, it has not proven useful in critically ill patients.

Similarly, while laboratory testing for D-dimer is very sensitive in outpatients and patients in the Emergency Department, it is rarely useful for critically ill patients. D-dimer detects the degradation product of cross-linked fibrin and although it seems to have a high sensitivity and specificity, the test has a very poor positive predictive value as an elevated D-dimer can be found in many conditions typical in hospitalized patients, including advanced age, systemic inflammation, trauma, surgery, and advanced liver or kidney disease. Use of the D-dimer as a diagnostic tool for VTE is further complicated by the heterogeneity of available assays. Comparisons of commercially available tests have shown significant variability in sensitivity, specificity, and optimal cut-off values [18]. Therefore, D-dimer is not routinely used in the diagnostic assessment for VTE in ICU patients.

Duplex ultrasonography has become the preferred test for diagnosis of symptomatic DVT of both upper and lower extremities. Duplex ultrasonography can be performed rapidly and is portable, non-invasive, very sensitive, and very specific. While it is very useful for symptomatic patients, its utility in screening asymptomatic patients for sub-clinical DVT is controversial. It also has lower sensitivity and specificity for the detection of calf vein thrombosis, although the clinical significance of calf DVT is uncertain.

Other imaging modalities used in the diagnostic assessment of DVT include contrast venography, computed tomography (CT) venography, and magnetic resonance imaging (MRI). *Contrast venography* is considered to be the gold standard and is performed by injecting contrast into a superficial vein on the dorsum of the foot followed by serial imaging of the extremity to track the travel of contrast through the venous circulation. A filling defect or abrupt termination is diagnostic for DVT. Contrast venography is currently rarely performed as it is invasive, requires IV contrast, and can cause post-injection phlebitis. As evaluation for DVT and PE are frequently performed concomitantly, pelvic and lower extremity *CT venography* (CTV) can be performed simultaneously with chest computed tomography (CT) scanning (also called CT pulmonary angiogram). CTV can potentially discover pelvic clots that are not easily diagnosed with ultrasound (US). In the PIOPED II (Prospective Investigation Of Pulmonary Embolism Diagnosis) study, CTV performed similarly to duplex US in diagnosing or excluding DVT [23]. CT does have the disadvantages of obligatory transport out of the ICU, radiation exposure, and IV contrast administration.

MRI can also be used for diagnosis of DVT but has not been as well studied as ultrasonography and CTV. Although current data demonstrate good sensitivity and specificity (both >90 %), the cost, time, and need for patient transport make it a less desirable option, especially in the critically ill [22].

Diagnosis of PE

Various scoring tools have been designed and validated for risk stratification of PE, the most popular being the Wells score and the revised Geneva score. However, as with DVT, both these scoring tools and D-dimer assessment are generally not as helpful in critically ill patients, as most ICU patients are in the moderate to high-risk stratification which obligates further diagnostic testing. Some ancillary studies performed in the critically ill may occasionally offer clues to the diagnosis of PE. For example, electrocardiogram (EKG) changes may be seen in up to 70 % of patients with PE. These changes can be quite variable and non-specific, however, and include tachycardia, ST changes, T-wave inversions, right bundle branch block, and a S1Q3T3 pattern. Arterial blood gas may reveal hypoxemia and an increased A-a gradient. The absence of hypoxemia or an A-a gradient, however, does not exclude the presence of PE.

Patients with PE may have chest X-ray abnormalities including atelectasis, pleural effusion, or cardiomegaly, but these findings are also quite variable and nonspecific. Several findings previously thought to be specific for PE such as the Westermark sign (focal area of decreased vascularity), Fleishner sign (prominent central pulmonary artery), and Hampton hump (pleural-based wedge-shaped opacity), lack diagnostic accuracy. Especially in critically ill ventilated patients, where interpretation of a single view chest radiograph is often difficult, abnormal findings on the radiograph are not sufficient for diagnosis and the lack of an abnormal finding does not rule out PE.

PE can cause increased dead space volume and thus can, if alveolar ventilation is not maintained or increased, result in an increase of exhaled CO_2. It has been proposed that bedside capnography might be a useful measure to evaluate dead space ventilation, and one study found that end tidal (et) $CO_2 < 36$ mmHg had a negative predictive value of 97 % for PE. This suggests that $etCO_2$ may be a useful tool for excluding embolism in low-risk patients, although further validation studies need to be performed before this is widely implemented in routine clinical practice. Furthermore, patients with hypercapneic respiratory failure, receiving mechanical ventilation, with neuromuscular weakness, and/or requiring >5 L/min O_2 were excluded from the study, thus limiting the generalizability of these results in all critically ill patients [22].

Computed Tomography Pulmonary Angiography

Computed tomography pulmonary angiography (CTPA) has become the imaging modality of choice in diagnosing PE. The PIOPED II trial is the largest study evaluating the diagnostic accuracy of CTPA and demonstrated a specificity of 96 % and sensitivity of 83 % when CTPA was used alone, increased to 90 % when CTV was added [23]. The positive predictive value (PPV) depended on the location: 97 % for a PE of the main or lobar arteries, 68 % for segmental PE, and 25 % for subsegmental PE. Given the relatively high false negative rate of 17 % when CTPA alone was used, it is reasonable to combine CTPA with either CTV or duplex ultrasonography, especially when clinical suspicion is moderate or high.

Ventilation Perfusion Lung Scanning

Ventilation perfusion (VQ) lung scanning is a valuable diagnostic imaging modality for PE, but has several limitations. A negative VQ scan rules out PE with similar accuracy as pulmonary angiography. A negative VQ scan has a higher negative predictive value than a negative CTPA. In the PIOPED I trial, a high probability VQ scan was associated with a PE 87 % of the time [24]. The only two definitive results of a VQ are "normal" (negative) and "high probability"; however, the majority of patients have a VQ scan that is interpreted as "low" or "intermediate" probability, which makes definitive diagnosis impossible. When examined specifically in the critically ill population, VQ scan was diagnostic (i.e., negative or high-probability) in only 18 % of patients, and in only 11 % undergoing mechanical ventilation. Even with these limitations, there are certain situations where VQ scanning might be preferred over CTPA, as no IV contrast is required, and with a portable gamma scintillation camera, the perfusion portion of the VQ scan can be performed at the bedside.

Bedside Echocardiography

Bedside echocardiography can be a valuable tool aiding in the diagnosis of PE. While not a primary confirmatory test, characteristics of right ventricular (RV) dysfunction that have been associated with PE can be appreciated: McConnell sign (RV hypokinesis with sparing of apical motion) and the "60/60" sign (pulmonary acceleration time <60 ms in the presence of echocardiographically derived pulmonary artery pressure ≤60 mmHg). Both signs have a very high specificity and PPV but lack sensitivity. RV dysfunction can also be present in patients with acute lung injury and those being mechanically ventilated, which limits the sensitivity of bedside echocardiography. As such, bedside echocardiography can be a useful adjuvant clinical tool, but cannot diagnose or definitively rule out PE.

Magnetic Resonance Angiography

The PIOPED III trial was the largest study to evaluate magnetic resonance angiography (MRA) in diagnosing PE, and it found a sensitivity and specificity of 78 % and 99 %, respectively. However, these values were calculated excluding the technically inadequate studies (approximately 25 % of all MRAs included in the trial) [25]. MRA has many limitations, especially in the critically ill, including the time it takes to perform, need for transport, and the risks of gadolinium in patients with renal failure. Furthermore, MRA is contraindicated in patients with MR-incompatible implantable devices. As such, MRA has limited utility in the diagnosis of PE with the exception of special populations such as pregnant women.

Pulmonary Angiography

Long considered to be the gold standard for diagnosing PE, pulmonary angiography currently is not routinely performed as it is invasive, is not universally available, and carries increased risk of major complications. Furthermore, it requires experienced personnel to both adequately perform and interpret the test, and, as it is being less frequently performed, experienced personnel are increasingly rare. Given these limitations, pulmonary angiography has a limited role in critical care.

Risk Stratification and Prognosis

In general, the pursuit of diagnosis of VTE in critically ill patients begins with a high clinical suspicion potentially triggered by changes in patients' clinical status. Common clinical changes include new unilateral extremity edema, new and otherwise unexplained tachycardia, hypoxia, hypotension, or an increase in minute ventilation and reduction of etCO$_2$. As mentioned, the use of scoring tools is not especially useful in the ICU and diagnostic approach should be tailored to the clinical status and feasibility of testing.

Risk stratification based on clinical features and markers of myocardial injury can help guide treatment. Shock and sustained hypotension are associated with high mortality (up to 60 %) and require an aggressive treatment approach, such as thrombolysis and/or thrombectomy. In hemodynamically stable patients with evidence of RV dysfunction by echocardiography, elevated levels of B-type natriuretic peptide (BNP or pro-BNP) or troponin indicate a higher risk for an adverse outcome, although there are no clear guidelines to assist with management in this subgroup of patients [26].

Treatment of DVT/PE

The treatment of VTE should focus on preventing further clot extension, PE, and late complications such as post-thrombotic syndrome and chronic thromboembolic pulmonary hypertension. The initial therapeutic goal in the ICU is to ensure hemodynamic stability.

Anticoagulation

Anticoagulation is the first line of treatment in most cases of VTE unless contraindicated. Treatment with parenteral unfractionated heparin (UFH) or low molecular weight heparin (LMWH), such as enoxaparin and fondaparinux, should be initiated in cases of high clinical suspicion while awaiting results of diagnostic tests [21].

UFH is usually delivered by continuous infusion and monitored by lab tests (aPTT or anti-Xa levels). In general, nomograms and protocols reduce the time to achieve therapeutic state [27]. After initiation, levels should be measured every 6 h until consistently in the desired range.

LMWHs are often preferred because of their ease of use, better bioavailability, longer half-life, and no requirement for monitoring; however, they are more costly and caution is necessary in patients with obesity or renal failure. Additionally, unlike UFH, they cannot be reversed (protamine reverses LMWH only partly), and the longer half-life of LMWHs can increase the risk of bleeding during urgent interventional procedures. Of note, fondaparinux is less likely to cause HIT when compared to UFH and enoxaparin.

Currently warfarin, a vitamin K antagonist, is the most widely used oral antico-agulant for long-term therapy and is recommended for this indication by the ACCP. It should be initiated on the same day as UFH or LMWH , unless there are contra-indications (such as pending procedures). UFH or LMWH bridging should be con-tinued for at least 5 days and until the international normalized ratio (INR) reaches 2.0 for at least 48 h. Warfarin interacts with many medications. Although newer oral agents including dabigatran and rivaroxaban have been shown to be non-inferior to Warfarin in clinical trials, have a similar side-effect profile as Warfarin, and do not require bridging with a parenteral anticoagulant, the ACCP does not recommend them as a first-line choice for oral anticoagulation because of paucity of long-term outcomes data. In addition, initiation of these agents in the ICU is not advisable because they, unlike Warfarin, cannot be rapidly reversed.

Other Treatment Considerations

Deep Vein Thrombosis

Surgical thrombectomy and catheter-directed or systemic thrombolysis are gener-ally not recommended as routine treatment for DVT, but should be considered in patients with massive iliofemoral or proximal femoral DVT where severe swelling and limb ischemia might occur. Inferior vena cava (IVC) filters are advised in patients where anticoagulant therapy is contraindicated due to active bleeding or high bleeding risk; however, once this risk is resolved via conventional anticoagula-tion therapy, the filter should be removed as soon as possible. Guidelines also advise against the routine use of IVC filters as a primary prophylaxis for VTE.

Pulmonary Embolism

Again, preference is given to LMWH over IV UFH, but for patients with renal fail-ure and patients who might be considered for systemic thrombolysis, IV UFH is preferred.

Current data do not demonstrate that systemic thrombolysis has a mortality benefit, but per ACCP guidelines thrombolysis should be considered in patients without con-traindications, who have a confirmed diagnosis of acute PE *and* associated hypoten-sion/shock where the mortality risk (considered to be >30 %) outweighs the possible risk of hemorrhage due to thrombosis. Thrombolytic agents should be given via peripheral vein and followed by conventional anticoagulation. In general, shorter infu-sion times are recommended (2 h or less). Contraindications to systemic thrombolysis include previous hemorrhagic stroke, intracranial pathology or trauma, recent surgery, bleeding diathesis, thrombocytopenia, and uncontrolled severe hypertension.

Catheter-directed thrombolysis for PE does not seem to be superior to systemic thrombolysis, but catheter-directed removal (aspiration, fragmentation, or ultra-sound) or a combined mechanical and pharmacological approach has demonstrated promising preliminary results. However, there are limited data from large randomized trials to support widely generalized catheter-directed therapies. As catheter-directed interventions require a great deal of technical expertise and support, catheter-based treatments are primarily offered at tertiary care centers on a patient-by-patient basis. Potential adverse effects include contrast nephropathy, bleeding, vessel dissection, arteriovenous fistula (AVF) formation, pseudoaneurysm, arrhythmias, and pericardial tamponade. Surgical embolectomy is usually recommended when all the above-mentioned therapies fail as a salvage option, as surgical thrombectomy carries a high morbidity and mortality.

In general, VTE in critically ill patients is considered to be provoked and thus testing for thrombophilia is not recommended. Oral anticoagulant therapy is recommended for a minimum of 3 months, with the need for continued anticoagulation then re-evaluated based on risk factors. In pregnant women and patients with cancer, long-term therapy with LMWH is recommended over oral anticoagulation [27].

Disseminated Intravascular Coagulation

Disseminated intravascular coagulation (DIC) occurs in critically ill patients due to a robust activation of the coagulation system, resulting in microvascular thrombosis and potential organ failure. As part of the ongoing activation of the coagulation cascade, consumption of clotting factors and platelets may occur, resulting in bleeding. DIC is a consumptive coagulopathy that is characterized by thrombocytopenia, decreasing fibrinogen levels, and increasing thrombin time (TT), prothrombin time (PT), activated partial thromboplastin time (aPTT) and fibrin degradation products (FDPs). An increasing D-dimer level, which represents fibrinolysis of cross-linked fibrin, is the most specific DIC parameter; whereas the other parameters are more sensitive in detecting early DIC. The incidence of DIC in the ICU ranges from 9 to 19 % and is associated with a mortality of 45–78 %. This incidence has decreased over the past decade, especially in men, although mortality appears unchanged [28].

Etiology

DIC can be caused by various conditions encountered in the critically ill, including infection and sepsis, trauma, burns, malignancy, obstetrical conditions, vascular abnormalities and severe allergic/toxic reactions [28]. These conditions can lead to activation of coagulation that may not result in clinical complications or be detected by routine laboratory parameters. DIC occurs when this activation of coagulation is ongoing and extreme. Laboratory data that may aid in the diagnosis include decreased platelet count, prolonged PT and aPTT, increased FDPs, and decreased protease inhibitors (protein C and S, and antithrombin). The specificity of increased FDPs is limited by other underlying conditions, such as trauma, recent surgery, thromboembolic disease, and inflammation. Low levels of protease inhibitors are commonly found in critically ill patients and in 90 % of DIC patients.

Management

Management of DIC includes treatment of the underlying disorder in addition to supportive care of the coagulopathy. Plasma or platelet transfusion should generally be reserved for patients with active bleeding or those requiring invasive procedures. Similar to other critically ill patients, patients with DIC and severe thrombocytopenia (platelet count of <10) should receive platelet transfusions to raise the platelet count to 20–30. Patients with DIC who are actively bleeding or undergoing an invasive procedure should be transfused with a goal of 50. Heparin therapy in patients with thrombotic manifestations of DIC is controversial, especially due to the risk of bleeding, and a benefit has not been demonstrated in controlled clinical trials. However, some feel that heparin is beneficial in certain conditions associated with DIC, such as metastatic cancer, purpura fulminans, aortic aneurysm, and thromboembolic complications. Given the contradictory data, initiation of heparin in DIC should be performed in consultation with a Hematologist.

Heparin-Induced Thrombocytopenia

HIT is caused by IgG antibodies that lead to activation of platelets, coagulation, monocytes and endothelium resulting in a prothrombotic state. Of the two types of HIT, type I is a non-immune process that occurs in 10–20 % of patients who receive UFH and leads to decreased platelet counts (usually not less than 100,000/μL) 1–4 days after heparin administration. Type I HIT is not associated with thrombotic or hemorrhagic complications, and most patients have resolution of thrombocytopenia despite continued heparin use [29]. In contrast, Type II HIT, or immune-mediated HIT occurs via an antibody-mediated mechanism in 1–3 % of patients receiving UFH and is characterized by thrombocytopenia that occurs 5–10 days after heparin administration. It occurs more often in women than men and more often in surgical than medical patients. In the ICU, Type II HIT occurs in 0.3–0.5 % of patients [30]. Thrombosis occurs in 30–80 % of patients with Type II HIT, with venous thromboses being more common. A more rapid onset Type II HIT can occur in patients who have received heparin in the prior 3–4 months. The classic presentation of Type II HIT includes a greater than 50 % drop in platelets, accompanied by venous or arterial thrombosis, with no other clinical explanation. LMWH is less likely to cause HIT when used as a first-line agent; however, it has cross-reactivity with UFH-induced antibodies, and may worsen thrombocytopenia and thrombosis if it is given after HIT has developed.

Type II HIT is characterized by heparin-induced platelet activation and release of platelet factor 4 (PF4) from platelet granules, resulting in formation of heparin-PF4 complexes and induction of IgG anti-heparin-PF4 antibodies. Platelet activation assays, such as the platelet serotonin release assay (SRA), have a high sensitivity for clinical HIT with a higher specificity than the PF4-dependent enzyme immunoassays (EIAs) [30]. Approximately 50 % of patients with a positive EIA will also have a positive SRA, and in the ICU, the probability of EIA-positive status indicating the presence of platelet-activating antibodies is 10–20 %. Although SRAs are the gold standard for diagnosis of HIT, the heparin-induced platelet aggregation assay and the enzyme-linked immunosorbent assay (ELISA) are more widely available.

Management of HIT includes stopping heparin, using a non-heparin alternative anticoagulant, avoiding warfarin, testing for HIT antibodies, imaging for DVT, and avoiding prophylactic platelet transfusions. Alternatives for anticoagulation include the direct thrombin inhibitors, lepirudin and argatroban.

Thrombotic/Thrombocytopenic Purpura and Hemoytic Uremic Syndrome (B)

TTP was initially defined by the presence of the following five features: thrombocytopenia, microangiopathic hemolytic anemia, neurological abnormalities, fever and renal failure. Due to the importance of making a timely diagnosis and expeditiously initiating treatment, the current diagnostic criteria include only thrombocytopenia and microangiopathic hemolytic anemia without an alternative cause [31]. Changes in the diagnostic criteria and the availability of effective treatment have led to an increase in the number of patients treated for TTP with plasma exchange. Acute idiopathic TTP, an autoimmune disease, is the most common form of TTP and is characterized by antibodies against ADAMTS13, a disintegrin and metalloproteinase also known as von Willebrand Factor Cleaving Protease [32]. Other subtypes of TTP include HIV-associated, pregnancy-associated (5–25 % of cases), and drug-associated TTP (<15 % of cases). The diagnostic term HUS is used to refer to children who have thrombocytopenia and microangiopathic hemolytic anemia in the presence of renal failure. Most children have a diarrhea prodrome, and plasma exchange is rarely used since supportive care is associated with good survival. The term HUS is not used to describe adults with the same criteria. Multiple disorders can occur similarly to TTP, such as disseminated carcinoma, infections, malignant hypertension, systemic lupus erythematosis (SLE), and renal disorders; therefore, it is important to consider and exclude alternative causes. ADAMTS13 activity <5 % is specific for TTP, but does not identify all patients that may relapse, whereas a level of <10 % may better capture patients at risk for relapse. However, an ADAMTS13 level of <10 % is not as specific for TTP and may also occur in patients with sepsis and cirrhosis.

Treatment with plasma exchange should be initiated within 4–8 h of diagnosis [32]. Response to therapy is monitored by normalization of platelet count. The number of plasma exchange treatments needed to achieve remission is variable. Adjunctive treatment with immunosuppressants, such as corticosteroids, is reserved for patients with suspected autoimmune ADAMTS13 deficiency. Plasma exchange in conjunction with highly active antiretroviral therapy (HAART) should be started in HIV-associated TTP, and HAART therapy should be continued after remission. Mortality is approximately 15 % for all patients with TTP; however, many deaths are attributed to complications of hospitalization or plasma exchange rather than TTP itself.

Liver Failure

Coagulopathy is a common complication of acute and chronic liver failure. Acute liver failure also results in decreased platelet function that may precipitate bleeding diathesis, infections, and end-organ dysfunction. Coagulopathy in the setting of liver failure occurs due to decreased liver protein synthesis. Correction of coagulopathy is recommended for invasive procedures or significant bleeding; otherwise, prophylactic infusion of fresh frozen plasma (FFP) or platelets increases intravascular volume and may increase the risk of non-hematologic complications, such as cerebral edema, in these patients [33].

HELLP Syndrome

HELLP syndrome is characterized by hemolysis (microangiopathic hemolytic anemia), elevated liver enzymes, and thrombocytopenia). HELLP syndrome occurs in 0.1–0.8 % of pregnancies and in 10–20 % of women with severe pre-eclampsia or eclampsia [34]. Most patients are diagnosed before 37 weeks gestation. Activation of the complement and coagulation cascades, increased vascular tone, and platelet aggregation play a role in the pathophysiology of the syndrome, resulting in generalized endothelial and microvascular injury. Laboratory data may reveal microangiopathic hemolysis with schistocytes, platelet count of less than 50,000/mm^3, serum total bilirubin >20 μmol/L, serum LDH >600 U/L, and serum aspartate aminotransferase (AST) >70 U/L. The differential diagnosis includes TTP and HUS, cold agglutinins disease, and acute fatty liver of pregnancy. Management includes administration of steroids to advance lung maturity of the fetus if the gestational age is <34 weeks. Delivery of the fetus results in significant improvement. Steroids are not beneficial if the syndrome develops in the postpartum period, which occurs in 30 % of patients. Major complications of HELLP syndrome include hepatic hemorrhage, subcapsular hematoma, liver rupture, and multiorgan failure.

Iatrogenic Coagulopathy

Coagulopathy encountered in critically ill patients may also be due to iatrogenic causes. This may be seen in the setting of hypervolemia, which results in dilution of effective clotting factors; heparin overdose, which inhibits factors II, IX, X and XII; and anticoagulation, such as with use of warfarin.

Transfusion Complications in the ICU

Administration of blood products is a common medical practice and many patients in the ICU will receive blood products during their stay. Transfusion medicine has advanced immensely over the past decades and while screening, obtaining, and storing of products has become progressively safer, there are still many controversies and knowledge gaps regarding the indications and efficacy of transfusion. In addition, administration of blood products can be associated with serious short- and long-term complications. These complications can generally be grouped as *non-infectious* and *infectious* (see Table 4.6).

Infectious Complications

In general, any pathogen that can exist in the blood stream can be transmitted via transfusion. With advances in donor screening and testing of blood products prior to administration, the risks have been reduced significantly and are now extremely low.

Table 4.6 Infectious and non-infectious complications of transfusion

Infectious
– Bacterial (risk 1 in 100,000-500,000)
– Viral
  • HIV (risk 1 in 1,800,000)
  • HCV (risk 1 in 1,600,000)
  • HBV (risk 1 in 220,000)

Non-infectious
– Immune-mediated
  • Hemolytic transfusion reactions
  • Febrile non-hemolytic transfusion reactions
  • Mistransfusion
  • Allergic/anaphylactic reactions
  • TRALI
  • TRIM
  • Alloimmunization
  • Post transfusion purpura
  • Transfusion associated graft vs. host disease (TA-GVHD)
– Non-immune-mediated
  • Septic transfusion reactions
  • Non-immune hemolysis
  • TACO
  • Metabolic derangements
  • Coagulopathy
  • RBC storage lesions
    Iron overload

Bacterial

Bacterial contamination can occur during phlebotomy or during processing of the blood products. Transfusion-related bacteremia has been estimated to occur at a rate of 1 in 3,000; however, very few of these transfusions lead to clinically apparent sepsis, which is estimated to occur in 1 for every 250,000 transfusions. Both gram-positive and gram-negative bacteria have been reported [35,36] with platelet transfusions being more susceptible to bacterial contamination than PRBCs. Techniques such as single-donor platelet apheresis (rather than pooling platelets from many donors), pathogen inactivation methods (such as photochemical treatment), and rapid testing prior to transfusion have decreased bacterial contamination. Presenting signs of septic transfusion reactions are usually fever, rigors, and tachycardia within 4 h of starting a transfusion [35]. If bacteremia due to a transfusion is suspected, the remaining blood product (in the bag or tubing) and the patient's blood should be sent for gram stain and culture, and treatment for sepsis should be initiated.

Viral

Unlike bacterial infections, viral infections usually do not manifest immediately. The most feared viral infections are hepatitis B (HBV), hepatitis C (HCV), and HIV. In the past, hepatitis B was the most serious transfusion risk, but the development of a sensitive and specific test for HBV (both antigen and antibody detection) has dramatically reduced the risk of acquiring HBV via transfusion. Nonetheless, it remains the highest among the transfusion-acquired viral infections (Table 4.6). The risk for acquiring HIV has also steadily decreased, and currently the only remaining real risk of infection would be transfusion of infected blood donated during the "window period" immediately after occurrence of infection but before development of detectable antibody response. This period is estimated to last an average of 8 weeks. Using the newest nucleic acid technology screening techniques, the risk of transfusion-related infection has decreased 10,000-fold in recent decades [36] and the window period during which infection is not detectable is now reduced to 11 days for HIV and 8–10 days for HCV [35].

Other more recently discovered potential transfusion risks include prion disease (new variant Creutzfeldt–Jakob disease [CJD]) and West Nile virus. Although to date no transfusion-related CJD has been reported, many countries have implemented precautionary donor exclusions.

Non-infectious Complications

With the declining risk and incidence of transfusion-related infections, the non-infectious serious hazards of transfusion (NISHOT) have emerged as leading complications of transfusion. Currently a patient is a 1,000-fold more likely to develop a NISHOT than an infectious complication. Some of the more common NISHOT include transfusion reactions (hemolytic, febrile, septic, allergic/anaphylactic, and mistransfusion). Other NISHOT include TRALI, TACO, post transfusion purpura, TRIM, alloimmunization, complications from red cell storage lesions, and iron overload [36].

The NISHOT can be further divided into *immune-mediated* and *non-immune* mediated.

Immune-Mediated NISHOT

One of the most preventable complications is *mistransfusion*, or giving an incorrect blood product to a patient. Many hospitals have implemented strategies to minimize this risk, but it still occurs.

Hemolytic transfusion reactions can occur when blood is given to a patient who has pre-existing antibodies against the donor's blood. Symptoms can be quite variable and non-specific, and include fever, chills, rigors, chest/back/abdominal pain, pain at the infusion site, nausea, vomiting, dyspnea, feeling of impending doom, and hypotension. The historic incidence of hemolytic transfusion reactions is estimated to be between 1 in 10,000 and 1 in 50,000 transfused blood components. If suspected, the transfusion should be stopped immediately and supportive care should be initiated. Hemolysis labs should be ordered, as well as a urine sample to test for hemoglobin. The blood bank should be notified immediately.

Delayed Hemolytic Transfusion Reactions

Delayed hemolytic transfusion reactions (DHTRs) typically occur 3–10 days after transfusion. The cause for these reactions is alloimmunization of the recipient from prior transfusions. The alloantibodies are usually present in such small quantities that they go undetected during the pre-transfusion screening. However, after transfusion there is a rapid anamnestic response. Decreases in hematocrit and increases in serum bilirubin can be noted. No targeted treatment is usually necessary. Delayed serologic transfusion reactions (DSTRs) indicate a reaction that is detectable serologically but not clinically. The incidence of DHTRS and DSTRs is estimated to be 1 in 1,500 transfusions. Obtaining good transfusion history and selecting offending antigen-negative PRBCs for transfusion in patients with a history of significant alloantibodies is crucial in reducing the risk of DHTR and DSTR.

Hyperhemolytic Reactions

Hyperhemolytic reactions have been observed in sickle cell patients. In these instances hemolysis occurs not only of the donor's PRBCs but also of the patient's own RBCs. The pathophysiology of hyperhemolytic reactions is not clear, but should be considered in patients where the post-transfusion hemoglobin not only fails to increase but actually decreases.

Febrile Non-hemolytic Transfusion Reactions

Febrile non-hemolytic transfusion reactions (FNHTR) are classically defined as an increase in body temperature by 1 °C (into the febrile range), but this diagnostic criteria can be masked if the patient received antipyretics. Other symptoms can include chills, rigor, and discomfort. The diagnosis of FNHTR can be made only after other reasons for fever have been excluded. Cytokines and recipient white cell alloantibodies have been implicated in FNHTRs. This type of transfusion reaction is also more commonly seen in platelets as opposed to RBC transfusions, but rates have declined significantly with universal leukoreduction. In cases of suspected FNHTR, the transfusion should be stopped and evaluation for possible hemolytic reaction should be undertaken. Pre-medication with acetaminophen and antihista-mines has not been proven beneficial in reducing these types of reactions, but these medications are still commonly provided in clinical practice regardless.

Allergic Reactions

Allergic reactions can occur with many symptoms and signs including urticaria, edema, pruritus, and angioedema. Urticarial reactions usually manifest with rash only (no other symptoms) and have been estimated to occur in 1–3 % of transfu-sions. They are presumably due to soluble antigens in the donor unit to which the recipient has been previously sensitized, and they tend to be dose-dependent. Major allergic reactions (anaphylaxis) are rare, estimated to occur in 1 in 20,000 to 1 in 50,000 transfusions and usually present with hypotension, bronchospasm, stridor, and gastrointestinal symptoms. If a severe allergic reaction occurs, the transfusion should be stopped immediately and fluid resuscitation should be started; mechanical ventilation and circulatory support with vasopressors may be necessary. IgA defi-ciency, HLA antibodies and anticomplement antibodies have been associated with anaphylactic reactions. Thus, the evaluation of an anaphylactic transfusion reaction includes testing the recipient for IgA deficiency. Patients known to be IgA-deficient should receive blood products either collected from IgA-deficient donors or washed to remove residual IgA containing plasma.

Transfusion-Related Lung Injury

Transfusion-related lung injury (TRALI) is an important cause of transfusion-related morbidity and mortality, and is defined as a new acute lung injury that occurs with a clear temporal relationship to transfusion (usually minutes to hours) in patients without alternative obvious causes of acute lung injury. Therefore, as ICU patients typically have cardiopulmonary disease, the diagnosis of TRALI in the ICU can be challenging. Anti-neutrophil and anti-HLA antibodies have been implicated in the pathogenesis of TRALI, as they can damage the pulmonary alveolar-endothelial barrier with resultant pulmonary edema. Transfusion of plasma (rather than PRBCs) and products from multiparous female donors is more frequently associated with development of TRALI. Treatment is supportive with supplemental oxygen and mechanical ventilation if required; patients usually do not respond to diuretics. Symptomatic improvement should be seen within 48 h. Mortality from TRALI is reported to be between 1 and 10 % [37].

Transfusion-Related Immunomodulation

Transfusion-related immunomodulation (TRIM) has been recognized since the 1970s. Although controversy remains regarding the role of transfusion in increasing cancer risk, blood transfusion has been clearly associated with higher rates of infection in hospitalized patients, longer ICU and hospital stays, and increased mortality.

Alloimmunization

RBC alloimmunization occurs in 2–8 % of chronically transfused patients who develop anti-D antibodies, and occurs in up to 40 % of sickle cell patients. This can make locating compatible, antigen-negative RBCs difficult, and can increase the risk for developing DHTR and DSTR (see above). HLA alloimmunization is the most common cause of platelet refractoriness, and, therefore, transfusion of HLA-matched platelet products can address platelet refractoriness in some cases.

Other rare forms of immune-mediated transfusion reactions include post-transfusion purpura resulting in destruction of transfused and autologous platelets after any blood product transfusion, and transfusion-related graft versus host disease (TA-GVHD) which includes engraftment of donor T-lymphocytes. TA-GVHD can occur 1–6 weeks after transfusion with fever, rash, diarrhea, liver abnormalities, and pancytopenia, and can be fatal. Prevention is essential so patients at risk (patients receiving chemotherapy or those status-post stem cell transplant) should receive gamma-irradiated cell products as this inactivates donor lymphocytes.

Non-immune-Mediated NISHOT

Transfusion-Associated Circulatory Overload

Transfusion-associated circulatory overload (TACO) is due to circulatory overload and unlike TRALI, is not antibody-mediated. The pathophysiology of TACO relates to the increased circulatory volume in the pulmonary vessels overwhelming the transvascular fluid filtration and absorption by the lymphatics, which leads to lung edema. Estimated to occur in up to 1 % of transfusions, it can manifest within 1–2 h of transfusion with tachycardia, dyspnea, cough, hypertension with widened pulse pressure, and distended neck veins. Patients at risk include those with pre-existing cardiac or renal failure. Measurement of B-type natriuretic peptide (BNP) can be helpful in establishing the diagnosis. Treatment is supportive and includes supplemental oxygen, diuretic therapy, and in severe cases, positive pressure ventilation. Future transfusions in patient with TACO should be administered at a slower rate [36]. Mortality rate is reported to be between 3.6 and 20 %.

Non-immune Hemolysis

Non-immune hemolytic reactions can occur in vitro (while the unit is stored) and may be secondary to improper blood warming, bacterial overgrowth, or transfusing through a small bore IV or through a line with a hypotonic solution or incompatible drug.

Complications of Massive Transfusion

Massive transfusion is occasionally required for patients with acute hemorrhage, and trauma centers commonly have massive transfusion protocols. Commonly observed complications from massive transfusion include metabolic derangements and coagulopathy, as well as development of acute respiratory distress syndrome (ARDS).

Metabolic Derangements

Metabolic derangements include citrate toxicity, hyperkalemia, acidosis, and hypothermia. *Citrate toxicity* manifests with hypocalcemia due to the anticoagulant sodium citrate binding to plasma calcium. Since citrate is metabolized in the liver, patients with liver failure and shock are at higher risk. Treatment includes correction of hypocalcemia and judicious use of blood products. *Hyperkalemia* occurs due to RBCs naturally leaking potassium during storage. Usually this is not a problem, unless the patient receives massive transfusion and has compromised cardiac, liver or renal function. Hypothermia (due to infusion of a large volume of cold blood products) can increase the toxicity of hypocalcemia and hyperkalemia leading to possible arrhythmias. In addition, hypothermia, together with acidosis, worsens coagulopathy. Blood warmers can prevent hypothermia but the temperature should be closely monitored since overheating blood products can induce hemolysis. Acidosis occurs due to the decreased pH of stored RBCs and tissue hypoperfusion in the setting of shock.

Coagulopathy

Coagulopathic complications usually occur when patients receive >10 units of PRBCs in a 24-h period, and manifest as reduced platelet count (<50,000/mm^3), prolonged PT and aPTT or decreased fibrinogen. This form of coagulopathy is usually dilutional and consumptive. In addition, hypothermia and acidosis may worsen the coagulopathy. The occurrence of coagulopathy and the associated mortality can be counteracted with simultaneous infusion of FFP and platelets, and many authors suggest a ratio of 1:1:1 of pRBCs:FFP:platelets for massive transfusion protocols [38].

RBC Storage Lesion

RBC storage lesion is a term referring to changes that RBCs undergo while in storage. Alterations include decreased pH, ATP, 2,3-DPG, or glutathione; increased lactate; and reduced deformability, which may explain why stored RBCs do not always increase oxygen delivery at the tissue level. There is still controversy regarding the relationship of age of PRBCs and clinical outcomes, and there are clinical trials underway to further clarify the role of storage lesion and define optimal storage practices.

Blood Product Alternatives

In acutely bleeding patients, alternatives that may reduce the need for blood products such as recombinant Factor VIIa (rFVIIa), prothrombin complex concentrate (PCC), and tranexamic acid (TA) [38] may be considered. rFVIIa is thought to be active at the site of vascular injury by activating platelets and inhibiting fibrinolysis. Most current data on rFVIIa are from trauma patients and suggest that while it can reduce the use of RBCs it does not change the need for FFP, cryoprecipitate or platelet products, and does not affect mortality. PCC contains coagulation factors II, VII, IX and X and the anticoagulation proteins C and S and may especially benefit patients with acute bleeding from coagulopathy related to vitamin K antagonism. Unlike FFP transfusion, which requires time to test for ABO compatibility, thawing and usually larger volumes to correct the coagulopathy, PCC can be administered very quickly and can correct the INR more predictably. TA is a synthetic derivative of lysine which inhibits fibrinolysis by blocking the lysine binding sites of plasminogen. TA has been successfully used in trauma patients and has been shown to reduce both the need for blood products and mortality. Additionally, it is often used off-label in hemophilia patients and perioperatively to reduce bleeding.

Summary

Blood product transfusion is a common medical practice but similar to other clinical interventions, it carries risks. Indications, risks, and efficacy of transfusion continue to be re-evaluated in the literature and there are emerging trends toward conservative transfusion strategies in which judicious use of blood products are associated with better clinical outcomes. Clinicians should attempt to address the underlying process (e.g., active GI bleeding, coagulopathy due to infection or trauma, or cytopenias due to drug effects) in addition to correcting the hematologic disorder.

Blood products should be administered only if absolutely necessary and one should be prepared to deal with the immediate possible complications. If an acute transfusion reaction occurs, stop the transfusion and ensure stability of patient (airway, hemodynamics). If the type of transfusion reaction is unclear, order hemolysis labs, notify the blood bank, and send the blood product and a sample of the patient's blood for serologic and microbiologic analysis. For suspected TRALI or TACO, chest X-ray, BNP and EKG can be helpful. Treatment will depend on the etiology of the reaction.

References

1. Hayden SJ et al. Anemia in critical illness: insights into etiology, consequences, and management. Am J Respir Crit Care Med. 2012;185(10):1049–57.
2. Asare K. Anemia of critical illness. Pharmacotherapy. 2008;28(10):1267–82.
3. DeBellis RJ. Anemia in critical care patients: incidence, etiology, impact, management, and use of treatment guidelines and protocols. Am J Health Syst Pharm. 2007;64(3 Suppl 2): S14–21.
4. Hebert PC et al. A multicenter, randomized, controlled clinical trial of transfusion requirements in critical care. Transfusion requirements in critical care investigators, Canadian critical care trials group. N Engl J Med. 1999;340(6):409–17.
5. Vincent JL et al. Anemia and blood transfusion in critically ill patients. JAMA. 2002;288(12): 1499–507.
6. Corwin HL et al. The CRIT study: anemia and blood transfusion in the critically ill–current clinical practice in the United States. Crit Care Med. 2004;32(1):39–52.
7. Lacroix J et al. The age of blood evaluation (ABLE) randomized controlled trial: study design. Transfus Med Rev. 2011;25(3):197–205.
8. Sloan SR et al. Current randomized clinical trials of red cell storage duration and patient outcomes. Crit Care Med. 2012;40(10):2927.
9. Villanueva C et al. Transfusion strategies for acute upper gastrointestinal bleeding. N Engl J Med. 2013;368(1):11–21.
10. Kremyanskaya M, Mascarenhas J, Hoffman R. Why does my patient have erythrocytosis? Hematol Oncol Clin North Am. 2012;26(2):267–83.
11. Reagan JL, Castillo JJ. Why is my patient neutropenic? Hematol Oncol Clin North Am. 2012;26(2):253–66.
12. Boxer LA. How to approach neutropenia. Hematol Am Soc Hematol Educ Program. 2012;2012:174–82.
13. Freifeld AG, Sepkowitz BE, et al. Clinical practice guideline for the use of antimicrobial agents in neutropenic patients with cancer: 2010 update by the Infectious Diseases Society of America. Clin Infect Dis. 2011;52(4):56–93.
14. Cerny J, Rosmarin AG. Why does my patient have leukocytosis? Hematol Oncol Clin North Am. 2012;26(2):303–19.
15. Hui P et al. The frequency and clinical significance of thrombocytopenia complicating critical illness: a systematic review. Chest. 2011;139(2):271–8.
16. Parker RI. Etiology and significance of thrombocytopenia in critically ill patients. Crit Care Clin. 2012;28(3):399–411.
17. Rice TW, Wheeler AP. Coagulopathy in critically ill patients: part 1: platelet disorders. Chest. 2009;136(6):1622–30.

18. Ho KM, Yip CB, Duff O. Reactive thrombocytosis and risk of subsequent venous thromboembolism: a cohort study. J Thromb Haemost. 2012;10(9):1768–74.
19. Schafer AI. Thrombocytosis. N Engl J Med. 2004;350(12):1211–9.
20. Vannucchi AM, Barbui T. Thrombocytosis and thrombosis hematology. ASH Educ. 2007;2007(1):363–70.
21. Guyatt GH et al. Executive summary: Antithrombotic Therapy and Prevention of Thrombosis, 9th ed: American College of Chest Physicians Evidence-Based Clinical Practice Guidelines. Chest. 2012;141(2 Suppl):7S–47S.
22. Magana M, Bercovitch R, Fedullo P. Diagnostic approach to deep venous thrombosis and pulmonary embolism in the critical care setting. Crit Care Clin. 2011;27(4):841–67.
23. Stein PD et al. Multidetector computed tomography for acute pulmonary embolism. N Engl J Med. 2006;354(22):2317–27.
24. PIOPED investigators. Value of the ventilation/perfusion scan in acute pulmonary embolism. Results of the prospective investigation of pulmonary embolism diagnosis (PIOPED). JAMA. 1990;263(20):2753–9.
25. Stein PD et al. Gadolinium-enhanced magnetic resonance angiography for pulmonary embolism: a multicenter prospective study (PIOPED III). Ann Intern Med. 2010;152(7):434–43. W142-3.
26. Agnelli G, Becattini C. Acute pulmonary embolism. N Engl J Med. 2010;363(3):266–74.
27. Tapson VF. Treatment of pulmonary embolism: anticoagulation, thrombolytic therapy, and complications of therapy. Crit Care Clin. 2011;27(4):825–39.
28. Singh B et al. Trends in the incidence and outcomes of disseminated intravascular coagulation in critically ill patients (2004–2010): a population-based study. Chest. 2013;143(5):1235–42.
29. Drews RE. Critical issues in hematology: anemia, thrombocytopenia, coagulopathy, and blood product transfusions in critically ill patients. Clin Chest Med. 2003;24(4):607–22.
30. Warkentin TE. Heparin-induced thrombocytopenia in critically ill patients. Crit Care Clin. 2011;27(4):805–23.
31. George JN. The thrombotic thrombocytopenic purpura and hemolytic uremic syndromes: overview of pathogenesis. (Experience of The Oklahoma TTP-HUS Registry, 1989–2007). Kidney Int. 2009;75 Suppl 112:S8–S10.
32. Scully M. Rituximab in the treatment of TTP. Hematology. 2012;17 Suppl 1:S22–4.
33. Trotter J. Practical management of acute liver failure in the intensive care unit. Curr Opin Crit Care. 2009;15(2):163–7.
34. Neligan PJ, Laffey JG. Clinical review: Special populations–critical illness and pregnancy. Crit Care. 2011;15(4):227.
35. Dellinger EP, Anaya DA. Infectious and immunologic consequences of blood transfusion. Crit Care. 2004;8 Suppl 2:S18–23.
36. Hendrickson JE, Hillyer CD. Noninfectious serious hazards of transfusion. Anesth Analg. 2009;108(3):759–69.
37. Sachs U. Side-effects of blood products. ISBT Sci Ser. 2010;5(1):267–70.
38. Dries DJ. The contemporary role of blood products and components used in trauma resuscitation. Scand J Trauma Resusc Emerg Med. 2010;18:63.

Chapter 5
Gastrointestinal Complications

Preeti Dhar and Eddy Fan

Abstract Gastrointestinal (GI) complications in the critically ill population are important to recognize and manage because of their implications not only on nutrition but also the endocrine and immunomodulatory functions of the GI system. An understanding of the anatomy and physiology of the peritoneal and retroperitoneal components of the GI tract is essential to appreciating their impact on morbidity and mortality for critical care patients. Addressing these issues often requires a multidisciplinary approach which includes nursing, pharmacy, nutrition and physician input in order to prevent, recognize and actively manage complications including malnutrition, infection and bleeding. Gastrointestinal physiology is sensitive to the hemodynamic shifts which are common in the critically ill patient. The following discussion will address the alterations in gastrointestinal physiology in the critically ill patient, followed by a review of GI complications in the intensive care unit using an anatomic-based approach. The pathophysiology, diagnosis and management of these complications will be discussed using an evidence-based approach.

Keywords Abdominal compartment syndrome • GI bleeding • Reflux • Feeding intolerance • Liver dysfunction • Diarrhea • Pneumoperitoneum

P. Dhar, M.D. (✉)
Interdepartmental Division of Critical Care, University of Toronto,
Toronto, ON, Canada
e-mail: preeti.dhar@utoronto.ca

E. Fan, M.D., Ph.D.
Interdepartmental Division of Critical Care, Mount Sinai Hospital,
University of Toronto, 600 University Avenue, Room 18-232, Toronto,
ON, Canada M5G 1X5
e-mail: efan@mtsinai.on.ca

J.B. Richards and R.D. Stapleton (eds.), *Non-Pulmonary Complications of Critical Care:* 105
A Clinical Guide, Respiratory Medicine, DOI 10.1007/978-1-4939-0873-8_5,
© Springer Science+Business Media New York 2014

Gastrointestinal (GI) complications in the critically ill population are important to recognize and manage because of their implications not only on nutrition, but also the endocrine and immunomodulatory functions of the GI system. The following discussion will address the alterations in gastrointestinal physiology in the critically ill patient, followed by a review of GI complications in the intensive care unit (ICU) using an anatomic approach. The pathophysiology, diagnosis and management of these complications will be discussed using an evidence-based approach.

Peritoneal-Based Complications

Intra-Abdominal Hypertension and Abdominal Compartment Syndrome

Intra-abdominal hypertension (IAH) is defined as a sustained intra-abdominal pressure greater than or equal to 12 mmHg, as measured by a trans-bladder measurement. Isolated clinical examination of the abdomen has been shown to be unreliable in diagnosing IAH and so serial objective measurement with a standardized trans-bladder approach is recommended in all patients with known risk factors for IAH (Table 5.1) [1]. There are several accepted techniques for measurement of trans-bladder pressure, with excellent inter-rater reliability when a single, standardized protocol is implemented within an institution [2] (see Fig. 5.1).

Diagnosis and management of IAH is important in preventing its progression to abdominal compartment syndrome (ACS) which is defined as a sustained intra-abdominal pressure greater than or equal to 20 mmHg with evidence of new end-organ dysfunction. The latter is thought to be a consequence of decreased abdominal perfusion pressure for delivery of blood flow to intra-abdominal organs. The incidence of ACS in the combined medical and surgical critically ill population is estimated at approximately 5–12 %, with a reported associated mortality of 40–100 % [2–4].

ACS is classified as primary or secondary. Primary ACS is a result of an injury or disease process that originates in the abdomen (e.g., abdominopelvic trauma, pancreatitis) whereas secondary ACS occurs when the inciting condition is not in the abdomen or pelvis (e.g., aggressive fluid resuscitation in sepsis and burns). Regardless of the classification, ACS has important physiologic consequences for not only the GI system, but the central nervous, cardiac, pulmonary and renal systems as well. Clinically, ACS often manifests as abdominal distension with worsening hemodynamic instability resulting from decreasing venous return and cardiac output, difficulty with ventilation secondary to decreasing respiratory system compliance (i.e., increasing peak airway pressures), and decreasing urine output. Management of ACS has been addressed comprehensively by the World Society for the ACS in their 2013 practice guidelines [1]. These recommendations can be categorized as noninvasive and invasive. Included in the noninvasive category is the use of sedation and analgesia, and if required as a temporizing measure, a trial of neuromuscular blockade with the objective of increasing abdominal wall compliance. Recommendations also include the use of nasogastric and rectal tubes for luminal decompression.

Table 5.1 Risk factors for intra-abdominal hypertension

Decreased abdominal wall compliance
Major burns
Abdominal surgery
Prone positioning
Increased abdominal volume
Intraluminal
Gastroparesis
Ileus
Bowel obstruction
Extraluminal
Pneumoperitoneum
Hemoperitoneum
Intra-abdominal fluid collections or abscess
Ascites
Tumor/mass
Pregnancy
Capillary leak and fluid resuscitation
Pancreatitis
Sepsis
Burns
Trauma
Hemorrhage and coagulopathy
Other
Obesity
Mechanical ventilation
PEEP > 10

Adapted from Kirkpatrick A, Roberts DJ, De Waele J, et al. Intra-abdominal hypertension and the abdominal compartment syndrome: updated consensus definitions and clinical practice guidelines from the World Society of the Abdominal Compartment Syndrome. Intensive Care Med 2013; 39:1190

As discussed later in this chapter, in patients with an established diagnosis of colonic pseudo-obstruction (where mechanical obstruction has been ruled out), consideration may be given to the use of neostigmine to affect colonic decompression. Targeting a negative fluid balance is an important feature in the management of IAH/ACS, but this can be challenging in the setting of end-organ dysfunction that often includes renal failure. The impact of diuretics versus renal replacement therapy on outcome in this population has not been clearly established. Indeed, goal-directed fluid resuscitation, with the objective of minimizing excessive fluid administration, should be carried out. The benefit of colloid over crystalloid resuscitation in limiting progression of IAH to ACS has only been demonstrated in burn patients thus far [5].

Invasive interventions for ACS include percutaneous drainage of ascitic fluid, and the more definitive decompressive laparotomy. Drainage of ascitic fluid should be undertaken if technically feasible. Early surgical consultation should be considered even as the less invasive therapies are being instituted. This is particularly important in the setting of primary ACS as there may be underlying intra-abdominal pathology (e.g., intraperitoneal hemorrhage) that may need to be addressed surgically. Surgical intervention in this patient population involves substantial risks, with mortality for patients with ACS requiring surgical decompression reported as high as 50 % [6].

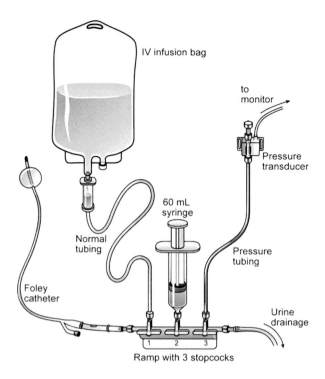

Fig. 5.1 Trans-bladder measurement of intra-abdominal pressure. Key features of trans-bladder pressure measurement: 1. Supine positioning, 2. Transducer placement, zeroed at the mid-axillary line, level of iliac crest, 3. Foley drainage tube clamped, with 25 mL sterile saline instilled into bladder. Measurement at end expiration, in absence of abdominal contractions. Reprinted from Desie N, Willems A, Da Iaet I, et al. Intra-abdominal pressure measurement using the FoleyManometer does not increase the risk for urinary tract infection in critically ill patients. Ann Intensive Care 2012; 2(Suppl 1):S10

Intra-abdominal pressure should be measured serially even after surgical decompression as patients can develop recurrent IAH even in the setting of an open abdomen. Other important considerations include careful management of fluid balance: a negative fluid balance facilitates subsequent abdominal closure, but this goal needs to be weighed against the ongoing fluid losses and redistribution (e.g., third space) that occur in the setting of an open abdomen. Other morbidity related to the open abdomen includes increased risk of infection, loss of abdominal domain, and the potential to develop enteric fistulae. Current recommendations target same-admission fascial closure when possible, as inability to complete primary closure is associated with increased morbidity and decreased quality of life in the post-ICU period [1].

Pneumoperitoneum

Pneumoperitoneum refers to extraluminal air within the peritoneal cavity. The most common cause of pneumoperitoneum is a perforated viscous, which is the case in almost 90 % of patients [7]. However, this radiological finding should be interpreted in clinical context, which may be challenging in ICU patients as clinical parameters and physical examination are confounded by medications and underlying disease. Establishing a timely diagnosis for the etiology of pneumoperitoneum is essential, because if perforated viscous is suspected, surgical intervention must be prompt.

Thoracic causes of pneumoperitoneum in the ICU include mechanical ventilation causing rupture of alveoli with dissection of air along peribronchial and perivascular tissues of the lung into the mediastinum. It is felt that mediastinal air travels into the peritoneum via microdefects in the diaphragm, or into the retroperitoneum along the esophageal or aortic hiatus. From the retroperitoneum, air travels into the peritoneum along the planes of the intestinal mesentery or perinephric vasculature. Most case reports describe peak inspiratory pressures averaging around 40 cm H_2O, with most positive end expiratory pressures of 10 cm H_2O or less, but it is felt that respiratory system compliance is the more important determinant of who develops this unusual complication of mechanical ventilation [7].

Another described phenomenon is post-cardiopulmonary resuscitation pneumoperitoneum. This can be related to difficult intubation (e.g., aggressive bag-mask with a mechanism similar to that of mechanical ventilation), rib fracture with pneumothorax tracking into the abdomen, or esophageal and gastric perforation as a result of either difficult intubation or chest compressions. In this setting, decisions regarding further management are complex and establishing whether pneumoperitoneum is truly benign is difficult: the patient is often unstable from the underlying cause of arrest and transport of the patient for further imaging studies may be precarious. Determining whether pneumoperitoneum is contributing to patient instability is of utmost importance, because this may prompt surgical exploration without attempts to obtain imaging first.

An X-ray demonstrating pneumoperitoneum in the critically ill is most often a postoperative finding. Free air is seen on an erect chest X-ray more commonly with open procedures, but can also be seen following laparoscopic procedures. This finding should resolve over the course of 2–5 days [8]. If there is any concern regarding the clinical exam at any point in a postoperative course, surgical review should be requested regardless of imaging findings.

Intra-abdominal causes of pneumoperitoneum also include endoscopic interventions such as percutaneous endoscopic gastrostomy (PEG) tube placement. A small amount of post-procedural free air may be encountered, and is related to insufflation of air during endoscopy as the tube is placed percutaneously through the anterior gastric wall. If clinical examination of the abdomen and hemodynamic parameters are stable with these imaging findings, intervention is not required. Serial exam and repeat X-ray can be considered. One of the complications of PEG placement is inadvertent injury to small bowel or colon, and any clinical concern should prompt imaging in the form of CT abdomen with water soluble contrast administered via the PEG. Progressive symptoms on clinical exam or suspicion of injury to other viscera on imaging should prompt surgical consultation.

Esophagus

Esophagitis

Esophageal mucosal injury in the ICU patient has important clinical implications, namely bleeding and infection. The mechanism of injury in this population is generally either mechanical or reflux-induced, with a small subset caused by infectious precipitants. Nasogastric tubes can cause mucosal injury via direct irritation, and perhaps more importantly, by the mechanical interference with normal motility and lower esophageal function. This results in increased rates of gastroesophageal reflux (GER).

Infectious etiology of esophagitis is a consideration in the ICU patient, who may be immunocompromised on the basis of underlying medical conditions or secondary to the relative immunosuppression from critical illness. Infectious esophagitis is a rare cause of symptomatic esophagitis and is usually seen in immunocompromised hosts, such as patients with human immunodeficiency virus (HIV) infection, hematologic malignancy, chemotherapy, or organ transplant. Risk factors for infectious esophagitis in the immunocompetent host include underlying conditions such as diabetes, adrenal insufficiency and alcohol abuse. The broad categories of infectious organisms include fungal (*Candida*, *Aspergillus*), viral (herpes simplex virus [HSV], cytolomegavirus [CMV]), and less commonly bacterial (*Staphylococcous*, *Streptococcus* species). Although some organisms have a typical appearance on endoscopy, histopathologic diagnosis is ideal for directing further management. The most commonly implicated infectious agent is fungal, specifically *Candida albicans* [9]. Systemic treatment is required for this condition, and usually consists of an azole for 14–21 days. Echinocandins and amphoterecin B are alternative treatment options if the patient fails to respond to treatment with an azole. Diagnosis of other fungal infections such as *Aspergillus* or *Blastomycoces* should prompt consideration of a primary mediastinal or pulmonary infectious source [9].

Independent of nasogastric tube placement, GER and the related duodenogastroesophageal reflux (DGER) (i.e., bile reflux) are important risk factors for the development of esophagitis in the critically ill population. These disorders are described in further detail in the sections below.

The diagnosis of esophagitis in the ICU is often made at the time of endoscopy, usually precipitated by bleeding complications. This is one of the most common findings at the time of upper endoscopy performed for upper gastrointestinal bleeding in the ICU [10, 11]. Treatment of esophagitis is generally supportive, with the majority of bleeding episodes being self-limited. More specific therapy is instituted only if the precipitant of esophagitis is apparent on direct visualization. If the precipitant is determined to be nasogastric tube placement, the tube is removed. Brushings or biopsies may be taken to rule out or demonstrate suspected infectious etiology based on appearance (e.g., candidiasis, CMV). Further treatment may be directed by histopathological findings. If no mechanical or obvious infectious precipitant is demonstrated at the time of endoscopy, patients are generally treated for reflux esophagitis including acid suppression and promotility agents. Tissue manipulation for diagnostic purposes is avoided in the setting of active bleeding. In general, severe hemorrhagic esophagitis is not amenable to endoscopic treatment because it tends to be diffuse. If, however, areas of focal, active hemorrhage are identified at the time of endoscopy they may be treated with epinephrine injection or topical ablative therapy.

Gastroesophageal Reflux

Retrograde movement of gastric secretions into the esophagus is a well-described problem in the critically ill, with important consequences including esophagitis and pulmonary aspiration. The mechanisms of GER all center on anatomic and physiologic lower esophageal sphincter (LES) dysfunction. Important pathophysiologic features include:

1. Transient Lower Esophageal Sphincter Relaxations (TLERs)
   TLERs are the most common cause of reflux in both normal subjects and GER patients with normal LES tone. LES relaxation occurs in two general scenarios: those in coordination with swallowing and peristalsis, and TLERs which are independent of swallowing and esophageal peristalsis but associated with relaxation of the diaphragm, an important part of the normal anti-reflux mechanism. TLERs are most frequent in the post-prandial period and are thought to be stimulated by gastric distension. Obesity is also associated with increased TLER frequency. The problem may be potentiated by the diaphragmatic dysfunction associated with these more frequent TLERs.
2. Diaphragmatic Hiatus Dysfunction
   Contraction of the diaphragm during inspiration increases LES tone by acting as an "external sphincter" at the level of the esophageal hiatus, and is therefore a component of the body's normal anti-reflux mechanism. This external sphincter relaxes in the setting of esophageal distension and both swallow-induced and transient LES relaxations. This mechanism is pathologically disrupted by the misalignment of crus and LES in the setting of hiatal hernia.
3. LES Hypotension
   While TLERs are the most frequent mechanism for reflux in the average patient population, in the critically ill impaired LES tone is the most important factor [12]. The normal LES is tonically contracted smooth muscle. Relative hypotension of the LES results in GER by both stress and free reflux. Stress reflux occurs when a sudden increase in intra-abdominal pressure overcomes the resting tone of the LES. In patients with lower resting tone of the LES, episodes of stress reflux become increasingly frequent. Therefore, episodes of increased abdominal pressure, (e.g., coughing during suctioning of the intubated patient), are more likely to result in GER. In contrast, free reflux is defined as a drop in esophageal pH without any detected change in LES resting tone, but occurs only in the setting of LES pressures less than half of normal (0–4 versus 10–30 mmHg) [12]. In addition to being common in critically ill patients, LES hypotension is found with increased frequency in diabetes, scleroderma, and pregnancy. Medications, many of which are used in the ICU, also can contribute to decreased LES tone, including beta-agonists, morphine, diazepam, and calcium channel blockers.

There is a substantial body of work that establishes the damage to esophageal mucosa that results from sustained exposure to an acidic milieu (e.g., pH < 4.0). At the cellular level, hydrogen ion diffusion into the mucosal cells and the subsequent acidity results in cell necrosis. This effect is potentiated by pepsin, secreted by the gastric chief cells as a zymogen which causes direct damage to the mucosal barrier, making it even more permeable to hydrogen ions. The mainstay of management of esophagitis secondary to esophageal reflux is acid suppression with proton pump inhibitors (PPIs). PPIs have been demonstrated to be more effective in healing esophagitis than H2 receptor antagonists [11, 13]. The role of prokinetic agents such as metoclopramide in this setting, however, remains unclear.

Duodenogastroesophageal Reflux

The term bile reflux has been used interchangeably with DGER in the past, but this is a misnomer because in addition to bile, duodenal secretions include hormones (e.g., secretin, cholecystokinin) as well as bicarbonate and digestive enzymes secreted by the pancreas. DGER is seen most frequently in the post-gastric resection population, where the mechanical barrier of the gastric pylorus is removed en bloc with the surgical specimen. However, there is some evidence to suggest that DGER occurs in the non-operative population as well, but a pure alkaline reflux is rare [12, 14]. In the last two decades the concept of DGER causing an "alkaline esophagitis" has been modified to suggest that combination acidic/alkaline reflux may result in higher rates of severe erosive esophagitis, strictures, and Barrett's esophagus. From a critical care perspective, the details of potential bile acid-mediated esophageal injury are less relevant in terms of acute reflux complications such as esophagitis: acid suppression therapy is the mainstay of treatment, because it is the acidic pH that causes most of the *acute* mucosal injury. The role of prokinetics for DGER in critically ill patients remains unclear, but there is some evidence to suggest prokinetics may have a role in patients who have previously undergone gastric resection [15]. However, the use of prokinetic agents in this setting needs to be weighed against the potential for adverse drug interactions and complications.

Stomach

Stress Ulcers

Most critically ill patients (75–100 %) have endoscopically detectable mucosal erosions within 24 h of ICU admission [10]. Stress ulcers fall into a broader category of what is referred to as stress-related mucosal disease (SRMD). This set of conditions represents an acute erosive gastritis ranging from superficial erosions to deep ulcerations penetrating the submucosa. Anatomically, most SRMD is found in the fundus and body of the stomach, although it can also be seen in the distal esophagus and duodenum. The two most important risk factors for this disease are mechanical ventilation greater than 48 h and coagulopathy [16]. The most significant implications are perforation (a rare event, occurring in less than 1 % of SRMD in ICU patients), and most commonly, bleeding. A recurring concept in the literature discussing this topic is the term "clinically-important bleeding", which has been defined as bleeding causing hemodynamic instability or requiring transfusion. Clinically-important bleeding is associated with increased morbidity, mortality, and length of ICU stay [17]. However, it is important to note that while there is a strong association between clinically-significant bleeding in SRMD and subsequent mortality, it is more a marker for severity of illness, with patients dying from their underlying disease, and not from GI bleeding per se [11, 17].

The pathophysiology of SRMD is related to an interaction between the acidic pH of gastric contents and impaired gastric barrier function secondary to mucosal ischemia and direct toxic insults from factors such as pepsin [18]. Most ICU patients with SRMD have normal gastric pH of around 2. Although gastric acid is part of the pathophysiology of SRMD, the only critical care populations that have demonstrated acid hypersecretion are patients with head trauma, traumatic spinal cord injury, or burns. The normal barrier function of gastric mucosa to hydrogen ions is affected by the glycoprotein layer which traps bicarbonate and allows for neutralization of intraluminal acid. This barrier is disrupted by two main mechanisms: mucosal ischemia likely secondary to splanchnic hypoperfusion, and direct toxins such as bile acids and pepsin, each of which compromises the ability of the mucosa to neutralize acid resulting in enhanced tissue necrosis.

The mainstay of treatment of SRMD is prophylaxis in the form of acid suppression. Guidelines from the American Society of Health-System Pharmacists were last published in 1998, with an update to be published in 2014 [19]. These guidelines were based on studies comparing rates of SRMD in patients with prophylaxis versus no prophylaxis, using clinically-important GI bleeding as an endpoint. Patients who warrant stress ulcer prophylaxis include the following:

1. Mechanical ventilation >48 h
2. Coagulopathy (platelets <50, INR >1.5)
3. History of ulcers or bleeding in the past 12 months
4. Patients at risk for hyperacidity (burn, traumatic brain injury, spinal cord injury)
5. Patients with two or more of the following "minor" risk factors: sepsis, ICU stay >1 week, steroid therapy, occult GI bleeding for at least 6 days

The main classes of medications used for stress ulcer prophylaxis in ICU patients include histamine-2 receptor antagonists (H2RAs) and PPIs. H2RAs inhibit histamine-stimulated acid secretion by blocking receptors on the parietal cells of the stomach. Considerations in the use of H2RAs include potential for tolerance after short duration of therapy and possible drug interaction secondary to interference with cytochrome P450 enzymes. Dose adjustments are also required in patients with renal dysfunction. PPIs inhibit the hydrogen–potassium ATPase enzyme at the parietal cell surface, thereby preventing H+ transport out of the cell. This inhibition of acid transport takes place irrespective of the cell stimulant (e.g., histamine, gastrin). In general, PPIs are well tolerated. Meta-analyses suggest that PPIs are associated with less bleeding than H2 blockers without affecting rates of nosocomial pneumonia or mortality [20]. In February 2012 the American Food and Drug Administration issued a warning that PPI use may predispose to Clotstridium difficile infection (CDI). Two meta-analyses published in 2012 attempted to address this association, but were based on a heterogenous group of observational studies that did not define the length of exposure or comorbidities. At this time a causal relationship cannot be established, but clinicians should be aware of the possible association and consider this risk in the context of comborbidities and concurrent risk factors for CDI including antibiotic use [21, 22].

Concern that acid suppression therapy may be associated with increased rates of nosocomial pneumonia has not been demonstrated conclusively. The suggested mechanism for this potential association is bacterial colonization secondary to a less acidic milieu in the stomach. Consideration of this risk may be more applicable to patients who do not meet the criteria for stress ulcer prophylaxis as outlined above but are being considered for prophylaxis because of clinical context. The role of enteral nutrition in stress ulcer prophylaxis is not well delineated. It is likely that enteral nutrition does have a protective effect on SRMD, but there is no good evidence to suggest feeding alone is sufficient in the populations warranting stress ulcer prophylaxis. Cost is another consideration in choosing appropriate agents. Enteral PPIs are a reasonable first choice for prophylaxis in critically ill patients who tolerate enteral intake.

Management of the patient with clinically-significant upper GI bleeding in the critical care setting should involve standard resuscitation interventions including fluids, transfusions as indicated, correcting coagulopathy, and intravenous infusion of PPIs until endoscopy can be performed to confirm the diagnosis and control the bleeding source. Further treatments are determined by findings at the time of endoscopy. There is no compelling evidence for the routine use of octreotide in nonvariceal upper GI bleeding.

Dysmotility and Feeding Intolerance

Delayed gastric emptying (DGE) occurs frequently in critically ill populations and is associated with impaired feeding tolerance. Consequences of DGE therefore include malnutrition and increased risk of aspiration pneumonia. For a population already under catabolic stress and with systemic inflammatory activation, the implications of malnutrition include immune dysfunction and an increased risk of infections, weakened skeletal and respiratory muscles and ventilatory drive, and GI dysfunction including GER and esophagitis. The pathophysiologic mechanisms involved in DGE are complex and an area of ongoing study. The main mechanisms associated with DGE in the ICU population are thought to be as follows:

1. Autonomic Nerve Dysfunction

   Parasympathetic supply to the stomach is mediated by the vagus nerve. Dysfunction of the vagal nerve interferes with normal fundic relaxation in response to distension; it also impairs pyloric relaxation. Medical issues including diabetes, Parkinson's disease, and multiple sclerosis are well-described risk factors for gastroparesis, likely secondary to their effect on the vagal nerve. Anticholinergic medications (e.g., atropine, diphenhydramine) are implicated in DGE through this mechanism.

2. Enteric Nerve Dysfunction

   The interstitial cells of Cajal (ICC) are considered the "pacemaker cells" of the gut, and are responsible for the slow wave electrical activity causing phasic contractions of smooth muscle. Histopathologic studies of DGE demonstrate qualitative (dysmorphic) or quantitative loss of ICC, as well as a loss of expression of neuronal nitric oxide synthase (nNOS) [23]. Nitric oxide is synthesized by nNOS, and plays an important role in smooth muscle relaxation. nNOS is expressed in enteric nerves and functions to control tone of the LES, pylorus and the peristaltic reflex of the small intestine. It is possible that the upregulation of the feedback loop that normally guides gastric emptying (through inhibition of antral motility and increased pyloric tone seen in response to nutrient exposure) may be mediated by enteric nerve dysfunction. Loss of ICC is seen in models of diabetes and hyperglycemia [23, 24]. Opioids, a class of medications frequently used in the ICU, are thought to mediate their dysmotile effects via endogenous opioid receptors of the enteric nervous system.

3. Smooth Muscle Cells

   The role of smooth muscle cells in the development of DGE is clear as the endpoint of the nerve dysfunction discussed above. Interestingly, loss of ICC is also associated with smooth muscle atrophy, possibly related to decreased expression of stem cell factors.

The development of dysmotility in the critical care patient is multifactorial and influenced by a combination of the patients' baseline medical issues with the superimposed electrolyte abnormalities, hemodynamic shifts and medications associated with critical illness.

Clinical evidence of DGE has typically been defined by vomiting/regurgitation, and what was thought to be a preceding factor, high gastric residual volume (GRV). The measurement of GRV is neither standardized nor validated, but nevertheless it is widely used in the ICU setting. The concern with vomiting, regurgitation, and high GRV is the perceived increased risk of aspiration pneumonia. Interestingly, a recent randomized controlled trial (RCT) evaluating mechanically ventilated patients receiving early enteral nutrition demonstrated no significant differences in the rates of ventilator-associated pneumonia when comparing routine measurement of GRV versus no measurement (17 versus 16 %) [25]. Moreover, there were no significant differences in other ICU-acquired infections, mechanical ventilation duration, ICU length of stay, or mortality rates between groups. In fact, many trials have implicated measurement of so-called "high" GRV in severe underfeeding in the ICU population because the common practice once high GRV is measured is to hold enteral feeding [26]. Indeed, in the recent RCT by Reignier and colleagues, the proportion of patients receiving 100 % of their caloric goal was significantly higher in the group without GRV measurements (odds ratio 1.77; 90 % confidence interval 1.25–2.51) [25]. If ongoing measurement continues while further research is done, enteral feeding should only be held if single GRV measurement is 250–500 mL or a cumulative 1,000 mL is measured in 24 h of feeding. In these cases, after ruling out a distal obstruction, consideration may be given to adding prokinetic agents (e.g., metoclopramide, domperidone, or erythromycin).

The prokinetic activity of domperidone and metoclopramide is mediated through their antidopaminergic activity, and in the case of metoclopramide, enhanced cholinergic transmission (via the $5\text{-}HT_4$ receptor) effects. The antidopaminergic effects include increased LES pressure, antral contractility, and antroduodenal coordination. Erythromycin enhances gastric emptying by binding to the motilin receptors in the antrum and duodenum.

There is reasonable evidence for postpyloric feeding for patients who demonstrate feeding intolerance in the form of recurrent aspiration, GER, and DGE. The reduction in rates of nosocomial pneumonia has not, however, been consistently demonstrated in patients who do not exhibit symptoms of feeding intolerance. In the 2013 Canadian Clinical Practice Guidelines, it is recommended that where post pyloric tube placement is feasible, routine small bowel feeding should be implemented. This is predicated on the likelihood that post pyloric feeding decreases rates of aspiration pneumonia, and studies based on previous guidelines demonstrate patients receive a greater percentage of their calculated caloric requirements [27]. Studies comparing enteral and parenteral feeding do not show a difference in terms of mortality, but do suggest a lower risk of infection with enteral feeding. A randomized multicenter trial published in 2011 demonstrated a lower rate of infectious complications without a significant difference in mortality in patients for whom parenteral nutrition was initiated after 8 days compared to within 48 h of ICU admission [28]. These results suggest that there may be an 8-day window for patients admitted to the ICU to be stabilized and optimized to attempt enteral feeding if appropriate. These studies do not address patients who are malnourished at the time of ICU admission.

In terms of management of nutrition in critically ill patients, recommendations can be summarized as follows:

1. Early enteral feeding (within 24–48 h of admission), when there are no contraindications.
2. Withholding of feeds only in extreme hemodynamic instability and suspicion of associated bowel ischemia, or clinical suspicion of other abdominal surgical pathology.
3. Routine use of post pyloric feeding where technically feasible.
4. Addition of prokinetics (preferred agent: metoclopramide) in the setting of feeding intolerance after ruling out distal obstruction, with a threshold for GRV of 250–500 mL to guide decisions regarding feeding tolerance.
5. Consideration of parenteral nutrition after 7 days of inadequate enteral nutrition intake.

Hepatobiliary

Acute Acalculous Cholecystitis

Acute acalculous cholecystitis is acute inflammation of the gallbladder in the absence of cholelithiasis. The incidence in the ICU population is between 0.5 and 3 % [29]. Although the pathogenesis of this disease is multifactorial, the common underlying pathway involves ischemia of the gallbladder wall and bile stasis. Risk factors for acute acalculous cholecystitis include mechanical ventilation greater than 72 h, systemic inflammatory response syndrome, and hemodynamic shifts that result in decreased splanchnic blood flow, including shock and use of vasopressors. Other important risk factors include prolonged fasting, dehydration, and total parenteral nutrition (TPN) (Table 5.2).

Clinical manifestations of acalculous cholecystitis are often non-specific in the critically ill patient, with inconsistent physical exam and laboratory findings. Diagnosis of this clinical entity relies on imaging studies, primarily that of ultrasound which is the modality of choice in initial imaging of the biliary system. Computed tomography (CT) is also useful in the diagnostic work-up of signs and symptoms suggestive of acalculous cholecystitis as it can help to rule out other intra-abdominal pathology.

Management of suspected acute acalculous cholecystitis should include blood cultures followed by prompt initiation of broad-spectrum antibiotics targeting enteric flora including gram-negative bacteria, anaerobes, and *Enterococcus* species. Surgical consultation is also warranted. The definitive management of cholecystitis is cholecystectomy, which may not be feasible or appropriate in unstable critically ill patients. In these cases consideration may be given to percutaneous drainage with a cholecystostomy tube. Risks of the procedure include tube dislodgement with bile peritonitis, hemobilia, and bowel injury. Patient selection for a less invasive approach (i.e., antibiotics with or without cholecystostomy tube) is very important. Patients with diabetes and immunosuppression, for example, have a higher rate of serious

Table 5.2 Risk factors for acute acalculous cholecstitis	Conditions promoting bile stasis
	Fasting
	TPN
	Ileus
	Conditions promoting gallbladder ischemia
	Mechanical ventilation
	Shock
	Burn
	Sepsis
	Trauma
	Vascular disease
	Other
	Immunodeficiency
	Chronic medical illness: diabetes, hypertension, obesity

complications from cholecystitis including gangrene or perforation. Clinical improvement should be expected within 24 h of drainage [29]. If no clinical improvement is seen within this time frame, surgical intervention is indicated.

Liver Dysfunction

Liver dysfunction is a frequent finding in the critically ill, typically occurring initially with abnormal laboratory values. Patterns of abnormal liver tests must be interpreted in the clinical context of the patient, and in the ICU population there are generally two patterns of dysfunction: cholestasis and ischemic hepatopathy ("shock liver"). Each of these entities has important implications in the management of ICU patients because of the hematologic, metabolic, and immunologic functions of this organ.

Ischemic Hepatopathy

Hepatic blood supply originates from a combination of the portal vein, with inflow from the superior mesenteric and splenic veins, and the hepatic artery, typically branching from the celiac axis. The hepatic artery response is the homeostatic mechanism that maintains blood flow to the liver, with an inverse change of flow as a response to portal venous flow. An important anatomic distinction of the hepatic artery is that it forms the sole blood supply of the bile ducts of the liver. At baseline the liver receives approximately 25 % of cardiac output, but this is significantly decreased at times of systemic stress as the body preferentially delivers blood flow to the cerebral and cardiac circulation. This can lead to hepatocellular hypoxia, which along with reperfusion injury results in hepatic injury. Passive venous congestion is another contributory factor in the development of ischemic hepatitis, and is most often seen in the setting of right-sided heart failure. Ischemic hepatopathy, then, refers to a diffuse pattern of injury resulting from decreased blood flow to the liver, passive venous congestion, or hypoxemia from a different primary source (e.g., lung injury).

Clinical diagnosis of this disorder is based primarily on abnormal liver tests that usually manifest within 24–48 h of an ischemic insult. The "hepatocellular" abnormalities include aminotransferase levels greater than 25 times the upper limit of normal with an early and precipitous rise in lactate, but only minimal evidence of synthetic dysfunction as measured by international normalized ratio (INR) and partial prothromboplastin time (PTT). The aminotransferases usually return to normal within 7–10 days of stabilized hemodynamics [30]. Hyperbilirubinemia may be present but rarely exceeds three to four times the upper limit of normal, and is generally the last abnormality to resolve. It is important to exclude an anatomic vascular cause of compromised hepatic flow by Doppler ultrasound of the liver. Depending on the clinical context, additional investigations may be required to address the differential diagnosis of a hepatocellular pattern of dysfunction including viral infection (e.g., hepatitis B or C), drug-induced toxicity (e.g., acetaminophen), or autoimmune hepatitis.

Management of ischemic hepatopathy focuses on restoring adequate cardiac output and addressing the underlying etiology of hemodynamic instability. Ischemic hepatopathy is typically self-limited (presuming the underlying insult is reversed), and morbidity and mortality are usually related to underlying systemic disease. Progression to fulminant hepatic failure is rare (2–5 %), with the majority of cases of fulminant hepatic failure having underlying baseline congestive or cirrhotic disease [30].

Cholestasis

Cholestasis is the most frequent hepatic abnormality noted in the critically ill, found in up to 40 % of ICU patients [30]. The implications of cholestasis include bacterial infections, hypotension secondary to the vasodilatory effects of bile acids, alterations of glucose and lipid metabolism, and renal toxicity leading to acute tubular necrosis. This diagnosis can be approached from an anatomic and physiologic perspective: prehepatic (e.g., hemolysis, hematoma resorption), hepatic (e.g., autoimmune and medication causes), and extrahepatic (e.g., biliary obstruction from gallstone, pancreatic head mass). In the ICU setting the most common causes of cholestasis fall into the intrahepatic category—shock, sepsis, medications, and parenteral nutrition—all have hepatotoxic effects leading to impairment in bile production and transport.

Shock and mechanisms of hepatocellular damage were discussed in the previous section. Sepsis has been implicated in impaired bile acid transport at a cellular level, likely mediated by cytokines. Gram-negative sepsis has been specifically identified, with a mechanism possibly related to endotoxin release. Several forms of cholestatic liver injury can be caused by medications, with variable mechanism and presentation (Table 5.3). The target of injury can vary from a mixed hepatocellular cholestatic injury to impairment of canalicular bile flow resulting in pure intrahepatic cholestasis [31]. The mechanism of TPN-related cholestasis is likely multifactorial including bacterial overgrowth secondary to gut hypomotility, leading to endotoxin absorption that impairs bile acid transport. Another contributory factor is excess nutrient delivery with accumulation of triglycerides in hepatocytes mediated by upregulation of insulin due to relative insulin resistance in critical illness [32].

Cholestasis is defined by hyperbilirubinemia and elevated alkaline phosphatase (typically greater than three times the upper limit of normal) with only mild associated elevation in aminotransferases. INR may be elevated because of the effect on vitamin K-dependent coagulation factors. The first step in management of ICU cholestasis is to address the underlying mechanism of injury. Restoring hemodynamic stability and treating underlying sepsis is critical. When drug-induced cholestasis is suspected, a careful review of any new medications in the past 3 months should be carried out, with removal of any potentially offending agents (Table 5.3). Addressing TPN-induced cholestasis requires adjustment of composition, assessment of energy balance, and consideration of metronidazole for bacterial overgrowth, which should be done in consultation with a dietician and gastroenterologist.

Table 5.3 Medications
frequently implicated in
cholestasis

| **Antimicrobials** |
| Amoxicillin–clavulanate |
| Nafcillin |
| Trimethoprim–sulfamethoxazole |
| Erythromycin |
| Rifampin |
| Ketoconazole |
| **Cardiac** |
| Captopril |
| Amiodarone |
| **Antiretrovirals** |
| Nevirapine |
| Efavirenz |
| **Endocrine** |
| Ezetimibe |
| Rosiglitazone |
| Troglitazone |
| Estrogens |
| Anabolic steroids |
| **Immunosuppression** |
| Azathioprine |
| Infliximab |
| **Other** |
| Chlorpromazine |
| Carbamazepine |

Intestinal

Hemorrhage

The majority of acute gastrointestinal hemorrhage originates in the foregut: esophagus, stomach and duodenum.

Upper GI Bleeding

The most common cause of acute upper GI bleeding (AUGIB) in hospitalized patients is peptic ulcer disease. In general, an approach to diagnosis and management of upper GI bleeding (UGIB) divides this problem into variceal hemorrhage versus nonvariceal bleeding, including peptic ulcer disease and stress-related mucosal hemorrhage. Although GI bleeding is a frequently encountered problem in the ICU, bleeding as a complication of ICU stay has become less common in an era of prophylactic acid suppression therapy, because the majority of bleeding seen in this context is secondary to SRMD. Since this topic has been addressed in a previous section, the following section will focus on the management of patients presenting with AUGIB.

Regardless of etiology, the first step in management of bleeding involves hemodynamic monitoring and adequate resuscitation with fluids and blood products as clinically indicated. A nasogastric tube can be placed to confirm an upper GI source of bleeding if it is clinically unclear; however, lack of bloody return does not reliably exclude upper GI bleeding. The tube can also be used to perform lavage to prepare the foregut for visualization during endoscopy, which should be performed within 24 h of the onset of bleeding. Erythromycin can also be used to attempt to clear the stomach of blood to improve visualization. Transfusion targets in the setting of AUGIB have been studied, and a recent RCT supports a relatively restrictive transfusion strategy (targeting a hemoglobin threshold of 7 g/dL compared to a more liberal strategy targeting a hemoglobin threshold of 9 g/dL) in patients with AUGIB. The results of this study suggest that a restrictive strategy is associated with decreased rates of rebleeding and mortality. This study excluded patients who were hemodynamically unstable with massive hemorrhage, and also noted that patients with unstable coronary artery disease were exceptions to this guideline [33]. Coagulopathy should also be corrected with appropriate blood products or replacement therapy.

The management of suspected variceal bleeding prior to endoscopy requires the addition of a somatostatin analogue such as octreotide, to affect splanchnic vasoconstriction and decrease portal pressures, to a PPI infusion. The PPI infusion is provided because patients with cirrhosis are also at high risk for peptic ulcer-related bleeding. Cirrhotics who present with UGIB should also be treated with propylactic third-generation cephalosporins or fluoroquinolones as up to 40 % develop a bacterial infection within one week of AUGIB, which is an independent risk factor for rebleeding and mortality [11]. Of note, in patients with cirrhosis and GI bleeding, platelet targets may be adjusted from the standard target of 50 with active bleeding, to a slightly lower target of 30, since thrombocytopenia is seen commonly in cirrhotics and does not necessarily convey risk of bleeding. Many cases of variceal bleeding will stabilize with vasoactive treatment alone, but endoscopy is still required for definitive management. Placement of an esophageal/gastric balloon (i.e., Sengstaken–Blakemore tube, Linton–Nachlas tube) can be considered in cases of massive UGIB that is inadequately controlled with endoscopic therapy. This should be considered a bridge to more definitive management of portal hypertension with variceal bleeding, such as transjugular intrahepatic portosystemic shunt (TIPS).

The management of non-variceal bleeding should involve the same initial steps of monitoring, supportive resuscitation with fluids and blood products to appropriate targets, and nasogastric (NG) tube placement. In this case, intravenous (IV) PPI infusion should be started pending endoscopy. The continuation of PPI infusion post-endoscopy is determined by the procedural findings: the Forrest classification is one system that designates endoscopic findings as high and low risk for rebleeding. Patients who are deemed to be a high risk of rebleeding (Forrest Ia + b, IIa + b) should be continued on PPI infusion for 72 h because this has been shown to decrease rates of rebleeding, surgery, and mortality [11]. In general, screening for *Helicobacter pylori* in the critically ill population is not necessary because there is no rebleeding prophylaxis advantage to treating *H. pylori* in the emergency setting. The long-term risk of rebleeding may be improved with *H. pylori* eradication, and

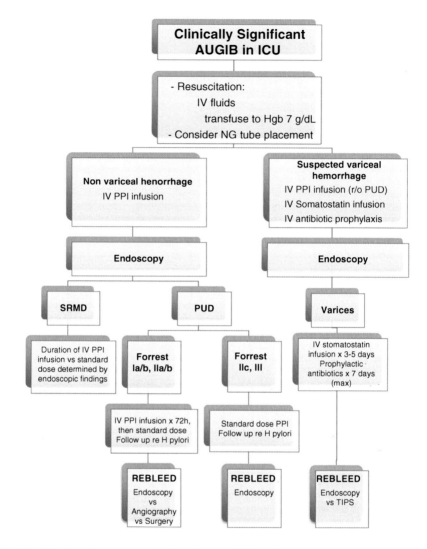

Fig. 5.2 Algorithm for management of acute upper GI bleeding

biopsy screening can be performed during initial endoscopy with little risk of increasing AUGIB [11]. Failure of endoscopic therapy to control non-variceal bleeding should be followed by surgical consultation and discussion with interventional radiology for potential embolization. Endoscopy is usually helpful in at least localizing the problematic area—if there is high-risk stigmata or clearly uncontrolled bleeding at the time of endoscopy, it is helpful if a member of the surgical team can be present at endoscopy (see Fig. 5.2 and Table 5.4).

Table 5.4 Forrest
classification of bleeding
peptic ulcer disease

Forrest I: Active bleeding
I (a)—spurting bleeding
I (b)—non spurting bleeding
Forrest II: Signs of recent hemorrhage
II (a)—visible vessel, no active bleeding
II (b)—non-bleeding ulcer with overlying clot
II (c)—flat ulcer with pigmented base
Forrest III:
III—clean ulcer base

Lower GI Bleeding

Traditionally lower GI bleeding (LGIB) refers to bleeding occurring distal to the ligament of Treitz (i.e., fourth part of the duodenum). In the ICU setting a hemodynamically-significant LGIB source is uncommon. The first step, in addition to standard resuscitation measures, is to place an NG tube to rule out a brisk UGIB source, which happens at least 10 % of the time. The NG tube can also be used to facilitate colon preparation once UGIB has been ruled out (e.g., with upper endoscopy). The most common causes of LGIB in adults originate in the colon and include diverticulosis, neoplasm, ischemia, and anorectal disease such as hemorrhoids. Small bowel sources of GI bleeding are relatively uncommon, and are identified only about 5 % of the time [11].

The most important diagnostic maneuver for hematochezia is colonoscopy. This also allows visualization of the terminal ileum, and if blood is visible proximally into the small bowel this suggests a source proximal to the colon. If significant diverticulosis is identified as the cause, management is generally supportive and bleeding is usually self-limited. Management of bleeding due to ischemia is discussed below. Neoplasm identified at the time of endoscopy warrants surgical consultation. Anorectal disease can be more challenging to treat, and is determined by endoscopic findings and consultation with Surgery. In general, ensuring regular bowel movements and minimizing the use of rectal tubes is recommended in managing problems such as hemorrhoids and ulceration caused by rectal tubes.

The diagnostic and management dilemma arises when a bleeding source cannot be identified clearly on upper and lower endoscopy, or if bleeding does not stop with endoscopic therapy. In the latter, surgical intervention is usually indicated. For the former, visualizing the small bowel can be done with terminal ileoscopy (i.e., colonoscopy with visualization of up to 30 cm of distal small bowel), and push enteroscopy which allows visualization of approximately 60 cm of small bowel distal to the ligament of Treitz. Other diagnostic maneuvers include capsule endoscopy, CT enteroscopy, and CT enteroclysis [11]. In the critically ill patient, investigation is usually prompted by ongoing hemodynamic instability or transfusion requirements. In this case, if bleeding is brisk enough (at least 0.5 mL/min), angiography is the modality of choice since it has both diagnostic and therapeutic potential. The limitation of this modality is that active bleeding must be seen in order to embolize the offending vessel and derive the therapeutic benefit. The technetium 99 m labeled red blood cell scan is highly specific and sensitive for active arterial or venous bleeding in the GI tract (it can detect bleeding rates of 0.1 mL/min) but is less specific about localization of bleeding [34]. The other obvious disadvantage is there is no therapeutic potential of the investigation, but it can be used to direct angiography and/or surgical intervention.

Ischemia

Ischemic intestinal injury is generally thought to be a consequence of hypoperfusion, but may also contribute to further hemodynamic instability through the release of inflammatory mediators and bacterial translocation as intestinal injury progresses. A thorough understanding of the risk and pattern of bowel ischemia requires knowledge of the anatomy and physiology of the intestine. The blood supply of the small and large bowel is summarized as follows:

1. Duodenum—supplied by branches of the celiac axis and the superior mesenteric artery.
2. Jejunum, ileum, ascending and proximal transverse colon—supplied by branches of the superior mesenteric artery.
3. Distal transverse, descending and sigmoid colon—supplied by branches of the inferior mesenteric artery.
4. Rectum—supplied by branches of the inferior mesenteric artery and internal iliac artery.

As noted above, the colon is supplied by branches of the superior and inferior mesenteric arteries. The collateral supply between these arteries are important when patients have significant atherosclerotic disease, or in the case of open abdominal aortic surgery, when the inferior mesentery is sometimes sacrificed. Points of transition of major arterial blood supply are referred to as watershed areas. Collaterals are smaller and less abundant at the watershed areas of the splenic flexure and sigmoid colon; these segments are therefore more vulnerable to periods of hypotension leading to colonic hypoperfusion and ischemia.

Small Bowel

There are four distinct pathophysiologic mechanisms that can lead to acute mesenteric ischemia:

1. Arterial embolus
2. Arterial thrombosis
3. Venous thrombosis
4. Non-occlusive mesenteric ischemia

The most common overall cause of acute mesenteric ischemia is arterial embolus, accounting for 50 % of ischemic bowel presentations. The most common embolic source is the heart. In contrast, the ischemic mechanism most often seen in the critically ill is non-occlusive, resulting from splanchnic hypoperfusion usually on a background of pre-existing atherosclerotic disease. Hypoperfusion results in mesenteric vasospasm, a homeostatic mechanism that redistributes blood flow to maintain cardiac and cerebral perfusion.

At a physiologic level, the bowel is vulnerable to ischemic injury because of relatively low mucosal oxygenation at the tips of intestinal villi, a consequence of countercurrent blood flow designed to maximize nutrient absorption. Interestingly, studies have shown splanchnic vasoconstriction to persist even after systemic hemodynamic stability has been restored. Injury to the bowel from ischemic insult is both a result of hypoxia and also free radical and inflammatory response in reperfusion injury. The duration and extent of injury is, therefore, difficult to measure with clinical information and investigations [10, 35].

Clinical presentation of small bowel ischemia in the critically ill population is usually insidious and difficult to diagnose early. The classic presentation of acute mesenteric ischemia is sudden onset of severe abdominal pain out of proportion to clinical exam, associated with nausea, vomiting and sometimes diarrhea, none of which are easy to assess in ICU patients who are often intubated and sedated. Unfortunately, abdominal distension, bloody enteral outputs (diarrhea or hematemesis), and peritonitis are relatively late clinical findings in the ischemia pathway, often once transmural ischemia and necrosis have occurred. For this reason, clinical suspicion should direct laboratory and imaging studies early on when a patient develops signs of sepsis with clinical change in either the abdominal examination or bowel function. Concurrent with fluid repletion and NG decompression, laboratory studies including complete blood count (CBC), lactate, and an arterial blood gas should be drawn. Blood cultures should also be collected and empiric broad-spectrum antibiotics covering for enteric pathogens initiated while awaiting diagnostic studies. Plain abdominal radiographs are generally not useful in the diagnosis of bowel ischemia, and will only precipitate intervention when demonstrating free intraperitoneal air. CT scan with IV contrast is the most useful test in diagnosing bowel ischemia, but unfortunately carries the risk of transport and contrast-induced nephropathy in a patient who likely already has compromised renal function. Surgical intervention is warranted when there is evidence of segmental infarction or free air. The most important consideration is whether there is a clear underlying occlusive lesion in the proximal vasculature which will need to be addressed either by angiography or surgery. If such a lesion is identified, therapeutic anticoagulation should be initiated while awaiting definitive management.

Large Bowel

Ischemic colitis is the most common form of large bowel ischemia, and the pathophysiologic mechanisms are identical to those seen in small bowel ischemia. The colon is more vulnerable to hypoperfusion than the small bowel because it receives less blood flow compared to the rest of the GI tract, and the microvascular supply at the level of the colon wall is less developed and robust than that of the small intestine [35].

Ischemic colitis usually occurs in elderly patients with a history of atherosclerotic risk factors and disease. Abdominal pain (usually less severe than in small bowel ischemia) typically localizes over the involved bowel segment. Commonly it is the left colon, and more specifically, the splenic flexure, which is involved because anatomically this is a "watershed area" of vascular supply. This is usually accompanied by hematochezia, fever, and leukocytosis. In its more severe form, this will progress to acidosis and peritoneal findings when there is full thickness ischemic insult to the bowel wall. As discussed above in the small bowel ischemia section, clinical symptoms are non-specific and difficult to interpret in ICU patients, and thus ancillary testing should be initiated when the diagnosis is suspected. CT findings of colitis in a watershed area are typically used to diagnose ischemic colitis. This can be supported with colonoscopy, which may be considered in the setting of hematochezia.

The course of ischemic colitis is usually self-limited and responds to supportive care with IV fluids and bowel rest. Antibiotics are typically started to treat potential bacterial translocation, and are usually stopped with resolution of fever, leukocytosis, and abdominal pain on clinical exam. If symptoms fail to respond to conservative management, or the patient becomes increasingly unstable, this may indicate progression to transmural ischemia and necrosis, warranting surgical intervention. The extent of resection, with or without diversion, is decided at the time of operation.

Pseudo-Obstruction

Colonic pseudo-obstruction (Ogilvie's syndrome) is a clinical entity characterized by gross cecal and colonic dilation without mechanical obstruction. The cecum is most vulnerable for this complication because of Laplace's law, which states that the pressure required to distend a pliable tube is inversely proportional to its diameter. The pathogenesis of this disorder is unclear and likely multifactorial. Risk factors for pseudo-obstruction include male sex, age >60, trauma, orthopedic or cardiovascular surgery, and immobilization. Chemotherapy is another emerging risk factor for the development of colonic pseudo-obstruction [36, 37].

Clinical manifestations of this disorder include abdominal distension, obstipation/constipation, and nausea/vomiting. There are no pathognomonic laboratory studies to diagnose this condition although there is an established association with electrolyte abnormalities (e.g., hypokalemia, hypocalcemia, hypomagnesemia). In the setting of abdominal distension and leukocytosis, impending perforation should be ruled out. The etiology of the pseudo-obstruction should also be considered (e.g., sepsis). The most important ancillary study in making the diagnosis is imaging with a CT scan or hypaque enema to rule out a mechanical cause of colonic dilation. The distinction is important because it guides further management.

In the absence of abdominal tenderness or severe colonic distension on imaging, a trial of conservative management is appropriate. This treatment involves making the patient nil per os (NPO or nothing by mouth), using NG and rectal tube decompression, IV fluid support, and addressing any precipitants (e.g., minimizing narcotics, correcting electrolyte abnormalities). Surgical consultation is appropriate upon failure of these conservative measures to address the problem.

The use of pharmacologic agents has been described, with the most studied agent being neostigmine, an acetylcholinesterase inhibitor. The standard dose of this agent is 1.5–2 mg IV in the setting of continuous cardiac monitoring. Co-administration with glycopyrrolate is useful in mitigating the bradycardic and bronchspastic effects of neostigmine, but atropine should also be available at the bedside. The time to onset of action has been reported in the literature to be on the order of 3–10 min [36, 38]. Contraindications to the use of neostigmine in this population include mechanical obstruction, underlying bradyarrhythmia, recent myocardial infarction, and a relative contraindication of concurrent use of beta-blockers. Trials of neostigmine suggest a success rate of 80–100 % in achieving decompression, with recurrence as high as 30 %. It is reasonable to repeat neostigmine treatment if an interval greater than 24 h has elapsed from the initial treatment [38]. Erythromycin has also been described in case reports as sometimes being effective in this disorder.

Should pharmacologic decompression fail or be contraindicated, evaluation for endoscopic decompression is appropriate. Success rates for this procedure are in the order of 60–90 % [37]. Recurrence rates after successful decompression can be as high as 40 %. Complications of endoscopy include bleeding and perforation, which is estimated at 1–3 % [37]. More invasive management options should be discussed in the context of a surgical consult. These include percutaneous tube cecostomy and colostomy. Surgical resection/decompression is usually performed in the setting of a serious complication of pseudo-obstruction (e.g., perforation). See Fig. 5.3 for the management algorithm of acute colonic dilatation.

Diarrhea

Up to 50 % of critically ill patients develop diarrhea during their ICU stay. The Working Group on Abdominal Problems of the European Society of Intensive Care Medicine defines diarrhea as the passage of three or more loose or liquid stool with volume greater than 250 mL daily [39]. This clinical problem can have significant implications on hemodynamics and nutrition, so it is important to understand how to determine its etiology and devise an appropriate management plan. The etiology of diarrhea as a complication of ICU stay can be divided into infectious and non-infectious causes.

Infectious: *Clostridium difficile*

The infectious category, assuming baseline immunocompetence, most commonly involves *Clostridium difficile*. The incidence of *C. difficile* infection (CDI) in the ICU population ranges from 10 to 60 % [40]. Mortality of ICU-acquired CDI is high, approximately 60–70 % [40]. The pathophysiology of *C. difficile*-associated

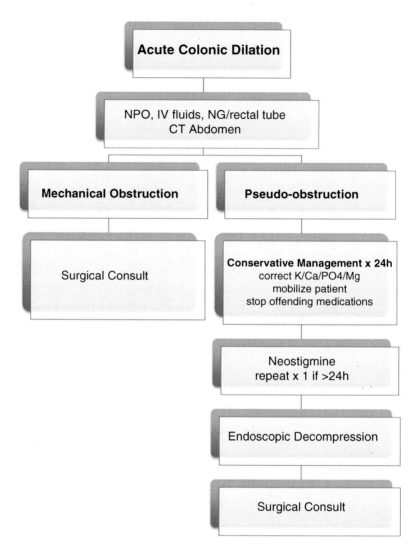

Fig. 5.3 Algorithm for management of acute colonic dilation. At any point if there is evidence of ischemia, perforation or peritonitis, a surgical consult should be requested. Adapted from Harrison ME, Anderson MA, Appalaneni V, et al. The role of endoscopy in the management of patients with known and suspected colonic obstruction and pseudo-obstruction. Gastrointest Endosc 2010; 71(4):669–79

diarrhea (CDAD) involves three major steps. The first includes alteration of normal gut flora, usually secondary to antibiotics. Although clindamycin, fluoroquinolones, and cephalosporins have been specifically implicated, any antibiotic can be associated with the development of CDI. Chemotherapeutic agents can also cause this alteration in gut flora. The next major step is acquisition of the microorganism. *C. difficile* is an anaerobic gram-positive bacillus. Outside the colon, the organism survives in a heat-, acid-, and antibiotic-resistant spore form. Once spores are in the colon, they convert into their virulent, toxin-producing form. Transmission of spores is fecal-oral and acquired in a healthcare setting through patient-to-patient transmission with healthcare workers as the vector. The final step in the pathway is clinical manifestation of disease. The symptoms of colitis and diarrhea are mediated by exotoxins released by the microbe. Both toxin A and B inactivate cell regulation pathways, activate a significant cytokine response, and disrupt intracellular tight junctions leading to increased vascular permeability and hemorrhage. Toxin A mediates inflammatory processes, but toxin B has been shown in studies to lend *C. difficile* its virulence [41].

Clinical manifestation of CDAD typically includes watery non-hemorrhagic diarrhea, accompanied by significant leukocytosis and fever. Abdominal distension and pain are also important clinical features and are often suggestive of complications such as fulminant colitis with megacolon or pre-perforation ischemic changes. The most common test used to diagnose CDI is an enzyme-linked immunosorbent assay (ELISA) for toxin A or both toxins A and B. The sensitivity of this test is estimated 65–85 %, with a specificity of more than 95 %. The traditional gold standard test is the tissue culture cytotoxic assay which measures toxin B and has a sensitivity of 80–90 % and a specificity of 99 %. This test requires tissue culture, is costly, and has a 24–48 h turnaround time which is why the ELISA test is used more commonly. A real-time polymerase chain reaction (PCR) study measuring both toxins A and B is also available in some hospitals, with sensitivity and specificity comparable to that of the cytotoxic assay [41]. If available, this is the diagnostic test of choice as it has comparable sensitivity and specificity but a rapid turnaround time of an hour. Sigmoidoscopy may also be considered to identify pseudomembranes and send tissue cultures if the diagnosis is unclear. Imaging studies are not required for diagnostic purposes, but they may used to monitor for signs of complications or progression. Computed tomography can be used to determine the extent of colonic involvement and rule out microperforations that may not be captured by plain abdominal radiographs.

The management of CDAD requires supportive care in the form of monitoring, IV fluid, and antimicrobial therapy. According to the most recent Infectious Disease Society of America guidelines, CDAD without signs of systemic toxicity can be managed with enteral or IV metronidazole, whereas severe CDAD should be managed with oral vancomycin [42]. Intravenous vancomycin has no role in the treatment of CDI, as it is not excreted into the colon. Patients exhibiting signs of toxic colitis warrant surgical consultation. Patients with megacolon or free air of any amount on imaging warrant surgical intervention. Note that a lower threshold for surgical consultation should be applied to immunocompromised patients as their clinical exam (e.g., for peritonitis) is often unreliable. Failure to respond to medical management is another indication for surgical intervention. The standard surgical procedure for serious complications of CDI is subtotal colectomy.

As one of the main pathophysiologic steps in developing CDI is altered gut flora secondary to antibiotic use, there is preliminary research suggesting there may be a role for probiotic use in the ICU, but results are not conclusive at this time.

Recurrence rates of CDI within 60 days after successful treatment with metronidazole or vancomycin are reported between 20 and 30 % [43]. Retreatment with metronidazole or vancomycin is sufficient in two-thirds of patients with recurrence. The remaining subset of patients poses a management dilemma. A randomized trial published in 2011 demonstrated lower rates of recurrence with fidaxomicin compared with vancomycin (15.4 versus 25.3 %, $p = 0.005$) in treatment of primary CDI [43]. Another recently published study compared vancomycin and duodenal fecal infusion in a RCT. This study suggests that duodenal infusion of healthy donor feces is significantly more effective in treating recurrent CDAD than vancomycin [44]. The presumed mechanism underlying the efficacy of fecal infusion is reestablishment of normal intestinal flora as a host defense against CDI [44].

Non-infectious: Enteral Feeding

The majority of patients receive enteral nutrition at some point in their ICU stay. The most common complication of enteral feeding is diarrhea, which occurs in up to 20 % of this population. The pathophysiology of diarrhea associated with enteral feedings is likely multifactorial. Altered gut motility, changes in intestinal flora, composition of feeds, and method of delivery are important factors in the development of diarrhea. A high caloric load in the stomach and proximal small bowel stimulates a gastrocolonic reflex that results in increased colonic contractility, whereas lower calorie loads have little to no impact on colonic contractility. The caloric load is likely an explanation for why continuous pump delivery to ensure a constant rate of feeding results in a decreased rate of diarrhea when compared to gravity delivery and intermittent/bolus feeds. Importantly, the location of nutrient delivery does not change the rates of diarrhea in the critically ill: gastric and post-pyloric feeding have a similar incidence. The composition of feeds has been implicated in the rates of feeding-associated diarrhea, with specific factors of feeding formula osmolarity, non-absorbable carbohydrates, and bacterial contamination all being implicated. The evidence to date suggests that isotonic or low osmolarity feedings enriched with fiber improve feeding tolerance, including decreasing rates of diarrhea. This effect is thought to be mediated by the release of short chain fatty acids (SCFAs) upon fermentation of fiber. These SCFAs are used by colonocytes as an energy source and therefore improve resorption of water and electrolytes by the colon. Water-soluble fibers have been shown to have greater potential trophic effects, likely secondary to the increased viscosity of feedings which therefore decreases transit time from stomach to colon.

The most important consideration when addressing enteral feeding associated diarrhea is ruling out other contributory causes. The presence of diarrhea alone should not prompt withholding of feedings, which results in further malnutrition and the potential for bacterial overgrowth in the dysmotile gut. It should be noted that hypoalbuminemia has also been associated with increased rates of diarrhea, but this has not been proven to be a causal effect. The use of pre- and probiotics for prevention of diarrhea is an area of ongoing study without any conclusive evidence to support their routine use at this time.

Non-infectious: Medications

The most easily modifiable cause of diarrhea in the ICU population is medication-related. The mechanism of diarrhea may be:

1. Osmotic—as seen with administration of medications containing sorbitol (e.g., liquid acetaminophen), laxatives (e.g., lactulose), and magnesium salts as used in antacids.
2. Secretory—stimulant laxatives, which increase intraluminal water and electrolytes by increasing secretion of decreasing reabsorption in the small and large bowel.
3. Exudative—mucosal disruption secondary to inflammation from chemotherapeutic agents.
4. Hypermotility—as seen with prokinetics such as erythromycin and metoclopramide.

Simple antibiotic-associated diarrhea is likely mediated by altered intestinal flora, leading to impaired fermentation of carbohydrates and therefore decreased production of SCFAs causing decreased fluid reabsorption by the colon. This type of antibiotic-associated diarrhea, unlike CDAD, usually resolves with withdrawal of the antibiotics.

Retroperitoneal-Based Complications

Spontaneous Retroperitoneal Bleeding

The literature discussing spontaneous retroperitoneal bleeding (SRB) is limited to observational studies and retrospective chart reviews. Of the larger studies, both published within the last 10 years, neither identifies the number of patients diagnosed with SRB as a complication of ICU stay, though 40–50 % of patients required ICU for management. The biggest risk factors for SRB were age greater than 60 and anticoagulation–antiplatelet combination therapy [45, 46]. Only 15 % of patients were not on any blood-thinning regimen. The problem with this diagnosis is its non-specific clinical presentation. In patients with the above risk factors, sudden hemodynamic shifts and complaints of abdominal or flank pain should prompt consideration of the diagnosis. Classically described flank ecchymosis is rare. Laboratory investigations should include CBC, coagulation profile, and crossmatch. Resuscitation with fluids and blood products should be carried out before CT imaging is performed. If the diagnosis is confirmed, further management is dictated by response to resuscitation measures. The majority of patients respond to supportive care with reversal of anticoagulation. In approximately 25 % of patients interventional radiology embolization or coiling of bleeding was carried out successfully. Surgery was required in less than 10 % of patients, and was either indicated because of failure of IR management or other complications requiring surgery including perforation or nerve compression symptoms [46].

Key Points

1. Intra-Abdominal Hypertension

   - Screen patients for IAH based on risk factors
   - Measure trans-bladder pressure using an institutionally standardized approach
   - Institute non-invasive and/or invasive measures to prevent progression of IAH to ACS, which is associated with high morbidity and mortality

2. Stress-Related Mucosal Disease

   - A preventable cause of ICU morbidity and mortality
   - Prophylaxis should be instituted for defined at-risk patients, ideally in the form of enteral PPIs
   - The risk of acid suppression causing nosocomial pneumonia is not well defined

3. Dysmotility and Feeding Intolerance

   - ICU patients are at risk for malnutrition and aspiration pneumonia secondary to GI dysmotility
   - Enteral feeding should be instituted as early as possible on ICU admission
   - GRVs of 250–500 mL should prompt assessment for possible dysmotility but should not automatically result in withholding of feeds
   - Post-pyloric feeding tubes should be used when feasible
   - Consider institution of parenteral nutrition after 7 days of inadequate enteral intake

4. GI Bleeding

   - Clinically important bleeding is a cause of increased morbidity, mortality and length of ICU stay
   - The initial pathway in managing any clinically significant bleeding includes resuscitation with IV fluids, blood products for correction of coagulopathy and targeting a hemoglobin above 7 g/dL
   - Adjuncts to initial resuscitation should be guided by suspected source: upper versus lower, non-variceal versus variceal

5. Diarrhea

   - Starting point is to rule out infectious etiology and discontinue potentially contributory medications
   - If *C. difficile* is diagnosed in the context of systemic toxicity, first line agent is vancomycin, with surgical consult if peritoneal findings or no clinical response within 24 h
   - Fidaxomicin is associated with reduced recurrence rates when used in the treatment of primary CDI
   - Low osmolarity feeds enriched with fiber are associated with decreased rates of diarrhea

References

1. Kirkpatrick A, Roberts DJ, De Waele J, et al. Intra-abdominal hypertension and the abdominal compartment syndrome: updated consensus definitions and clinical practice guidelines from the World Society of the Abdominal Compartment Syndrome. Intensive Care Med. 2013;39:1190.
2. Katsios C, Ye C, Hoad N, et al. Intra-abdominal hypertension in the critically ill: interrater reliability of bladder pressure measurement. J Crit Care. 2013;28(5):886.e1–6
3. Malbrain ML, Chiumello D, Pelosi P, et al. Prevalence of intra-abdominal hypertension in critically ill patients: a multicentre epidemiological study. Intensive Care Med. 2004;30(5):822.
4. Malbrain ML, Chiumello D, Pelosi P, et al. Incidence and prognosis of intraabdominal hypertension in a mixed population of critically ill patients: a multiple-center epidemiological study. Crit Care Med. 2005;33(2):315.
5. O'Mara MS, Slater H, Goldfarb IW, et al. A prospective, randomized evaluation of intra-abdominal pressures with crystalloid and colloid resuscitation in burn patients. J Trauma. 2005;58(5):1011.
6. De Waele J, Hoste E, Malbrain ML. Decompressive laparotomy for abdominal compartment syndrome – a critical analysis. Crit Care. 2006;10(2):R51.
7. Mularski RA, Sippel JM, Osborne ML. Pneumoperitoneum: a review of nonsurgical causes. Crit Care Med. 2000;28(7):2638.
8. Gayer G, Hertz M, Zissin R. Postoperative pneumoperitoneum: prevalence, duration, and possible significance. Semin Ultrasound CT MR. 2004;25(3):286.
9. Mulhall BP, Wong RK. Infectious esophagitis. Curr Treat Options Gastroenterol. 2003;6(1):55.
10. Mutlu GM, Mutlu EA, Factor P. GI complications in patients receiving mechanical ventilation. Chest. 2001;19(4):1222.
11. Osman D, Djibre M, Da Silva D, et al. Management by the intensivist of gastrointestinal bleeding in adults and children. Ann Intensive Care. 2012;2(1):46.
12. Nind G, Chen WH, Protheroe R, et al. Mechanisms of gastroesophageal reflux in critically ill mechanically ventilated patients. Gastroenterology. 2005;128(3):600–6.
13. Wang WH, Huang JQ, Zheng GF, et al. Head-to-head comparison of H2-receptor antagonists and proton pump inhibitors in the treatment of erosive esophagitis: a meta-analysis. World J Gastroenterol. 2005;11(26):4067.
14. Koek GH, Tack J, Sifrim D, et al. The role of acid and duodenal gastroesophageal reflux in symptomatic GERD. Am J Gastroenterol. 2001;96:2033.
15. Vaezi MF, Sears R, Richter JE. Placebo-controlled trial of cisapride in postgastrectomy patients with duodenogastroesophageal reflux. Dig Dis Sci. 1996;41(4):754–63.
16. Cook DJ, Fuller HD, Guyatt GH, et al. Risk factors for gastrointestinal bleeding in critically ill patients. N Engl J Med. 1994;330(6):377.
17. Cook DJ, Griffith LE, Walter SD, et al. The attributable mortality and length of intensive care unit stay of clinically important gastrointestinal bleeding in critically ill patients. Crit Care. 2001;5(6):368.
18. Stollman N, Metz DC. Pathophysiology and prophylaxis of stress ulcer in intensive care unit patients. J Crit Care. 2005;20(1):35–45.
19. ASHP therapeutic guidelines on stress ulcer prophylaxis. ASHP commission on therapeutics approved by the ASHP board of directors on November 14, 1998. Am J Health Syst Pharm. 1999;56(4):347.
20. Barkun AN, Bardou M, Pham CQ, et al. Proton pump inhibitors vs histamine 2 receptor antagonists for stress-related mucosal bleeding prophylaxis in critically ill patients: a meta-analysis. Am J Gastroenterol. 2012;107(4):507.
21. Janarthanan S, Ditah I, Adler DG, Ehrinpreis MN. Clostridium difficile-associated diarrhea and proton pump inhibitor therapy: a meta-analysis. Am J Gastroenterol. 2012;107(7):1001–10.
22. Kwok CS, Arthur AK, Anibueze DG, et al. Risk of Clostridium difficile infection with acid suppression agents and antibiotics: meta-analysis. Am J Gastroenterol. 2012;107(7):1011–9.

23. Oh JH, Pasricha PJ. Recent advances in the pathophysiology and treatment of gastroparesis. J Neurogastroenterol Motil. 2013;19(1):18.
24. Corke C. Gastric emptying in the critically ill patient. Crit Care Resucs. 1999;1:39.
25. Reignier J, Mercler E, Le Gouge A, et al. Effect of not monitoring residual gastric volume on risk of ventilator-associated pneumonia in adults receiving mechanical ventilation and early enteral feeding: a randomized controlled trial. JAMA. 2013;309(3):249–56.
26. Montejo JC, Minambres E, Bordeje L, et al. Gastric residual volume during enteral nutrition in ICU patients: the REGANE study. Intensive Care Med. 2010;36(8):1386–93.
27. Strategies to optimize deliver and minimize risks of enteral nutrition: small bowel feeding vs gastric. Canadian Clinica Practice Guidelines 2013
28. Casaer MP, Mesotten D, Hermans G, et al. Early versus late parenteral nutrition in critically ill adults. N Engl J Med. 2011;365(6):506.
29. Huffman JL, Schenker S. Acute acalculous cholecystitis: a review. Clin Gastroenterol Hepatol. 2010;8:15–22.
30. Horvatits T, Trauner M, Fuhrmann V. Hypoxic liver injury and cholestasis in critically ill patients. Curr Opin Crit Care. 2013;19:128–32.
31. Padda MS, Sanchez M, Akhtar AJ, et al. Drug induced cholestasis. Hepatology. 2011;53(4): 1377–87.
32. Jeejeebhoy KN. Management of parenteral nutrition-induced cholestasis. Pract Gastroenterol. 2005;24:62.
33. Villanueva C, Colomo A, Bosch A, et al. Transfusion strategies for acute upper gastrointestinal bleeding. N Engl J Med. 2013;368:11.
34. Syed MI, Shaikh A. Accurate localization of life threatening colonic hemorrhage during nuclear medicine bleeding scan as an aid to selective angiography. World J Emerg Surg. 2009;4:20.
35. Rosenblum JD, Boyle CM, Schwartz LB. The mesenteric circulation. Anatomy and physiology. Surg Clin North Am. 1997;77(2):289.
36. Eisen GM, Baron TH, Dominitz JA, et al. Acute colonic pseudo-obstruction. Gastrointest Endosc. 2002;56(6):789–92.
37. Harrison ME, Anderson MA, Appalaneni V, et al. The role of endoscopy in the management of patients with known and suspected colonic obstruction and pseudo-obstruction. Gastrointest Endosc. 2010;71(4):669–79.
38. Ponec RJ, Saunders MD, Kimmey MB. Neostigmine for the treatment of acute colonic pseudo-obstruction. N Engl J Med. 1999;341(3):137.
39. Blaser AR, Malbrain ML, Starkopf J, et al. Gastrointestinal function in intensive care patients: terminology, definitions and management. Recommendations of the ESICM working group on abdominal problems. Intensive Care Med. 2012;38:384.
40. Wiesena P, Van Gossumb A, Preisera JC. Diarrhea in the critically ill. Curr Opin Crit Care. 2006;12:149–54.
41. Kuehne SA, Cartman ST, Heap JT, et al. The role of toxin A and toxin B in Clostridium difficile infection. Nature. 2010;467(7136):711.
42. Cohen SH, Gerding DN, Johnson S, et al. Clinical practice guidelines for Clostridium difficile infection in adults: 2010 update by the Society for Healthcare Epidemiology of America (SHEA) and the Infectious Diseases Society of America (IDSA). Infect Control Hop Epidemiol. 2010;31(5):431–55.
43. Louie TJ, Miller MA, Mullane KM, et al. Fidaxomicin versus vancomycin for Clostridium difficile infection. N Engl J Med. 2011;364(5):423.
44. Van Nood E, Vrieze A, Nieuwdorp M, et al. Duodenal infusion of donor feces for recurrent Clostridium difficile. N Engl J Med. 2013;368(5):407.
45. Ivascu FA, Janczyk RJ, Bair HA, et al. Spontaneous retroperitoneal hemorrhage. Am J Surg. 2005;189(3):345.
46. Sunga KL, Bellolio MF, Gilmore RM, et al. Spontaneous retroperitoneal hematoma: etiology, characteristics, management and outcome. J Emerg Med. 2012;43(2):157–61.

Chapter 6
Non-pulmonary Infectious Complications

Pamela Paufler and Robert Kempainen

Abstract Critically ill patients are especially vulnerable to healthcare-associated infections and these infections substantially increase the expense, morbidity, and possibly mortality associated with critical care. This chapter focuses on the epidemiology, pathophysiology, diagnosis, and treatment of catheter-associated urinary tract infections, catheter-related bloodstream infections, *Clostridium difficile* colitis, nosocomial sinusitis, and acalculous cholecystitis. Medical literature has convincingly demonstrated the ability to markedly reduce the risk of nosocomial infections, and accordingly, rates of infection now play a central role in measuring the quality of care. This chapter also highlights interventions that have, and have not, proven effective in reducing nosocomial infections.

Keywords Health care associated infections • Catheter associated urinary tract infections • Catheter related bloodstream infections • Central line associated bloodstream infections • *Clostridium difficile* • Acalculous cholecystitis • Nosocomial sinusitis

P. Paufler, M.D. (✉)
Division of Pulmonary and Critical Care Medicine, Hennepin County Medical Center, 701 Park Avenue, Minneapolis, MN 55415, USA
e-mail: pamela.paufler@gmail.com

R. Kempainen, M.D.
Division of Pulmonary and Critical Care Medicine, Hennepin County Medical Center, University of Minnesota School of Medicine, 701 Park Avenue, Mail Code G5, Minneapolis, MN 55415-1829, USA
e-mail: kempa001@umn.edu

J.B. Richards and R.D. Stapleton (eds.), *Non-Pulmonary Complications of Critical Care:*   135
A Clinical Guide, Respiratory Medicine, DOI 10.1007/978-1-4939-0873-8_6,
© Springer Science+Business Media New York 2014

Introduction

The combination of baseline comorbidities, acute organ failure, prolonged hospital-ization, and need for indwelling catheters make critically ill patients especially vul-nerable to healthcare-associated infections and, in particular, infections caused by multidrug-resistant organisms. The evaluation for, and treatment of, nosocomial infections substantially increases the expense, morbidity, and possibly mortality associated with critical care. This chapter focuses on the epidemiology, pathophysi-ology, diagnosis, and treatment of catheter-associated urinary tract infections (CAUTIs), catheter-related bloodstream infections, *Clostridium difficile* colitis, nosocomial sinusitis, and acalculous cholecystitis. Medical literature has convinc-ingly demonstrated the ability to markedly reduce the risk of nosocomial infections, and accordingly, rates of infection now play a central role in measuring the quality of care. This chapter also highlights interventions that have, and have not, proven effective in reducing nosocomial infections.

Catheter-Associated Urinary Tract Infections

Epidemiology

Urinary tract infection is one of the most common nosocomial infections in the intensive care unit (ICU) and is largely secondary to widespread use of urinary catheters. Cather-associated urinary tract infection (CAUTI) is associated with fre-quent antimicrobial use, may contribute to rising antimicrobial resistance, and serves as a reservoir of multidrug-resistant pathogens. The definition of CAUTI has evolved over time and is now distinct from asymptomatic bacteriuria (ASB). CAUTI currently is defined as the presence of compatible signs or symptoms and $\geq 10^3$ colony forming units (cfu)/mL of ≥ 1 bacterial species from a single culture in the absence of another source. In contrast, ASB is defined as a urine culture with $\geq 10^5$ cfu/mL of uropathogenic bacteria in the absence of symptoms [1]. Historically, both ASB and symptomatic urinary tract infection were reported as CAUTI. However, the National Healthcare Safety Network (NHSN) changed the definition in 2009 such that patients with ASB are no longer considered to have CAUTI [2]. In this review every attempt has been made to be consistent with the new definition such that an episode of CAUTI represents only symptomatic infection.

Burton et al. reported a significant decline in rate of CAUTI from 1990 to 2007 with an estimated decline of between 19 and 67 % depending on the ICU type. This decline may be a result of improvements in aseptic techniques and adherence to general infection control principles. Although encouraging, CAUTI rates still occurred at a rate of 2–3 per 1,000 catheter days [3]. Each episode of CAUTI adds $600 to the hospital stay but if secondary bacteremia occurs, then the additional cost is $2,800 [1, 4]. Only 1–4 % of urinary tract infections progress to bloodstream infections but these bear an estimated 13 % mortality [1].

Pathophysiology

The urinary system has multiple innate defenses against invading pathogens. Although more effective in men, the length of the urethra provides a physical barrier. The urinary tract mucosa secretes inhibitors that prevent bacterial adhesion and micturition washes bacteria out. In addition, osmolality, pH, and the presence of organic acids prevent growth of microorganisms. The urinary catheter not only disrupts these innate defense mechanisms but also prevents complete drainage of the bladder and forms a nidus for biofilm formation [5].

Biofilms, heterogeneous compositions of bacterial cells and extracellular matrix, form on both the intraluminal and extraluminal surfaces of the urinary catheter. Antimicrobials tend to penetrate the biofilm poorly and organisms grow more slowly within the biofilm, making them more resistant to antibiotics that work by attacking cell growth. Some common urinary pathogens such as *Proteus* are able to hydrolyze urea which leads to precipitation of minerals within the biofilm and can cause catheter obstruction [1, 6].

Bacteruria is the precursor to infection and develops at a rate of 3–8 % per day of catheterization [1]. Most commonly, endogenous bacteria from the perineum or rectal area ascend through the biofilm on the extraluminal surface of the urinary catheter. Alternatively, a break or failure of a closed drainage system or contamination of the drainage bag allows exogenous, often multidrug-resistant bacteria to ascend on the intraluminal surface. Bacteria may also be inoculated into the bladder at the time of catheter insertion. Hematogenous spread with secondary seeding of the urinary catheter is also reported [7].

Consistent with the above mechanisms, *Escherichia coli* and other *Enterobacteriaceae* are the most often isolated [1, 5]. In the ICU, *Enterococcus* species, *Candida* species, and *Pseudomonas aeruginosa* are also common. Also of importance, *Staphylococcus aureus* is a rare cause of urinary infection but is more likely to be associated with bacteremia [8].

Risk Factors

The most important risk for urinary tract infection is the urinary catheter. Specific risks related to the catheter include duration of catheterization, errors in catheter care, and bacterial colonization of the drainage bag [5]. In the latest NHSN report, both medical and surgical teaching hospitals reported higher rates of infection than their non-teaching counterparts [9]. This suggests that admission to a teaching hospital also places a patient at higher risk. Whether this is due to errors in catheter care of patients is unknown.

Specific patient populations also have higher risk. Due to anatomic differences, females are more prone to urinary infection. Older age, diabetes mellitus, severity of illness, and creatinine >2 are all potential risk factors [5]. In addition, the highest reported rates of 4.1 and 4.5 per 1,000 catheter days for burn and neurosurgical critical care units, respectively, suggests that these populations are at particularly high risk [9].

Risks for secondary bloodstream infection are less well known. In a study comparing 298 cases of CAUTI with secondary bacteremia against 667 cases of CAUTI without secondary bacteremia, Greene et al. reported neutropenia, renal disease, and male sex as risk factors for secondary bacteremia. Also of interest, the percentage of *Enterococcus* species and coagulase-positive *Staphylococcus* were also statistically higher in patients with secondary bacteremia [10].

Clinical Presentation

Signs and symptoms are defined broadly and include new onset or worsening fever, rigors, altered mental status, malaise, or lethargy. A patient may report flank pain, costovertebral angle tenderness, acute hematuria, and pelvic discomfort. If the catheter has been removed, the traditional urinary tract symptoms of dysuria, urgency, frequency, or suprapubic pain may be present. Patients with spinal cord injury may experience increased spasticity, autonomic dysreflexia, or a sense of unease [1].

Urinalysis is widely used as a screening tool. Of the individual components of a urinalysis, nitrite is the most specific indicator of infection [11]. Pyuria is not a reliable indicator as up to 30 % of patients with pyuria do not have bacteriuria. Gram-negative pathogens are more often associated with pyuria as compared to gram-positive pathogens or yeasts [1, 8]. In one study, the sensitivity, specificity, positive predictive value, and negative predictive value of the urinalysis were 100, 65.1, 15.5, and 100 %, respectively [12]. This suggests that the urinalysis is an excellent screening tool and, if negative, infection is highly unlikely.

Diagnosis

As stated above, a diagnosis of CAUTI is made by urine culture with $\geq 10^3$ cfu/mL of ≥ 1 bacterial species in the presence of compatible signs or symptoms and in the absence of another source. However, in the ICU, patients are often unable to report their symptoms, which can obscure the diagnosis. A patient may have ASB and a fever from another source making it difficult to distinguish between ASB and CAUTI. Pyuria is not diagnostic of ASB or CAUTI, should not be used to differentiate between the two, and should not be used as an indication for antimicrobial treatment. Likewise, the presence of cloudy or malodorous urine should not be used to differentiate between ASB and CAUTI, nor as an indication to obtain a urine culture or start antimicrobial therapy [1].

Differentiating infection from colonization with *Candida* is a commonly encountered challenge in the ICU. Although most often a contaminant or colonization, candiduria may be a potential marker for invasive candidiasis. Colony counts are not helpful in distinguishing between colonization and infection. The first step is to replace the catheter and then obtain a new sample. If the candiduria resolves, then no further work-up is needed. Microscopy may be able to distinguish *Candida glabrata* from other Candida species. Although rarely seen, casts are indicative of upper tract infection. In a symptomatic patient in the ICU, ultrasound is the preferred initial imaging study and may show focal lesions consistent with pyelonephritis. However, if ultrasound is negative yet suspicion remains high, computed tomography is more definitive for Candida-related pyelonephritis and perinephric abscess [13].

Treatment

Although in the literature ASB and CAUTI are sometimes used interchangeably, as noted above, these two entities are clinically distinct and should be treated differently. With few exceptions, no treatment is recommended for ASB. Treatment of ASB can lower the risk of pyelonephritis in pregnancy and is also recommended for patients undergoing invasive genitourinary procedures. Treatment should also be considered for patients with diabetes mellitus, severe immunosuppression, or recent renal transplant as these patients are at higher risk of developing bloodstream infection. Bacteriuria may persist after removal of the urinary catheter and it is reasonable to screen patients 48 h after catheter removal and then treat if bacteriuria is present [1].

Empiric treatment for CAUTI should be based on the patient's prior history as well as the local prevalence of pathogens and antibiotic resistance. Treatment can be narrowed as results of the urine culture and sensitivity data become available. If a catheter has been in place for >2 weeks (with some authors suggesting >1 week), then the catheter should be removed or, if unable to be removed, it should be replaced. If there is prompt resolution of symptoms with treatment, the Infectious Diseases Society of America (IDSA) recommends a 7 day course of antimicrobials. If there is a delayed response to treatment, the IDSA recommends 10–14 days even if the catheter remains. In a patient who is not severely ill, 5 days of levofloxacin may be sufficient. For women ≤65 years without upper urinary symptoms and in whom the catheter has been removed, duration of 3 days may suffice [1].

Prevention

Multiple authors suggest that urinary catheters are used without appropriate indications and duration of placement is commonly excessive. In one study, only half of the catheters placed in the emergency department had a physician documented order, and of those, only half had an appropriate indication [14]. Results of a survey at four university hospitals suggested that physicians were unaware that their patients had urinary catheters more than 25 % of the time. More striking, if the catheter was deemed inappropriate, physicians were even less aware of the catheter [15]. It follows that, the most effective method of prevention is to restrict use to patients with clear indications and remove the catheter when no longer needed.

Appropriate indications of urinary catheters include the need for close monitoring of urine output in critically ill patients, urinary retention or obstruction, during selected surgical procedures, when incontinence adversely affects adjacent wounds, and comfort at the end of life. Though often cited as a reason, placement of a catheter to manage incontinence alone is not considered appropriate [1, 8]. As catheters are often placed in the emergency department or operating room, education on appropriate use that targets these areas may be helpful. Other proposed strategies to limit catheter use include considering alternatives such as condom catheters or intermittent catheterization, having a protocol or checklist for removal, and empowering the nursing team to lead the prevention effort.

Prevention efforts specific to the catheter include using an aseptic technique for insertion, having a closed drainage system, limiting disconnection of the catheter junction, and using appropriate care after insertion. Maintenance of the collecting bag and tubing below the level of the bladder prevents reflux of potentially contaminated urine into the bladder. The IDSA does not recommend bladder irrigation, instillation of antiseptic or antimicrobial agents to the collecting bag, the use of antimicrobial catheters, or routine exchange [1]. General strategies are also important. Colonized patients may serve as a reservoir for multidrug-resistant organisms. Therefore, reducing the use of broad spectrum antimicrobials may reduce the selective pressure for pathogenic organisms. Most outbreaks of urinary pathogens are linked to inadequate hand hygiene [7]. For this reason, and central to all infection prevention efforts, hand hygiene is essential.

Summary of Key Points

- Urinary tract infection is one of the most common nosocomial infections in the ICU and is largely secondary to widespread use of urinary catheters.
- ASB and CAUTI are clinically distinct. With few exceptions, no treatment is recommended for ASB.
- The most effective method of prevention is to restrict catheter use to patients with clear indications and remove the catheter when no longer needed.

Catheter-Related Blood Stream Infections

Epidemiology

Maintaining good vascular access is essential in an ICU. Although rates vary by type of device, any vascular access is a potential source of infection. A systematic review of 200 studies by Maki and colleagues found rates of 0.5 infections per 1,000 device days for peripheral plastic catheters, 1.7 for arterial catheters, 2.7 for non-cuffed non-medicated non-tunneled central venous catheters (CVCs), and 4.8 for temporary non-cuffed hemodialysis catheters [16]. With greater than 150 million intravascular devices used each year in the United States, even these small rates of infection are significant.

With excellent stewardship and bundled prevention practices, the incidence of central line infections is decreasing. The NHSN reports published in 2009 and 2013 show a drop in the pooled average central line-associated bloodstream infection (CLABSI) rate for major medical teaching hospitals from 2.6 to 1.2 per 1,000 central line days [2, 9]. Catheter-related bloodstream infections (CRBSIs) are not necessarily an independent cause of increased mortality but even a single case of CRBSI can cost $45,000 and increase duration of hospitalization by >1 week [17, 18].

Of note, though often used interchangeably, the terms CRBSI and CLABSI are distinct. Intended for use when diagnosing and treating patients, CRBSI requires laboratory testing that identifies the catheter as the source of the bloodstream infection. Often used for surveillance, CLABSI is a primary bloodstream infection in a patient with a central line not related to an infection at another site. The simpler definition of CLABSI may overestimate the true incidence of CRBSI.

Pathophysiology

Catheter colonization is not simply individual bacteria on the catheter surface but a rather more complex process of biofilm formation. Biofilms are nearly universally present on CVCs within 3 days of insertion [6]. Colonization and biofilm formation starts from four recognized sources. Most commonly, bacteria on the skin, either at the time of insertion or from later migration along the outer surface of the catheter, colonize the catheter tip. Alternatively, bacteria either from the hands of healthcare workers or again from the skin of the patient are seeded into the catheter hub and then migrate along the intraluminal catheter surface. Less commonly, hematologic spread from other foci of infection may result in catheter colonization. Most rare, infusate contamination can lead to colonization of the catheter and to bloodstream infection [17].

Biofilms are heterogeneous compositions of bacterial cells and extracellular matrix and differ profoundly from their free floating counterparts. Of importance to the medical community, bacteria within biofilms are more resistant to antibiotics and to host clearance. For example, the minimum inhibitory concentration (MIC) for bacteria within biofilms is reported to be 10–1000 times higher than for detached bacteria [6]. Consistent with the mechanism of colonization, the most commonly isolated bacteria are those often found on the skin and those ubiquitous in a hospital environment. The most prevalent bacteria associated with CVCs are coagulase-negative *Staphylococci* followed by *S. aureus*, *Candida* species and enteric gram-negative bacilli. For surgically implanted catheters and peripherally inserted central venous catheters (PICCs), coagulase-negative *Staphylococci*, enteric gram-negative bacilli, *S. aureus*, and *P. aeruginosa* are most common [19].

Some patient populations may be more susceptible to specific pathogens. Among burn patients, *S. aureus*, *Enterococcus* species, *Pseudomonas* aeruginosa, *E. coli*, coagulase-negative *Staphylococci*, and *Candida* species are all common [20]. *E. coli* and other enteric gram negative bacilli predominate in patients with malignancies, possibly related to greater susceptibility to translocation of gut bacteria [21]. Fungal infections are a concern in patients receiving total parenteral nutrition.

Risk Factors

Risk factors for infection are related to the site, the catheter, and the host. The density of the skin flora is a major risk for infection. Femoral catheters, which are presumably exposed to the perineal flora, have consistently higher rates of infection as opposed to subclavian or internal jugular catheters. This effect may be accentuated in obese patients. Similarly, a higher rate of infection is seen with internal jugular catheters that are closer to the oral flora as opposed to subclavian catheters. However, the risk of infectious complications must be weighed against the risk of mechanical complications when choosing the catheter site [17].

As mentioned above, the rate of infection varies by catheter type. Traditionally, PICCs have been thought to have a lower rate of infection than CVCs. Maki et al. reported the rate of infection to be 1.0 and 2.1 per 1,000 catheter days for inpatient and outpatient PICCs, respectively [16]. In accordance, a recent meta-analysis by Chopra et al. reported a lower relative risk for CRBSI with PICCs as opposed to CVCs (relative risk [RR], 0.62; 95 % confidence interval [CI], 0.40–0.94). However, the difference was less pronounced among hospitalized patients (RR [95 % CI], 0.73 [0.54–0.98]) [22]. Other catheter-related factors associated with higher risk include use for total parental nutrition (TPN) or dialysis, increased manipulation, longer duration of use, and some types of needleless access.

Immune deficiency, presumably due to loss of natural defenses, predisposes a patient to a higher risk of infection. Patients with malignancies are at risk not only from a depressed immune status but also due to treatments that destroy protective flora. A prior history of bloodstream infection, extremes of age, skin breakdown from burns or wounds, and septic foci elsewhere are other host factors associated with increased risk.

Clinical Presentation

In the ICU, persistent fever often raises suspicion for line infection. However, a multitude of etiologies lead to fever and though a fever may be a sensitive marker for line infection, it is not specific. Additional non-specific signs and symptoms of CRBSI include hemodynamic instability, encephalopathy, catheter malfunction, and clinical improvement with line removal. In contrast, inflammation or purulence around the insertion site is more specific but is often absent in catheter infections. In the absence of another source of infection, positive blood cultures with *S. aureus*, coagulase-negative staphylococci, or *Candida* species raise the possibility of CRBSI [17].

Diagnosis

The IDSA guidelines recommend only performing catheter cultures when the catheter is removed for suspected bloodstream infection. Definitive diagnosis of CRBSI requires 1 of the following [19]:

(1) Growth of the same organism from both a percutaneous blood culture and the catheter tip.
(2) Two blood cultures, 1 from a percutaneous site and 1 from the catheter, that meet the criteria for quantitative blood cultures or differential time to positivity.
(3) Two cultures from different catheter lumens that demonstrate a three-fold colony count difference.

To avoid contamination and false positives, the IDSA recommends skin preparation with alcohol, alcoholic chlorhexidine, or tincture of iodine rather than povidone–iodine. Of note, blood samples obtained through catheters have a higher false-positive rate compared to percutaneous blood samples, likely due to catheter colonization. Negative cultures obtained from either catheters or obtained percutaneously have high negative predictive values and reliably rule out bloodstream infection [19].

Treatment

A full review of treatment of CRBSI is beyond the scope of this chapter, and the reader is referred to the IDSA guidelines for more complete recommendations about antimicrobial coverage [19]. Often it is necessary to start antimicrobials empirically and this should be based on local prevalence and susceptibility data. Vancomycin is a reasonable choice for settings with a high prevalence of methicillin-resistant *S. aureus* (MRSA) but daptomycin should be used if the MIC for vancomycin is >2 μg/mL. Fourth-generation cephalosporins, carbapenems, and B-lactam/B-lactamase combinations are reasonable choices for empiric gram-negative coverage. For infections involving femoral catheters, empiric coverage should include gram-positive, gram-negative, and possibly *Candida* species [19].

Double empiric coverage for gram-negative organisms should be used in neutropenic patients, those with severe sepsis, and also patients known to be colonized with a multidrug-resistant organisms, until susceptibility data are available. Empiric coverage of *Candida* species with an echinocandin is recommended in septic patients with any of the following risk factors: TPN, prolonged use of broad-spectrum antibiotics, hematologic malignancy, bone marrow or solid organ transplant, or colonization with *Candida* at multiple sites. Fluconazole is an acceptable alternative in select patients at low risk of infection with *C. krusei* and *C. glabrata* [19].

Duration of therapy is dependent on the severity of illness, organism, the catheter type, and whether or not the catheter can be removed. In general, removal of the catheter is recommended. Therapy should be continued for the recommended duration after the first negative culture [19].

Prevention

Effective strategies that are bundled together and novel technologies that directly target the pathogenesis of infection promise to reduce infection rates further. This section briefly discusses a few prevention strategies and some of the supporting studies. Table 6.1 provides a partial adaptation of IDSA guideline recommendations with a focus on central line infections. For a more complete discussion and list of recommendations, the reader is referred to the guidelines [17].

The cornerstones of prevention are education and training of healthcare personnel, as well as providing the necessary time and tools. Understanding and being able to weigh the risk of infection against the risk of mechanical complications are essential in choosing an appropriate site. In the hands of an experienced operator, placing lines with ultrasound guidance has been shown to reduce mechanical complications. Creating a line cart with all the necessary supplies increases compliance with recommended insertion practices. Lower patient-to-nurse ratios allow time for catheter care and are associated with reduced CRBSI [17].

The use of aseptic techniques inclusive of maximum sterile barrier precautions consistently lowers infection rates. Maximum sterile barrier precautions include the use of a cap, mask, sterile gown, sterile gloves, and a sterile full body drape. Berenholtz et al. demonstrated that a group of five interventions aimed at promoting adherence to aseptic techniques decreased infection rate in a single ICU from 11.3 to 0 per 1,000 catheter days. The five interventions included educating the staff, creating a catheter insertion cart, assessing catheter need daily, implementing a checklist to ensure adherence to evidence-based aseptic guidelines, and empowering nurses to stop the catheter insertion procedure if a violation was observed [23]. In a landmark study by Pronovost et al., bundled use of evidence-based interventions yielded a decline in the average rate of catheter infection from 7.7 at baseline to 1.4 per 1,000 catheter days at 16–18 months across 103 ICUs in Michigan. Hand washing, using full sterile barrier precautions during the insertion, cleaning the skin with chlorhexidine, avoiding the femoral site if possible, and removing unnecessary catheters as soon as possible were all included in the bundle. Strategies to increase use of and adherence to the bundle encompassed the same five interventions used in the prior study by Berenholtz et al. [24]. Based on these studies, the current guidelines for infection prevention recommend implementation of a comprehensive strategy that includes all three of the following: educating persons who insert and maintain

Table 6.1 Prevention of catheter-related bloodstream infections

General recommendations	Strength of evidence
Educate healthcare personnel regarding indications for use, proper insertion technique, and maintenance of intravascular devices	IA
Ensure appropriate nursing staff levels in ICUs	IB
Weigh the risks and benefits of placing a central venous device at a recommended site to reduce infectious complications against the risk for mechanical complications	IA
Avoid using the femoral vein for central access	IA
Use a subclavian site, rather than a jugular or a femoral site to minimize infection risk	IB
Avoid subclavian site for dialysis catheter due to the risk of stenosis	IA
Use ultrasound guidance to place CVCs to reduce the number of cannulation attempts and mechanical complications	IB
Promptly remove any intravascular catheter that is no longer essential	IA
Aseptic techniques and hygiene	
Maintain aseptic techniques for the insertion and care of intravascular catheters. When adherence to aseptic techniques cannot be ensured (during an emergency), replace the catheter within 48 h	IB
Hand hygiene should be performed before and after palpating catheter insertion sites as well as before and after inserting, replacing, accessing, repairing, or dressing an intravascular catheter	IB
Use maximal sterile barrier precautions, including the use of a cap, mask, sterile gown, sterile gloves, and a sterile full body drape, for the insertion of CVCs, PICCs, or guidewire exchange	IB
Prepare clean skin with a >0.5 % chlorhexidine preparation with alcohol before CVC and peripheral arterial catheter insertion and during dressing changes. When chlorhexidine is contraindicated, tincture of iodine—an iodophor—or 70 % alcohol are acceptable alternatives	IA
Change the dressing of CVC insertion site at least weekly	IB
If CLABSI rate is not decreasing despite education, chlorhexidine skin preparation, and maximal sterile barrier precautions, then	
Use a chlorhexidine-impregnated sponge dressing for temporary short-term catheters	IB
Use a 2 % chlorhexidine wash for daily skin cleansing	II
Use chlorhexidine/silver sulfadiazine or minocycline/rifampin-impregnated CVC in patients when the catheter is expected to remain in place >5 days	IA
Not recommended	
Do not use topical antibiotic ointments or creams on insertion sites, except for dialysis catheters, because of their potential to promote fungal infections and antimicrobial resistance	IB
Do not administer systemic antimicrobial prophylaxis routinely before insertion or during use of an intravascular catheter to prevent catheter colonization or CRBSI	IB
Do not routinely replace CVCs, PICCs, hemodialysis catheters, or pulmonary artery catheters	IB
Do not remove CVCs or PICCs on the basis of fever alone	II
Do not use guidewire exchanges to replace a non-tunneled catheter suspected of infection	IB

Category IA: Strongly recommended for implementation and strongly supported by well-designed experimental, clinical, or epidemiologic studies; *Category IB*: Strongly recommended for implementation and supported by some experimental, clinical, or epidemiologic studies and a strong theoretical rationale; or an accepted practice supported by limited evidence; *Category IC*: Required by state or federal regulations, rules, or standards; *Category II*: Suggested for implementation and supported by suggestive clinical or epidemiologic studies or a theoretical rationale catheters, use of maximal sterile barrier precautions, and a >0.5 % chlorhexidine preparation with alcohol for skin antisepsis during CVC insertion [17].

If, despite a comprehensive prevention strategy, the CRBSI rate remains unacceptably high, then the guidelines recommend consideration of chlorhexidine-impregnated sponge dressings, daily skin cleansing with chlorhexidine, and antimicrobial/antiseptic catheters [17]. In a large randomized controlled trial, Timsit et al. found that a chlorhexidine gluconate-impregnated sponge dressing decreased the incidence of CRBSI from 1.3 to 0.4 per 1,000 catheter days. Of note, several cases of contact dermatitis were reported in the study [25]. This trial suggests that chlorhexidine impregnated sponges may reduce the rate of infection even when it is already low. At Cook County Hospital, Bleasedale et al. showed that bathing with 2 % chlorhexidine gluconate-impregnated washcloths as compared to soap and water reduced the rate of primary bloodstream infections from 10.4 to 4.1 per 1,000 patient days [26]. Both of these interventions add relatively little cost and are easy to implement.

More expensive catheters coated with chlorhexidine silver sulfadiazine (CSS) or minocycline rifampin (MR) also reduce the rates of catheter-related infections. Though theoretical concern about resistance exists, studies thus far suggest that the risk is low. The guidelines recommend the use of these catheters when the CRBSI rate remains above the goal based on national benchmark rates, for patients with limited venous access and a history of CRBSI, and for patients at high risk for severe sequelae such as patients with recently implanted intravascular devices [17].

A number of other interventions have proven to be ineffective in reducing the risk of CRBSI. The use of systemic antibiotics immediately prior to or during line placement, the use of antiseptic/antibiotic ointments in non-dialysis CVCs, and removal of a CVC on the basis of fever alone are not recommended. Scheduled catheter changes are also not recommended. CRBSI is associated with duration of catheter use and several studies have attempted to prevent line infections by scheduled replacement. Cobb et al. performed a randomized controlled trial of scheduled replacement of CVCs. The trial consisted of 4 arms: replacement every 3 days at a new site, replacement every 3 days over a guidewire, replacement when clinically indicated at a new site, and replacement when clinically indicated over a guidewire. In this study there was no difference in the rate of infection with scheduled replacement. Replacing catheters over a guidewire resulted in a higher rate of infection but a lower rate of mechanical complications [27]. Eyer et al. conducted a randomized trial of replacement every 7 days at a new site, no weekly change, and guidewire exchange every 7 days. In concordance, this trial showed no difference in infectious risk between the three groups [28]. At this time, scheduled replacement is not recommended. If infection is suspected, then placement of a catheter at a new site is recommended [17].

To reduce the risk of needlestick injuries, the use of needleless connectors has been implemented widely in clinical practice. Like catheters, multiple types of needleless connectors are available and are associated with varied infection rates. Multiple reports suggest lower rates of infection with the split septum devices as compared to those with mechanical valves. The new prevention guidelines state a preference for split septum devices [17].

Clearly, a multitude of options that decrease the incidence of CRBSI exist. Providers must balance the available resources against the potential risk for CRBSI in their ICU.

Summary of Key Points

- Catheter-related bloodstream infections are associated with increased cost and longer hospital stays.
- Rates of infection vary by site, catheter-related factors such as device type and use, as well as by host-related factors including immune deficiency, malignancy, extremes of age, and wounds.
- The current guidelines for infection prevention recommend implementation of a comprehensive strategy including educating persons who insert and maintain catheters, use of maximal sterile barrier precautions, and a >0.5 % chlorhexidine preparation during CVC insertion.
- If the rate of line infection remains unacceptably high after implementation of a comprehensive strategy, consider chlorhexidine impregnated sponge dressings, chlorhexidine baths, and antimicrobial/antiseptic impregnated catheters.
- Empiric antimicrobial coverage should take into consideration the severity of illness as well as local prevalence and susceptibility data.

Clostridium difficile Colitis

Epidemiology

C. difficile is the leading cause of nosocomial infectious diarrhea. Not only is the incidence of *C. difficile* infection rising, but infections have also become more severe and refractory to therapy. Given their severe underlying disease and high likelihood of treatment with antimicrobials, critically ill patients are at particular risk of acquiring infection during their ICU stay. *C. difficile* infection adds to both the mortality and the cost of hospitalization. Mortality is estimated at 6 %, but can be as high as 17 % in outbreaks and 38 % in severe complicated disease [29, 30]. The estimated additional cost of *C. difficile* infection in the ICU is approximately $5,000 [29].

Pathophysiology

C. difficile is a gram-positive, anaerobic, spore-forming, toxin-producing bacillus. Transmission is via the fecal-oral route. The most widely accepted mechanism of infection is that antibiotics destroy the normal colonic flora, thereby opening a niche for *C. difficile*. Although rare, antibiotic-associated diarrhea is also attributed to other pathogens such as *S. aureus*, *Klebsiella oxytoca*, and *Clostridium perfringes* [29]. Inside the colon, the *C. difficile* spore germinates into its vegetative toxin-producing form. Two exotoxins, toxin A (enterotoxin) and toxin B (cytotoxin), incite the body's inflammatory response. In addition, the toxins interfere with intracellular regulation and signal transduction, thereby leading to apoptosis of the enterocytes and ulceration of the bowel wall. The body's response to the ulcers is to flood the area with proteins, mucus, and inflammatory cells, thus forming pseudomembranes. The resulting inflammation of the bowel wall causes albumin and other proteins to leak into the lumen. The loss of protein in combination with the inflammation results in profuse watery diarrhea.

External to the body, *C. difficile* exists as a heat-, acid-, alcohol-, and antibiotic-resistant spore. *C. difficile* can be cultured from nearly any surface in a room of an infected patient as well as from the hands, clothing, and stethoscopes of healthcare workers. Of note, the risk of contamination when entering the room of an infected patient is independent of whether or not the provider has direct patient contact [29]. Flushing the toilet of an infected patient can aerosolize *C. difficile* spores. Recurrent disease is felt to be from either persistent germination of spores within the colon or failure to re-establish normal colonic microflora, thereby resulting in secondary re-infection.

The majority of *C. difficile* strains are toxigenic. Earliest cases, identified as the J strain, were associated with clindamycin use. With the increasing use of fluoroquinolones, a new more virulent, fluoroquinolone-resistant strain, B1/NAP1/027, has emerged. The increased virulence of this strain is attributed to increased production of toxins.

Risk Factors

Antibiotic use is the most widely recognized and modifiable risk factor for *C. difficile* infection. The incidence of *C. difficile* increases with longer antibiotic exposure as well as with exposure to multiple antibiotics. Even perioperative antibiotic dosing can increase the risk in an epidemic setting. Although essentially any antibiotic can predispose a patient to *C. difficile* infection, clindamycin, broad-spectrum penicillins, second and third generation cephalosporins, and, increasingly, fluoroquinolones, are the most frequently implicated. Aside from antibiotics, any disruption of the normal colonic mucosa can open a niche for *C. difficile*. Chemotherapy, radiation, intestinal stasis, and abdominal surgery are all well-known risks. Of concern in the ICU, nasogastric tubes, enemas, and steroids also disrupt the normal colonic flora and are considered risk factors. Proton pump inhibitors and H2 blockers are often cited as a risk but this remains controversial. Patients with inflammatory bowel disease have altered gut mucosa, frequent hospital contacts, and frequent antibiotic usage, placing them at increased risk. Disease in healthy peripartum women is increasingly recognized and can be particularly severe including maternal and fetal death. Immunocompromised patients are another high-risk group, including those with human immunodeficiency virus/acquired immunodeficiency syndrome (HIV/AIDS), malignancy, or solid organ transplant. Older patients and those with chronic kidney disease on hemodialysis may have altered immunity, but the associated greater incidence of *C. difficile* infection may simply be related to increased health-care contact [31].

Presumably because of continued exposure, risk of infection is proportional to the duration of hospitalization. Up to 20 % of hospitalized patients and up to 50 % of patients in long-term care facilities are asymptomatically colonized [29]. Patients who remain asymptomatic longer have decreased, rather than increased, risk of developing infection. This paradox may be explained by asymptomatic colonization with nontoxigenic strains promoting antibody production. With advancing age, antibody production wanes which may partially explain the greater risk associated with older age [31].

Clinical Presentation

Clinical infections range in severity from self-limited watery diarrhea to life-threatening colitis. Common symptoms include profuse, watery diarrhea with a horse-barn odor, as well as lower abdominal pain, cramping, and mucus in the stool. Fever is limited to about a third of patients. Leukocytosis is the most common laboratory finding but is present in only about 50 % of patients [29]. Extracolonic manifestations, such as appendicitis, small bowel involvement, cellulitis, soft-tissue infection, and reactive arthritis are rare [31].

Signs and symptoms of severe colitis include severe pain with abdominal distention, temperature >38.5 °C, hypovolemia, lactic acidosis, hypoalbuminemia, marked leukocytosis, and occasionally ileus rather than diarrhea. Abdominal X-ray and computed tomography (CT) may show bowel dilatation, thickening of the colon wall, air-fluid levels, and thumb-printing due to submucosal edema. Direct visualization may show pseudomembranes [31]. Complications of severe *C. difficile* colitis include dehydration, electrolyte abnormalities, hypoalbuminemia, toxic megacolon, bowel perforation, hypotension, renal failure, systemic inflammatory response syndrome, sepsis, and death. Toxic megacolon is a clinical diagnosis made in the setting of severe systemic toxicity and is based on the presence of colonic dilatation >7 cm [31].

Given that treatment varies based on disease severity, knowledge of predictors of a severe clinical course would be helpful. Unfortunately, prediction tools have not yet been validated. Reported risk factors for severe disease include, but are not limited to, older age, white blood cell (WBC) count >20,000/L, renal insufficiency, immunosuppression, hypoalbuminemia, and any organ system failure. Independent predictors for more fulminant colitis in one study were age >70, WBC >35,000/L or <4,000/L, bandemia >10 %, and cardiorespiratory failure (intubation or vasopressors) [31].

Table 6.2 Stool tests for *C. difficile*

Test	Advantages	Disadvantages	Comments
Cell cytotoxin assay	Specificity 100 % Allows for strain typing during epidemics	Labor intensive—takes up to 2 days for results Sensitivity 67–100 %	Detection of toxin activity in stool was the initial observation that led to discovery of *C. difficile* as the cause of infection
Polymerase chain reaction for toxins A and B	Sensitivity 84–95 % Specificity 97–99 % Quick results	Requires technical expertise Does not differentiate between asymptomatic carriage and symptomatic infection	SHEA–IDSA guidelines do not recommend use until more data on utility is available
Enzyme Immunoassay for toxins A or toxins A and B	Specificity 75–100 % Quick results	Sensitivity 63–94 %	Toxin A/B assay preferred because 1–2 % of strains in the USA are negative for toxin A
Enzyme immunoassay for common antigen glutamate dehydrogenase (GDH)	Sensitivity 85–95 % Specificity 89–99 % Quick results	Does not differentiate between toxigenic and non-toxigenic strains	Two step algorithms recommended—GDH testing used for screening—positive results then confirmed by either cytotoxin assay or enzyme immunoassay for toxins A/B
Anaerobic culture	Good for epidemiology Sensitivity 94–100 % Specificity 84–100 %	Too slow and time-intensive for clinical practice High cost	Gold standard

SHEA–IDSA: Society for Healthcare Epidemiology of America and the Infectious Diseases Society of America

Diagnosis

The diagnosis of *C. difficile* infection requires the presence of moderate to severe diarrhea or ileus plus either a positive stool test or endoscopic or histologic findings of pseudomembranous colitis. Given the high rate of asymptomatic carriage, testing should only be done in the presence of signs and symptoms, including unexplained leukocytosis [31].

The optimal strategy for testing is controversial. As listed in Table 6.2, multiple stools tests are available, each with advantages and disadvantages. The optimal sample is a loose watery stool because toxin testing is less reliable with formed stool. Given the high rate of colonization in hospitalized patients, evaluation of formed stools also decreases the specificity of testing [31].

Clinical judgment may need to override a negative assay in patients for whom there is a high suspicion. In a patient with ileus, it may be possible to do a toxin assay or culture on a non-diarrheal stool, and therefore it is important to discuss testing options with the laboratory. Imaging may also aid in the diagnosis of severe or complicated disease. Due to its low sensitivity and the risk of rupture, endoscopy is not recommended in the diagnostic evaluation unless there is a high clinical suspicion combined with negative lab assays or ileus. Visualization with either sigmoidoscopy or colonoscopy can reveal patchy mild erythema, shallow ulcerations on the mucosal surface, or yellow to off-white plaques (pseudomembranes). Direct visualization will detect pseudomembranes in only about 50 % of *C. difficile* cases that are diagnosed by clinical and lab criteria. If direct visualization does not reveal pseudomembranes, biopsy is recommended [31].

Based on expert opinion, the IDSA guidelines propose definitions for severe and severe complicated *C. difficile* infection. Severe disease is defined by either leukocytosis of ≥15,000 cells/μL or a serum creatinine level ≥1.5 times the premorbid level. The presence of hypotension or shock, ileus, or toxic megacolon indicates severe complicated disease [31].

Treatment

Treatment includes supportive care with intravenous fluids and electrolytes as well as antibiotics based on the severity of disease. Table 6.3 lists preferred antibiotic choices categorized by severity of disease. In high-risk patients, it is often necessary to initiate empiric antibiotics while awaiting lab confirmation. Antimotility agents are not recommended as they may result in more severe colitis. If possible, it is highly recommended to discontinue all antibiotics beyond those to treat the *C. difficile* infection. Continued antibiotic treatment is associated with prolonged disease and increased risk of recurrence. If antibiotics must be continued, therapy for *C. difficile* infection should be administered concomitantly and extended for 1 week beyond the course of antibiotics. Treatment is not indicated for asymptomatic patients [31].

Based on 2 randomized controlled trials that demonstrated non-inferiority, the Food and Drug Administration (FDA) approved fidaxomicin for treatment of *C. difficile* infection in 2011. Fidaxomicin is a narrow spectrum macrocyclic antibiotic that inhibits RNA polymerase and has the potential to inhibit expression of genes responsible for sporulation. The drug reaches a high fecal concentration but has minimal activity against normal colonic flora such as bacteroides and minimal systemic absorption. It is bactericidal to *C. difficile* whereas metronidazole and vancomycin are bacteriostatic. Of note, patients with fulminant colitis were excluded from the clinical trials and it is as yet unclear if fidaxomicin should be considered in the ICU population. However, subsequent analysis of the two trials showed higher cure rates for those patients requiring concomitant antibiotic therapy, which is true of many ICU patients [32].

Patients with fulminant colitis are generally poor surgical candidates but surgery may be life-saving. The indications and optimal timing for surgery remain unclear.

Table 6.3 *C. difficile* treatment

Severity	Oral treatment options	If oral therapy not possible	Comments
Mild	1st line: metronidazole 500 mg orally three times per day for 10–14 days Alternative if contraindications to metronidazole: Vancomycin 125 mg orally four times per day for 10–14 days	Metronidazole 500 mg IV three times per day for 10–14 days	Adverse effects of metronidazole: peripheral neuropathy, nausea Metronidazole not recommended for use in pregnant or lactating women Currently, metronidazole substantially less expensive than oral vancomycin
Severe	First Line: Vancomycin 125 mg orally four times per day for 10–14 days Alternative: Fidaxomicin 200 mg orally twice per day for 10–14 days	Metronidazole 500 mg IV three times per day for 10–14 days AND Vancomycin 500 mg in 100 mL of normal saline every 6 h as a retention enema	Metronidazole is inferior to vancomycin for severe disease 200 mg PO fidaxomicin —approved by the FDA but not yet recommended in the guidelines To reduce costs some hospitals use the generic intravenous vancomycin formulation by mouth. IV vancomycin is NOT a treatment for *C. difficile*
Severe complicated	Vancomycin 500 mg orally four times per day AND Metronidazole 500 mg IV every 8 h AND Surgical consult	Vancomycin 500 mg in 100 mL of normal saline every 6 h as a retention enema AND Metronidazole 500 mg IV every 8 h AND Surgical consult	The IDSA guidelines recommend higher dose vancomycin and IV metronidazole to get therapeutic antibiotics to the colon as quickly as possible. PO vancomycin in general is not absorbed systemically but can be absorbed through a severely inflamed colon and can cause toxicity in patients with renal failure. Appropriate to obtain a trough serum level.

The IDSA guidelines recommend consideration of colectomy in cases of fulminant colitis, rising lactate, and WBC approaching 50,000/μL. Indications for immediate surgical intervention include bowel perforation, refractory shock, and peritonitis with impending perforation. Surgery after 12–24 h of medical therapy is recommended for toxic megacolon (>6 cm), severe colitis in older patients (age >65), coexisting inflammatory bowel disease, or progressive organ dysfunction. In a recent meta-analysis of patients undergoing emergency surgery, the strongest mortality predictors were preoperative cardiorespiratory failure (intubation or vasopressors), acute renal failure, and multiple organ failure. If surgical management is necessary, subtotal colectomy with preservation of the rectum is recommended [31].

There is growing interest in the use of fecal transplantation for patients with recurrent or persistent infection. In a recent meta-analysis that encompassed 317 patients, fecal transplantation led to disease resolution in 92 % of cases [33]. A recent randomized controlled trial was stopped early after finding infusion of donor feces resulted in substantially better outcomes than the use of oral vancomycin alone or in combination with rectal vancomycin [34]. However, critically ill patients were largely excluded from prior clinical trials and the published experience of fecal transplantation in fulminant colitis, while positive, is extremely limited.

The IDSA guidelines do not include a recommendation regarding either intravenous immunoglobulin (IVIG) or monoclonal antibodies. Some experts suggest that IVIG 200–500 mg/kg be used in patients with fulminant colitis. There are no randomized controlled trials reporting benefit of IVIG. A recent phase 2 randomized clinical trial of monoclonal antibodies used in conjunction with vancomycin or metronidazole suggests a decreased recurrence rate (7 % vs. 25 %, $p < 0.001$) of infection [35], but did not include critically ill patients. As yet, there is no randomized controlled trial of antibodies reporting benefit in severe or fulminant disease.

Prevention

With the rising incidence of infection, prevention is of utmost importance. Minimizing the duration and frequency of antimicrobials helps avoid disruption of the protective colonic flora and, thereby decreases risk. Gowns and gloves, patient placement in a private room, and environmental cleaning all disrupt the spread of *C. difficile*.

Compliance with hand hygiene is important. Although it is recommended to preferentially wash hands with soap and water rather than alcohol-based antiseptics in an outbreak setting, the benefit of doing so in a non-outbreak setting is unclear. To date, no studies show decreased rate of infection with soap and water [31].

A recent meta-analysis of probiotics showed a relative risk reduction of 66 % and no increase in adverse events. In addition, a recent randomized double-blind placebo-controlled trial for the use of probiotics to prevent ventilator-associated pneumonia, showed a significant reduction in *C. difficile* infection without adverse events. However, multiple reports of fungemia and sepsis with probiotics have also been reported and hence, use of probiotics remains controversial [31].

The most proven effective approach to infection control is a bundled approach including early recognition, implementation of contact precautions (gloves and gowns), placement of the patient in a private room, environmental cleaning, hand hygiene, education, evidence-based treatment, and antimicrobial stewardship [29].

Summary of Key Points

- *C. difficile* is the leading cause of hospital-associated infectious diarrhea, is an increasingly important cause of morbidity and mortality, and substantially increases the cost of care.
- Clinical presentation is non-specific and widely variable, ranging from self-limited diarrhea to life-threatening colitis.
- The diagnosis of *C. difficile* infection requires compatible symptoms plus either a positive stool test or endoscopic or histologic findings of pseudomembranous colitis.
- The optimal use of the many available diagnostic stool tests is unclear. Knowledge of the operating characteristics of the tests available at one's institution is imperative.
- Keys to treatment include early recognition, management of risk factors (discontinue offending antibiotics whenever possible), and, if evolving toward a more fulminant course, early surgical consult.
- Oral vancomycin is superior to metronidazole for treatment of severe disease.

Nosocomial Sinusitis

Epidemiology

Nosocomial sinusitis is an important occult source of fever in endotracheally intubated patients. Estimates of the incidence of radiologic and clinical sinusitis vary widely based on the patient population, route of intubation, radiographic technique used, diagnostic criteria, and whether or not the radiologic protocol required active search for sinusitis or if evaluation was prompted by fever. Opacification of the sinuses by computed tomography is frequently encountered and it is a challenge to discern which patients have actual infection requiring treatment. The reported range for clinical sinusitis in intubated patients is 2–26 % [36]. Nosocomial sinusitis is not directly reported to increase mortality but does place the patient at increased risk of ventilator-associated pneumonia and sepsis. Clinical sinusitis may be the sole cause of or a contributor to fever with unknown etiology [37].

Pathophysiology

Though not well delineated in the literature, nosocomial sinusitis may be the end result of a continuum starting from normal sinus tissue to mucosal edema and congestion that leads to fluid within the sinus cavity and finally to superinfection. The pathophysiology of nosocomial sinusitis is likely multifactorial with nasal congestion, compromise of host defense, and colonization or biofilm formation all playing a role. Increased central venous pressure, positive pressure ventilation, and supine position can also all induce sinus congestion. Additionally, any foreign body, inclusive of nasotracheal tubes, nasogastric tubes, and nasal packing, can cause mucosal irritation, inflammation, and nasal obstruction that lead to fluid retention within the sinus cavity [36, 38].

The presence of a foreign body may also alter mucociliary transport. In theory, inhalation anesthetics, atropine, and anticholinergics may also decrease mucociliary clearance. Bacteria such as *Haemophilus influenzae*, *Streptococcus pneumoniae*, *S. aureus*, and *P. aeruginosa* produce toxins that disrupt the epithelial cells leading to loss of the ciliary field. Another contributor to impaired host defense is decreased nitric oxide (NO) production. NO is involved in the stimulation of ciliated epithelium. Its absence may contribute to impairments of ciliary activity and thereby lead to decreased mucous and bacterial clearance. Additionally, NO directly inhibits microbial growth [36].

Normally, the paranasal sinuses are colonized with endogenous flora, but in the ICU, this protective flora can be rapidly replaced by exogenous pathogens from the environment [36]. Consistent with this, *S. pneumoniae* and *H. influenzae* often cause community-acquired sinusitis whereas *Pseudomonas* species, *Streptococcus* species, *S. aureus*, and *E. coli* are more often implicated in the ICU. Although more rare, fungi and anaerobes are also isolated [38]. Biofilms can form on either the intra- or extraluminal surfaces of endotracheal and feeding tubes and can serve as a reservoir of colonization for antibiotic-resistant nosocomial pathogens.

Risk Factors

Early studies that focused on the nasotracheal route of intubation as a risk factor yielded conflicting results [39]. More convincing evidence comes from a prospective study of 162 intubated patients by Rouby et al. [40]. In this study, all patients had a CT scan within 48 h of admission and cultures were obtained from all patients with radiologic maxillary sinusitis via transnasal puncture. Based on culture, 38 % were diagnosed with infectious sinusitis. Logistic regression identified four independent risk factors for the presence of infection: nasal placement of the endotracheal tube, nasal placement of the gastric tube, duration of intubation, and duration of gastric tube placement. This study not only reveals nasal instrumentation as a risk factor for nosocomial sinusitis but also suggests the continuum of disease with mucosal thickening and radiologic sinusitis as steps between normal sinuses and nosocomial infection. In a prospective observational cohort study, George et al. attempted to elucidate risk factors for infectious sinusitis other than nasotracheal intubation [41]. Twenty eight patients with sinusitis based on CT scan and positive cultures were compared to 338 patients without sinusitis. Sedative use, nasoenteric feeding, Glasgow coma score (GCS) ≤ 7, and nasal colonization with enteric gram-negative bacteria were all identified as risk factors.

Clinical Presentation

Common presenting symptoms of acute sinusitis include nasal drainage and congestion, facial pain or pressure, and headache. However, these symptoms are often absent in the intubated, sedated patient. Nasal discharge is reported to occur in just more than a fourth of cases [39]. The most often cited symptom in the ICU is fever of unclear etiology. In a study by van Zanten et al., orotracheally intubated patients with fever of unclear origin underwent a standardized infectious work-up (physical exam, blood cultures, WBC count, chest X-ray, central lines changed if in place for >1 week or any signs of local infection) and then underwent sinus radiography if no source of fever was elucidated or if fever persisted >48 h after initiation of appropriate antibiotics. In this study, sinusitis was implicated as the sole cause of fever of unknown origin in 16.2 % and a contributing cause in 13.8 % of patients. Of the patients with radiographic sinusitis, 84 % had positive cultures. Given that radiography was not performed in all patients, this study may underestimate the contribution of sinusitis to fever in the ICU [37].

Infectious sinusitis is reported to be associated with both pre- and post-septal orbital cellulitis, intracranial infections, pneumonia, and sepsis. Rouby et al. reported concomitant pneumonia in 67 % of patients with infectious sinusitis but only 43 % of patients with non-infectious sinusitis ($p < 0.02$). The same organism was isolated from the lung and sinuses in 59 % of cases. Although associated, causality is not yet established for either pneumonia or sepsis [40].

Diagnosis

In the appropriate clinical situation, radiologic evidence, including the presence of mucosal thickening, opacification, or an air fluid level, is suggestive of sinusitis. However, with plain radiographs, it may take up to five views to achieve adequate sensitivity. This is often not practical with portable equipment in the ICU. CT scanning is more sensitive and can evaluate the ethmoid and sphenoid sinuses in addition to the maxillary sinus, but typically requires transport of the patient. Ideal for use in the ICU, ultrasound may be a viable alternative. Although suggestive, radiologic findings are often present without infection [39, 42]. For instance, in the aforementioned study by Rouby et al., 75 % of patients had radiographic evidence of sinusitis within 48 h of ICU admission, but only a minority was subsequently diagnosed with infectious sinusitis [40]. Microbial analysis of fluid obtained by minimally invasive sinus puncture under aseptic conditions is definitive for the diagnosis. Equally important, sampling allows for pathogen identification and susceptibility testing [42].

Holzapfel et al. assessed whether the intensive care practitioner should actively search for sinusitis. In a randomized trial, febrile patients were divided into a standard work-up or a standard work-up plus sinus CT. In the active search group, 40 %

of patients were diagnosed with infectious sinusitis based on purulent aspiration and positive culture whereas no patients in the control group were identified. Of note, mortality was statistically lower in the study group. Although the effect on mortality needs verification, this trial suggests evaluation for sinusitis in intubated patients without a clear source of fever is indicated [43].

In 2008, the American College of Critical Care Medicine and the Infectious Diseases Society of America (ACCCM/IDSA) published guidelines for evaluation of new fever in critically ill adult patients. The ACCCM/IDSA recommend the following: obtaining a CT scan of the facial sinuses if clinical evaluation suggests that sinusitis may be a cause of fever, aspiration of the sinus using aseptic techniques if the patient has not responded to empiric therapy, and gram stain and culture of the aspirated fluid [42].

Treatment

A consensus on therapeutic intervention has not been established. Recommendations include removal of nasotracheal and nasogastric tubes and semi-recumbent positioning. Topical decongestants, alpha-agonists, and antihistamines may all be used to promote drainage. In many institutions where sinus aspiration is not routinely available, empiric antibiotic therapy is initiated after a sinus CT indicates that sinusitis may be present. Broad spectrum antibiotics that cover *Pseudomonas* species and methicillin-resistant *S. aureus* are recommended. If the patient does not improve, therapeutic aspiration with irrigation or placement of an irrigation catheter through the maxillary sinus ostia may be warranted. Formal surgical drainage and debridement is seldom required but may be needed in cases of invasive fungal disease [39].

Prevention

Relatively few studies address prevention. Duration of endotracheal intubation should be minimized. Simultaneous nasogastric and nasal endotracheal intubation should be avoided. Other interventions include aggressive mobilization of the patient, daily interruption of sedation, and avoiding fully supine recumbency. Pneumatikos et al. randomized 79 multiple trauma patients to either a combination of nasal decongestants (xylometazoline and budesonide) or placebo. Radiographic sinusitis developed in significantly fewer patients in the decongestant group (54 %) versus the control group (82 %) ($p < 0.01$). However, clinical sinusitis was not statistically different, occurring in 8 % of the decongestant group and 20 % of controls ($p = 0.11$) [44]. At the current time there is no updated consensus on prevention measures, and clinical practice likely varies from one ICU to another.

Summary of Key Points

- The pathophysiology of nosocomial sinusitis is likely multifactorial with nasal instrumentation, compromise of host defense, colonization and biofilm formation, and host immunity all playing a role.
- Nosocomial sinusitis is an important consideration in patients with fever of unclear etiology.
- When suspected, CT scan along with microbial analysis of fluid obtained by minimally invasive sinus puncture under aseptic conditions is definitive for the diagnosis.

Acute Acalculous Cholecystitis

Epidemiology

Acute acalculous cholecystitis (AAC) is defined as acute inflammation and necrosis of the gallbladder in the absence of gallstones. AAC is a known complication of critical illness, major surgery, and trauma. With increased awareness and improved diagnostic ability, the reported incidence is rising [45]. Two recent studies, one in a mixed ICU and the second in a trauma ICU, recently reported the incidence of AAC to be 1 and 1.1 %, respectively [46, 47]. The high mortality, estimated at 30 %, reflects the underlying disease process and multiple co-morbidities in this patient population [45, 48].

Pathophysiology and Risk Factors

Although the pathophysiology of AAC is likely multifactorial, gallbladder ischemia is believed to be the central mechanism [49]. Either systemic hypotension or increased intraluminal pressure may lead to decreased perfusion pressure and secondary ischemia. Systemic hypoperfusion may stem from volume depletion, left ventricular dysfunction, sepsis, or any other cause of hypotension. Alternatively, narcotics, nothing per os (NPO) status and TPN can all lead to biliary stasis which, in turn, increases the intraluminal pressure of the gallbladder and thereby decreases the perfusion pressure. Positive pressure ventilation, especially with high levels of positive end expiratory pressure (PEEP), can also increase venous pressure and decrease portal perfusion pressure [45]. In one study in a mixed surgical and medical ICU, sepsis was the most prevalent predisposing factor to AAC [46]. In a trauma center, the highest incidence was reported in patients with severe multiple injuries [47]. Reports of AAC complicating surgery and burn injury are common. Suspicion should be especially high in the setting of prolonged hypotension or jaundice.

Although the underlying cause is non-infectious, secondary infection is common. Bacteria may reach the gallbladder via translocation from the gut lumen or via hematogenous seeding. Alternatively, opportunistic infection may be a direct cause of AAC in immunocompromised patients.

Clinical Presentation

Clinical signs and laboratory findings are neither sensitive nor specific in the general population and become even less so in the critically ill. Classic symptoms of cholecystitis such as right upper quadrant pain, epigastric pain after a fatty meal, anorexia, nausea, and vomiting are obscured in the intubated, sedated patient. The most consistent, but unfortunately non-specific, signs are fever and leukocytosis. Other physical exam findings include jaundice, abdominal distention, loss of bowel sounds, and rarely a palpable gallbladder. Elevated liver enzymes and increased bilirubin in the absence of another cause of biliary stasis are suggestive, but the presence of normal liver function tests does not exclude the diagnosis [50]. Advanced cases may present with gangrene, perforation, abscess formation, and empyema.

Given the lack of a specific diagnostic test or finding and the relatively high mortality, the clinician will do well to have a high suspicion for AAC when caring for critically ill patients.

Diagnosis

The diagnosis of AAC is based upon a combination of clinical, lab, and radiologic criteria. As discussed above, clinical and lab findings are non-specific, thereby necessitating radiologic confirmation. However, radiologic tests also have suboptimal sensitivity and specificity, and there is no clear consensus on the optimal use of imaging studies in critically ill patients. Each option has advantages and disadvantages.

There is a relatively large published experience on the use of ultrasound and given that it can be performed at the bedside with minimal risk to the patient, it is generally recommended as the first-line radiologic test. As no single finding is both sensitive and specific, a constellation of findings, 2 major or 1 major and 2 minor, is required for diagnosis. Major findings include gallbladder thickening >3 mm, gallbladder wall edema, sonographic Murphy's sign, pericholecystic fluid, mucosal sloughing, and intramural gas. Minor findings include transverse diameter >5 cm and echogenic bile. False positives can occur even in patients with multiple radiographic signs of cholecystitis; this is especially common in patients with ascites, hypoalbuminemia, and portal hypertension. Sensitivity and specificity are widely variable depending on the criteria selected, with ranges of 30–92 % and 89–100 %, respectively [48].

Some clinicians recommend a radioisotope hepatobiliary iminodiacetic acid (HIDA) scan when the diagnosis of AAC remains uncertain based on clinical and ultrasound findings. The absence of gallbladder filling at 1 h after administration of technetium-labeled iminodiacetic acid is considered a positive test and is consistent with AAC. Of concern in the ICU population, false positives are associated with fasting, liver disease, analgesics, and TPN. However, when used with morphine sulfate, the time of testing is shortened and diagnostic accuracy improved. This test requires that a patient spend extended periods in the radiologic suite, which is often not feasible in the critically ill population [45, 48].

CT scans are valuable for identifying other potential causes of acute abdomen. The patient often must still leave the ICU but for a much shorter time than for an HIDA scan. The CT findings suggestive of AAC are comparable to those used for ultrasound; and as with ultrasound, the specificity improves when multiple findings are present [48]. Even when used in combination, making a confident diagnosis with imaging studies is often challenging.

Treatment

Antibiotics, analgesia, and early consultation with a surgeon are required. Antibiotics should target the most common intra-abdominal pathogens including *E. coli*, *Klebsiella* species, and *Enterococcus faecalis* [45]. If the patient has previously been on antibiotics or has had recent healthcare exposure, broader coverage is warranted. The most definitive treatment is cholecystectomy. However, ICU patients may be too ill to undergo this procedure and cholecystostomy has been established as an effective alternative therapy. One potential complication is catheter dislodgement with resultant bile leakage and peritonitis. Some patients improve with cholecystostomy such that subsequent cholecystectomy is unnecessary, in which case the tube can be removed in 3 weeks. In other patients, cholecystostomy serves as a bridge to definitive management with cholecystectomy once the patient has recovered from critical illness. However, patients with frank gangrene, transmural necrosis, emphysematous cholecystitis, or who have already sustained a perforation are not suitable candidates for cholecystostomy [48] and should proceed directly to surgical intervention.

Prevention

Many of the suspected triggers for acalculous cholecystis are unavoidable in critically ill patients, but presumably optimal management of hypotensive states, invasive mechanical ventilation, and nutritional support will mitigate the risk. Administration of intermittent cholecystokinin and deoxycholic acid are proposed preventive measures, but currently their efficacy is not well established.

Summary of Key Points

- Acalculous cholecystitis is an infrequent but important cause of fever in critically ill patients.
- The diagnosis of acalculous cholecystistis is often challenging as the signs, symptoms, and radiographic findings are usually non-specific.
- The mainstay of treatment for acalculous cholecystitis consists of antibiotics combined with cholecystectomy or cholecystostomy.

Conclusion

Non-pulmonary nosocomial infections are especially common in the ICU and are associated with increased morbidity and expense. The growing emphasis on prevention will likely translate into further reductions in the rate of hospital-acquired infections. However, a thorough knowledge of the pathophysiology, presentation, and diagnosis of ICU-acquired infection remains vital to ensure patients receive prompt, appropriate treatment when infection does occur.

References

1. Hooton TM, Bradley SF, Cardenas DD, Colgan R, Geerlings SE, Rice JC, et al. Diagnosis, prevention, and treatment of catheter-associated urinary tract infection in adults: 2009 international clinical practice guidelines from the infectious diseases society of America. Clin Infect Dis. 2010;50:625–63.
2. Edwards JR, Peterson KD, Mu Y, Banerjee S, Allen-Bridson K, Morrell G, et al. National Healthcare Safety Network (NHSN) report: data summary for 2006 through 2008, issued December 2009. Am J Infect Control. 2009;37:783–805.
3. Burton DC, Edwards JR, Srinivasan A, Fridkin SK, Gould CK. Trends in catheter-associated urinary tract infections in adult intensive care units – United States, 1990–2007. Infect Control Hosp Epidemiol. 2011;32:748–56.
4. Saint S, Meddings JA, Calfee D, Kowalski CP, Krein SL. Catheter-associated urinary tract infection and the medicare rule changes. Ann Intern Med. 2009;150:877–84.
5. Chenoweth CE, Saint S. Urinary tract infections. Infect Dis Clin North Am. 2011;25:103–15.
6. Donlan RM, Costerton JW. Biofilms: survival mechanisms of clinically relevant microorganisms. Clin Microbiol Rev. 2002;15:167–93.
7. Chenoweth CE, Saint S. Preventing catheter-associated urinary tract infections in the intensive care unit. Crit Care Clin. 2013;29:19–32.
8. Shuman EK, Chenoweth CE. Recognition and prevention of healthcare-associated urinary tract infections in the intensive care unit. Crit Care Med. 2010;38(Suppl):S373–9.
9. Dudeck MA, Horan TC, Peterson KD, Allen-Bridson K, Morrell G, Anttila A, et al. National healthcare safety network report, data summary for 2011, device-associated module. Am J Infect Control. 2013;41:286–300.
10. Greene MT, Chang R, Kuhn L, Rogers MAM, Chenoweth CE, Shuman E, et al. Predictors of hospital-acquired urinary tract-related bloodstream infection. Infect Control Hosp Epidemiol. 2012;33:1001–7.

11. Schwartz DS, Barone JE. Correlation of urinalysis and dipstick results with catheter-associated urinary tract infections in surgical ICU patients. Intensive Care Med. 2006;32:1797–801.
12. Stovall RT, Haenal JB, Jenkins TC, Jurkovich GJ, Pieracci FM, Biffl WL, et al. A negative urinalysis rules out catheter-associated urinary tract infection in trauma patients in the intensive care unit. J Am Coll Surg. 2013;217:162–6.
13. Kauffman CA, Fisher JF, Sobel JD, Newman CA. Candida urinary tract infections – diagnosis. Clin Infect Dis. 2011;52(S6):S452–6.
14. Fakih MG, Pena ME, Shemes S, Rey J, Berriel-Cass D, Szpunar SM, et al. Effect of establishing guidelines on appropriate urinary catheter placement. Acad Emerg Med. 2010;17:337–40.
15. Saint S, Wiese J, Amory JK, Bernstein ML, Patel UD, Zemencuck JK, et al. Are physicians aware of which of their patients have indwelling urinary catheters? Am J Med. 2000;109:476–80.
16. Maki DG, Kluger DM, Crnich CJ. The risk of bloodstream infection in adults with different intravascular devices: a systematic review of 200 published prospective studies. Mayo Clin Proc. 2006;81:1159–71.
17. O'Grady NP, Alexander M, Burns LA, Dellinger P, Garland J, Heard SO, et al. Guidelines for the prevention of intravascular catheter-related infections. CID. 2011;52:e1–e32.
18. Daniels KR, Frei CR. The United States' progress toward eliminating catheter-related bloodstream infections: Incidence, mortality, and hospital length of stay from 1996 to 2008. Am J Infect Control. 2013;41:118–21.
19. Mermel LA, Allon M, Bouza E, Craven DE, Flynn P, O'Grady NP, et al. Clinical practice guidelines for the diagnosis and management of intravascular catheter-related infection: 2009 update by the infectious diseases society of America. CID. 2009;49:1–45.
20. Brussalaers N, Monstrey S, Snoeij T, Vandijck D, Lizy C, Hoste E, et al. Morbidity and mortality of bloodstream infections in patients with severe burn injury. Am J Crit Care. 2010;19:e81–7.
21. Norgaard M, Larsson H, Pederson G, Schonheyder HC, Rothman KJ, Sorensen HT. Short-term mortality of bacteraemia in elderly patients with haematologic malignancies. Br J Haematol. 2005;132:25–31.
22. Chopra V, O'Horo JC, Rogers MAM, Maki DG, Safdar N. The risk of bloodstream infection associated with peripherally inserted central catheters compared with central venous catheters in adults: a systematic review and meta-analysis. Infect Control Hosp Epidemiol. 2013;34: 908–18.
23. Berenholtz SM, Pronovost PJ, Lipsett PA, Hobson D, Earsing K, Earley JE, et al. Eliminating catheter-related bloodstream infections in the intensive care unit. Crit Care Med. 2014–2020;2004:32.
24. Pronovost P, Needham D, Berenholtz S, Sinopoli D, Chu H, Cosgrove S, et al. An intervention to decrease catheter-related bloodstream infections in the ICU. NEJM. 2006;355:2725–32.
25. Timsit JF, Schwebel C, Boudadma L, et al. Chlorhexidine-impregnated sponges and less frequent dressing changes for prevention of catheter related infections in critically ill adults: a randomized controlled trial. JAMA. 2009;301:1231–41.
26. Bleasedale SC, Trick WE, Gonzalez IM, Lyles RD, Hayden MK, Weinstein RA. Effectiveness of chlorhexidine bathing to reduce catheter-associated bloodstream infections in medical intensive care unit patients. Arch Intern Med. 2007;167:2073–9.
27. Cobb DK, High KP, Sawyer RG, Sable CA, Adams RB, Lindley DA, et al. A controlled trial of scheduled replacement of central venous and pulmonary artery catheters. NEJM. 1992;327:1062–8.
28. Eyer S, Brummitt C, Crossley K, Siegel R, Cerra F. Catheter-related sepsis: prospective, randomized study of three methods of long-term catheter maintenance. Crit Care Med. 1990;18:1073–9.
29. Bobo L, Dubberke E, Kollef M. Clostridium difficile in the ICU the struggle continues. Chest. 2011;140(6):1643–53.
30. Bassetti M, Pecori D, Righi E. Update on Clostridium difficile. In: Vincent JL, editor. Annual update in intensive care and emergency medicine 2013. Berlin: Springer; 2013.

31. Cohen S et al. Clinical practice guidelines for Clostridium difficile infection in adults: 2010 update by the society for healthcare epidemiology of America (SHEA) and the infectious diseases society of America (IDSA). Infect Control Hosp Epidemiol. 2010;31(5):431–55.
32. Cornely OA. Current and emerging management options for Clostridium difficile infection: what is the role of fidaxomicin? Clin Microbiol Infect. 2012;18 Suppl 6:28–35.
33. Gough E, Shaikh H, Manges A. Systematic review of intestinal microbiota transplantation (fecal bacteriotherapy) for recurrent Clostridium difficile infection. Clin Infect Dis. 2011;53(10):994–1002.
34. Van Nood E et al. Duodenal infusion of donor feces for recurrent Clostridium difficile. N Engl J Med. 2013;368:407–15.
35. Lowry I et al. Treatment with monoclonal antibodies against Clostridium difficile toxins. N Engl J Med. 2010;362:197–205.
36. Riga M, Danielidis V, Pneumatikos I. Rhinosinusitis in the intensive care unit patients: a review of the possible underlying mechanisms and proposals for the investigation of their potential role in functional treatment interventions. J Crit Care. 2010;25:171.e9–171.e14.
37. van Zanten AR, Dixon JM, Nipshagen MD, de Bree R, Girbes ARJ, Polderman KH. Hospital-acquired sinusitis is a common cause of fever of unknown origin in orotracheally intubated critically ill patients. Crit Care. 2005;9:R583–90.
38. Agrafiotis M, Vardakas KZ, Gkegkes ID, Kapaskelis A, Falagas ME. Ventilator-associated sinusitis in adults: systematic review and meta-analysis. Respir Med. 2012;106:1082–95.
39. Talmor M, Li P, Barie PS. Acute paranasal sinusitis in critically ill patients: guidelines for prevention, diagnosis, and treatment. Clin Infect Dis. 1997;25:1441–6.
40. Rouby JJ, Laurent P, Gosnach M, Cambau E, Lamas G, Zouaoui A, et al. Risk factors and clinical relevance of nosocomial maxillary sinusitis in the critically ill. Am J Respir Crit Care Med. 1994;150:776–83.
41. George DL, Falk PS, Umberto Meduri G, Leeper Jr KV, Wunderink RG, Steere EL, et al. Nosocomial sinusitis in patients in the medical intensive care unit: a prospective epidemiologic study. Clin Infect Dis. 1998;27(3):463–70.
42. O'Grady NP, Barie PS, Bartlett JG, Bleck T, Carroll K, Kalil AC, et al. Guidelines for evaluation of new fever in critically ill adult patients: 2008 update from the American college of critical care medicine and the infectious diseases society of America. Crit Care Med. 2008;36:1330–49.
43. Holzapfel L, Chastang G, Demingeon G, et al. A randomized study assessing the systematic search for maxillary sinusitis in nasotracheally mechanically ventilated patients. Influence of nosocomial maxillary sinusitis on the occurrence of ventilator-associated pneumonia. Am J Resp Crit Care Med. 1999;159:695–701.
44. Pneumatikos I, Konstantonis D, Tsagaris I, Theodorou V, Vretzakis G, Danielides V, et al. Prevention of nosocomial maxillary sinusitis in the ICU: the effects of topically applied alpha-adrenergic agonists and corticosteroids. Intensive Care Med. 2006;32:532–7.
45. Barie PS, Eachempati SR. Acute acalculous cholecystitis. Gastroenterol Clin North Am. 2010;39:343–57.
46. Laurila J, Syrjala H, Laurila PA, Saarnio J, Ala-Kokko TI. Acute acalculous cholecystitis in critically ill patients. Acta Anaesthesiol Scand. 2004;48:986–91.
47. Hamp T, Fridrich P, Mauritz W, Hamid L, Pelinka L. Cholecystitis after trauma. J Trauma. 2009;66:400–6.
48. Huffman JL, Schenker S. Acute acalculous cholecystitis: a review. Clin Gastroenterol Hepatol. 2010;8:15–22.
49. McChesney JA, Northup PG, Bickston SJ. Acute acalculous cholecystitis associated with systemic sepsis and visceral arterial hypoperfusion, a case series and review of pathophysiology. Dig Dis Sci. 2003;10:1960–7.
50. Tisherman SA. Calculous and acalculous cholecystitis. In: Vincent JL, editor. Textbook of critical care. 6th ed. Philadelphia: Elsevier; 2011. p. 780–4.

Chapter 7
Nutritional and Endocrinologic Complications

Eoin Slattery, Dong Wook Kim, and David S. Seres

Abstract Nutrition support plays an important role in the management of critical illness. Our understanding of the difference between the impact of catabolism and that of nourishment in critical illness continues to evolve. In this chapter we will discuss the new diagnostic criteria for malnutrition in the setting of uncontrolled catabolism of critical illness.

Numerous recent studies have investigated the role that adjunctive nutritional therapies may play in ameliorating the metabolic response to stress as seen in critical illness. We will discuss the role of micronutrient deficiencies and attempts at supplementation, and critically analyze their effectiveness.

Both parenteral and enteral nutrition have important roles to play in the ICU. The route, timing and potential risks of each strategy will be discussed in depth. Particular attention will be made to refeeding syndrome, a potentially life-threatening condition when not recognized or anticipated.

E. Slattery, M.D. (✉)
Division of Preventative Medicine and Nutrition, Department of Medicine,
Columbia University Medical Center, 630 West 168th Street, P&S 9-501,
New York, NY 10032, USA
e-mail: slattery.eoin@gmail.com

D.W. Kim, M.D.
Boston Medical Center, Nutrition and Weight Management Center, Boston University
of Medicine, 88 East Newton Street, Robinson 4400, Boston, MA 02118, USA
e-mail: mdwook@gmail.com

D.S. Seres, M.D., Sc.M., P.N.S.
College of Physicians and Surgeons and Institute of Human Nutrition, Columbia University,
630 West 168th Street, New York, NY 10032, USA

Medical Nutrition and Nutrition Support Service, Division of Preventative Medicine
and Nutrition, Department of Medicine, Columbia University Medical Center,
630 West 168th Street, P&S 9-501, New York, NY 10032, USA
e-mail: dseres@columbia.edu

J.B. Richards and R.D. Stapleton (eds.), *Non-Pulmonary Complications of Critical Care:*   165
A Clinical Guide, Respiratory Medicine, DOI 10.1007/978-1-4939-0873-8_7,
© Springer Science+Business Media New York 2014

Lastly, we will address aspects of the management of endocrine-related issues in the critically ill patient. Management of blood glucose, thyroid disease and adrenal insufficiency will be discussed at length.

Keywords Malnutrition • Parenteral nutrition • Enteral nutrition • Catabolism • Refeeding syndrome • Hyperglycemia • Thyroid disease • Adrenal insufficiency

Introduction

The nutritional and metabolic care of critically ill patients is extremely important but complex, challenging, and often underappreciated with regard to their impact on patient outcomes. It is vital that the practitioner develop expertise at identifying nutritional and endocrine complications of critical illness as they are often overlooked opportunities to improve outcomes in these patients.

Malnutrition in Critical Illness

Malnutrition is not uncommon. Inpatient prevalence of malnutrition has been reported to be between 20 and 50 % [1]. For critically ill patients, malnutrition may not only exist at the time of admission but may also develop as a consequence or complication of critical illness.

Malnutrition has been variably defined, combining and confusing the impact of disease on body compartments with that due to imbalance (e.g. inadequate intake or uptake). It can be broadly defined as an inadequate or imbalanced nutritional state, which increases morbidity and mortality, causes higher health care costs, and requires nutritional therapy to improve outcomes. But much of what is called malnutrition includes phenomena such as muscle wasting or low serum protein, which are solely due to systemic inflammation and not responsive to alterations in nourishment. Therefore, patients with malnutrition may or may not be malnourished.

In critical illness, protein catabolic rates are significantly increased by systemic inflammation, which can induce a severely negative protein balance. Patients in this condition may develop malnutrition, regardless of how much nourishment they receive. Previously, this state was called "protein-calorie malnutrition." In 2012, the Academy of Nutrition and Dietetics and the American Society for Parenteral and Enteral Nutrition (ASPEN) proposed etiologic-based definitions that take the degree of inflammatory response into consideration. These etiologic-based definitions were classified into three categories: (1) starvation-related malnutrition, (2) chronic disease-related malnutrition, and (3) acute disease-related malnutrition. Among the three types of malnutrition, acute disease-related malnutrition (previously designated protein-calorie malnutrition) is commonly associated with critical illness, and is due to high-grade systemic inflammatory reaction.

Micronutrient Deficiencies in the Critically Ill Patient

Micronutrient deficiencies are uncommon complications for critically ill patients. However, daily requirements for certain vitamins and trace elements are thought to be much greater during critical illness due to alterations in metabolic demands. For instance, increased levels of oxidative stress result in concern about endogenous antioxidant defenses. While supplementation is often recommended, there are scant data that supplementation, even in the face of low measured levels of nutrients, results in improved outcomes. In fact, decreased levels of several vitamins have been documented in critically ill patients, despite daily supplementation of micronutrients [2]. Given the conflicting data, the true role for supplementation of most micronutrients remains controversial and poorly understood.

Symptoms and signs associated with micronutrient deficiencies are somewhat non-specific and often unrecognized and under-diagnosed. Supplementation of micronutrients is included in guidelines and recommended for critically ill patients to prevent depletion [3]. Outcomes studies are needed to better clarify which specific micronutrient(s) results in better outcomes [3]. We will separately discuss thiamine, selenium, glutamine, vitamin D and antioxidant vitamins, which are promoted as key micronutrients in critical illness.

Thiamine

Thiamine is a critical co-factor in the catabolism of carbohydrates and the oxidative decarboxylation of pyruvate for generation of adenosine triphosphate (ATP). Thiamine deficiency can lead to life-threatening conditions such as Wernicke–Korsakoff syndrome and beriberi. Mortality rates of up to 20 % have been described in patients with untreated Wernicke's encephalopathy [4]. Because of complexity of both illness and care provision, reliable recognition of the classical triad of confusion, ophthalmoplegia and ataxia is often not possible in critical illness. Therefore, clinicians should be aware of risk factors for thiamine deficiency so prophylactic supplementation can be initiated. Risk factors for thiamine deficiency include severe sepsis, burns, alcoholism, starvation, chronic disease or acute disease-related malnutrition, long-term parenteral feeding, chronic vomiting (or high gastric tube output) and a history of bariatric surgery [4]. Early thiamine supplementation is recommended for critically ill patients who have one of those risk factors [3]. It should be provided during the first 3 days in the intensive care unit (ICU) and it should not be delayed for confirmation of blood test results as complications may be irreversible once triggered (even by providing small amounts of dextrose, such as in 5 % dextrose intravenous fluids). Guidelines recommend doses of between 100 and 300 mg/day to prevent neurological complications [3]. It is worth noting that the evidence for this practice is supported only by case reports and expert consensus [5]. The only clinical trial to address this issue used intramuscular thiamine at varying doses, but no conclusive recommendations could be taken from this study [6].

Selenium

Selenium is an endogenous antioxidant and an essential component of glutathione peroxidases, which can reduce free hydrogen peroxide and protect against oxidative damage. Utilization of selenium is thought to increase in critically ill patients because critical illness is associated with generation of oxygen free radicals and decreased selenium plasma concentrations. This has led some to postulate an increased requirement for selenium in critical illness. Patients from Europe and parts of Australasia are known to be prone to low pre-morbid levels of selenium due to low soil content. It has been suggested that this deficiency may predispose these patients to increased risk of oxidative damage and thus worsen clinical outcomes. This notion has (in part) been supported by animal models of sepsis and brain injury that worsen in the selenium-deficient state [7]. Several investigators have tested the hypothesis that outcomes in sepsis could be improved with selenium supplementation with variable results.

Earlier smaller studies demonstrated that selenium supplementation may improve clinical outcomes by reducing illness severity, infectious complications, and decreasing mortality in critically ill patients [8–10]. However, a larger subsequent trial using high dose selenium (4,000 µg on the first day, 1,000 µg/day for the nine following days) failed to show any improvement in clinical outcomes [11]. Two more recent studies using lower doses of selenium (500 µg/day) have shown some conflicting results. A Scottish multicenter prospective randomized control trial in which critically ill patients received selenium suggested a decrease in "new" infections if selenium was given for more than 5 days [12]. In contrast, an international multicenter trial found no benefit to administration of selenium [13]. Both trials were well-designed, large multicenter trials using a 2×2 factorial design. However, the international trial recruited twice as many patients.

Unsurprisingly, questions remain about the appropriateness of provision of selenium supplementation. The European Society for Parenteral and Enteral Nutrition (ESPEN) recommended initiating selenium supplements (350–1,000 mcg/day) with an initial bolus followed by continuous infusion in critically ill conditions in their 2009 guidelines [3]. ASPEN, on the other hand, included no such recommendation in their most recent guideline for nutrition support of the critically ill. Expert consensus remains divided [14, 15]. It has been suggested that supplementation of selenium in the deficient state is beneficial, but potentially harmful for patients with normal/adequate selenium status [15]. In any event, further work is required to clarify the role of selenium supplementation.

Glutamine

Glutamine is the most abundant non-essential free amino acid in the human body. It plays an important role in nitrogen transport and provides the fuel for rapidly dividing cells (immune cells, enterocytes, hepatocytes, and others). Low glutamine levels have been demonstrated in patients with critical illness [16, 17]. This observation led to the suggestion that replenishment of this amino acid may be beneficial in critical illness, and may ultimately lead to improved outcomes. A meta-analysis published in 2002 of six randomized trials which examined the role of glutamine in critical illness suggested a trend towards better outcomes with supplementation [18]. While initially encouraging, some concerns were raised about the quality of the data.

Recently two large trials have refuted the suggestion that glutamine supplementation may be beneficial. The first study randomized patients in multiple Scottish centers to receive 20 g of glutamine per day, with and without selenium [12]. They found no benefit with respect to mortality or infections. The second study, a large multicenter blinded prospective randomized controlled study recruited more than 1,200 patients [13]. Patients were randomized in a 2×2 factorial design to receive glutamine (0.35 g/kg/day), a mixture of antioxidants (including selenium, zinc, beta-carotene, vitamin E and vitamin C), both glutamine and antioxidants, or placebo. Surprisingly, a statistically significant increase in mortality was seen at 6 months in the patients randomized to receive glutamine (with and without antioxidant supplementation).

Both ASPEN and ESPEN recommend consideration of supplementary glutamine in their latest consensus guidelines; however, in the light of new data, these recommendations are likely to be rescinded.

Vitamin D

Vitamin D, and its associated endocrine system effects (calcium, PTH), is known to have effects on innate and adaptive immunity as well as lung, muscle, endothelial and mucosal function. Deficiency of vitamin D is recognized as one of the most common mild medical conditions worldwide. Recent reports have demonstrated that vitamin D levels are decreased in patients in the ICU [19]. It is unclear, however, if low vitamin D levels are a surrogate of disease activity or represent true functional depletion. Given the relative ease and lack of expense of repletion of vitamin D, supplementation has unsurprisingly become of interest in the critical care setting. However, few data exist at present as to the utility or safety of such an approach. Additionally, decrements in critically ill patients may be due entirely to systemic inflammation-related decreases in vitamin D carrier proteins.

Anti-Oxidants (Including Vitamins E and C)

Vitamins E and C serve as important endogenous antioxidants. Therefore, like other antioxidants, it has been proposed that daily requirement of vitamins E and C are increased in critically ill conditions due to increased rates of biological oxidation in critical illness. An early randomized trial revealed that early administration of vitamin C and E reduces the incidence of organ failure and shortens ICU length of stay in the surgical ICU (1,000 unit α-tocopherol given enterally every 8 h and 1,000 mg ascorbic acid given parenterally daily) [20]. More recent randomized studies, however, have questioned this finding [12, 13]. As with other micronutrients the role and effectiveness of routine supplementation remains unclear.

How and When to Feed

Patients diagnosed with "acute disease-related malnutrition" should receive appropriate nutritional assessment as soon as possible, as guidelines recommend provision of enteral nutrition early in the course of their illness [21]. Enteral nutrition is preferred to parenteral and should be considered first for critically ill patients [22]. If enteral feeding is not feasible for an extended period, parenteral nutrition should be considered [21].

Enteral Nutrition

Enteral nutrition (EN) is favored as the first line in nutritional support therapy. This is based, primarily, on safety data. In addition, there are putative physiologic benefits of EN. It is believed that EN supports functional integrity of the gut by maintaining tight epithelial junctions, stimulating blood flow and maintaining villous height [21, 22]. Moreover, early enteral nourishment may enhance gut immune function and reduce inflammation, which in turn can result in a reduction of oxidative stress and potential improvement of patient outcomes in the ICU.

It is recommended that enteral feeding should be initiated within the first 24–48 h following admission to the ICU and then advanced to the goal rate. Guidelines recommend goal rate be achieved within 48–72 h [21]. However, a recent study suggests that a period of as long as a week of trophic (low dose) enteral feeding results in similar outcomes, at least in patients with acute respiratory distress syndrome (ARDS) [23]. If patients are hemodynamically unstable, and requiring multiple catecholamine agents or large volume resuscitation of fluid or blood products, enteral nutrition should be withheld to minimize a theoretical risk for bowel ischemia.

Standard nasogastric sump tubes, which are larger and stiffer (14–16 French) are generally used for gastric decompression and are not preferred as feeding tubes. The smaller and more flexible nasogastric tubes (8–10 French) are preferred. A case review of 2000 feeding tube insertions showed a malposition rate of 1.3–2.4 % when tubes were placed blindly at the bedside [24]. Malposition of feeding tubes into the trachea can be asymptomatic in critically ill patients (due to sedation and other causes of decreased consciousness). Therefore, feeding tube position should be confirmed by X-ray, or other well-validated methods, before being used [25]. Forcing air through the tube and listening for bubbles is extremely insensitive for detecting malposition and this practice should be abandoned [26]. Case reports of pneumothorax due to a tube puncturing through the lung into the pleural space [27], puncture of a tube through the roof of the mouth into the brain in the setting of craniofacial trauma [28], and other complications, serve as the basis for these concerns.

Nosocomial pneumonia is a source of much concern for clinicians, particularly in the management of the critically ill patient. It has been noted to occur in between 10 and 20 % of mechanically ventilated patients, and is associated with a two-fold increase in risk of mortality [29]. Older observational studies found a relationship between gastric colonization and gastric acid modifying drugs with nosocomial pneumonia [30]. Experimental studies have also demonstrated a potential gastro-pulmonary route of infection. In these studies radioactively labeled enteral nutrition suggested the occurrence of intra-tracheal aspiration [31]. However, while the presence of EN and nasogastric tubes are associated with aspiration pneumonia, a causal relationship has never been proven. In one report, H2 blockers and presence of tracheostomy were associated with development of pneumonia to a similar magnitude as the presence of nasogastric tube feeding [32]. Despite this, observational data continues to recognize nasogastric tube feeding as an independent risk factor for pneumonia after multivariate analyses [33, 34]. In one report the presence of a nasogastric feeding was associated with a three-fold increased risk of pneumonia [34].

Aspiration is not a complication of EN, unless it leads to pneumonitis or impaired respiration. It is a fervently held belief that aspiration of small amounts of gastric contents is something to be greatly feared in tube-fed patients. Undoubtedly the incidence of aspiration is likely to be increased in critically ill patients receiving EN. This may be due to retrograde regurgitation of gastric contents due to the impact of medications, positioning, or hemodynamics on protective mechanisms against reflux, and the inability to protect the airway due to decreased sensorium. It is our opinion that the increased incidence of pneumonia described in tube-fed patients is largely due to these and other phenomena resulting from the critical illness, rather than resulting from the feeding or the tubes themselves. However, it is unlikely that patients deemed to need tube feeding will be subject to a non-feeding arm in randomized trials in the near future. Such studies would be required to determine causality.

Historically, gastric residual volume has been used as a surrogate marker for risk of regurgitant aspiration (i.e., the larger the residual volume the higher the likelihood of aspiration and thus pneumonia). It has been common practice to measure residual volumes and use arbitrary cutoff values to stop or hold enteral nutrition in an attempt to minimize risk of pneumonia. Recent studies have strongly questioned this approach. An adequately powered prospective randomized trial has shown that checking gastric residuals and holding feeding in response does not decrease the incidence of pneumonia. Further, there was no increase in pneumonia despite a statistical increase in vomiting [35]. These data would suggest that continuing to measure residual volumes is of dubious clinical benefit. Further, fewer calories were delivered in the patients in whom residuals were checked. Despite this finding, patients with large gastric residuals (in excess of 500 ml) should be considered potentially at risk for regurgitation and pneumonia, and monitored closely.

Some authors postulate that recurrent micro-aspiration of gastrointestinal (but particularly pharyngeal) contents is the true risk factor for the development of pneumonia. A recent meta-analysis of 13 trials demonstrated that continuous aspiration of retained fluid from above the inflated cuff (containing predominantly oropharyngeal secretions) of the endotracheal tube can reduce ventilator-associated pneumonia by 45 % [36]. This is further supported by the observation that ventilator-associated pneumonia can be lowered by topically applied oropharyngeal decontamination [37]. Conversely, teeth brushing has no effect on the incidence of pneumonia [38].

Other strategies that may prove useful for reducing pneumonia include elevation of the head of the bed to 45°. This may help to reduce the risk of reflux and

Table 7.1 Potential complications of enteral feeding

Malposition of nasogastric tube
Vomiting
Diarrhea
Refeeding syndrome
Possible bowel ischemia when bowel is hypoperfused (theoretical)

aspiration and has been adopted as a standard of care for tube-fed and/or ventilated patients. When an elevation of 45° is not possible, the head of the bed should be elevated as much as possible.

Post-pyloric feeding can be considered in patients at highest risk for aspiration. A number of trials have shown that this can reduce gastroesophageal regurgitation [39, 40]. However, meta-analyses have failed to prove a reduction of mortality and incidence of aspiration pneumonia by using post-pyloric tubes [41, 42]. Given the technical difficulties, wholesale placement of post-pyloric tubes is not recommended.

Continuous tube feeding, as opposed to bolus feeding, has been suggested as another method to diminish risks of aspiration and improve tolerability [21, 43]. While bolus feeding is an intriguing concept and would seem to make sense by more closely matching normal meals from a physiological perspective, evidence to support this approach is lacking. Studies in both healthy volunteers and critically ill patients have not found any difference between these two modes of feeding when outcomes such as calorie provision, aspiration and diarrhea have been examined [44, 45]. Prokinetic agents such as metoclopramide and erythromycin should be considered for patients with high gastric residual volumes. Although there is no strong evidence to show that prokinetic agents can improve clinical outcomes and decrease aspiration pneumonia, they can improve gastric emptying and enteral feeding tolerance [46]. Metoclopramide should be avoided for patients with head injury because it can increase intracranial pressure [47].

Diarrhea is a potential adverse event in patients receiving EN [48] (Table 7.1). In critically ill patients, it can be associated with significant negative clinical outcomes, including fluid and electrolyte abnormalities, fecal incontinence, and pressure sores. Diarrhea also frequently results in cessation of enteral nutrition, which may exacerbate starvation in acute disease-related malnutrition.

The etiology of diarrhea in tube-fed critically ill patients should be carefully and thoroughly evaluated, as it is rarely due solely to tube feeding. Infectious or antibiotic-related diarrhea is a more common and serious cause of diarrhea in the critically ill. Critically ill patients, not uncommonly, also receive medications that can cause diarrhea (e.g., antibiotics, antifungal medications, proton pump inhibitors, laxatives, etc.), and the carrier for liquid medications is commonly highly hypertonic 70 % sorbitol. Therefore, the medications must be reviewed and evaluated prior to consideration of changes to enteral feeding regimes. In addition, calculation of stool osmotic gap may help differentiate osmotic diarrhea.

Fiber is frequently added to correct diarrhea in patients who already receive enteral nutrition. ASPEN ICU guidelines discuss the benefit of using soluble fiber-containing formulation for preventing enteral nutrition-associated diarrhea [21]. However, there is no conclusive evidence, and many studies have failed to prove the reduction of diarrhea by their administration [49]. Moreover, fiber or feeding formulas which contain fiber should be avoided for patients who receive catecholamine agents because bezoar formation and bowel obstructions have been reported [50, 51]. Predigested formula may be tried for patients experiencing diarrhea. Evidence for this approach is also lacking, however, and the cost is significant [21].

Parenteral Nutrition

As described above, EN is associated with fewer complications than parenteral nutrition (PN) and is cost-effective to deliver nutrition to critically ill patients [52]. Therefore, PN is indicated only when enteral nutrition is not feasible for an extended period of time. The appropriate timing for initiation of PN remains controversial, primarily due to a lack of high-quality data. Consensus guidelines from ASPEN have recommended that for adequately nourished patients who have contraindications to enteral nutrition, PN should be initiated only after 7 days of ICU admission [21]. On the other hand, for patients with clinical signs of protein-calorie malnutrition on admission to the ICU, ASPEN guidelines recommend that it is appropriate to start PN as early as possible, once adequate fluid resuscitation has been completed. In contrast, ESPEN has advocated commencing PN in patients within 2 days of ICU admission to meet 100 % of estimated calorie and protein needs not met by EN [3]. Much of the discrepancy between the professional societies guidelines appears to relate to a flawed and highly criticized systematic review which suggested that early PN was associated with a significant reduction in mortality when compared to delayed EN (i.e., for between 2 and 5 days) [53].

A large randomized trial from Australia and New Zealand has attempted in part to address some of these issues [54]. They found no benefit to early PN (i.e., <24 h) in patients with short-term relative contraindications to EN compared to "standard of care." In fact, of the patients in the "standard of care" group only 51 % ever required PN at all. Interestingly 40 % of the "standard of care" patients received no supplemental nutrition (PN or EN) during their ICU stay (median 3.72 days) and no adverse outcomes were observed. A post hoc analysis of a subgroup of patients from the Early Parenteral Nutrition to Supplement Insufficient Enteral Nutrition in Intensive Care (EPaNIC) study (discussed in more detail below) also examined the role of early vs. late initiation of PN in patients who had a contraindication to EN (i.e., where calories were derived from PN only, with no enteral component), and found a statistically significant reduction in infection and a trend towards early discharge in the late initiation arm [55]. These results seem to clarify that at least in the first 48 h of critical illness there is no benefit to early provision of PN. Indeed, the EPaNIC trial suggested that early PN may in fact be harmful.

Combining both PN and EN has been seen by some as an attractive alternative to provision of nutritional support by only one route. While recognized as the preferred source of nutrition by most, EN does of course have limitations. Primary among these is the ability to deliver adequate calories. Previous studies have documented that in some circumstances patients may only receive between 50 and 80 % of their prescribed calories during their ICU stay [56, 57].

Supplemental use of PN for patients has been suggested as a solution. A recent large multicenter prospective trial from Belgium (EPaNIC) investigated this approach [55]. In this study, early PN was used to reach 100 % of calories (within 48 h) in patients unable to receive all their required calories enterally (for whatever reason) and was compared to late initiation of PN (i.e., 7 days). There was no associated effect on mortality. On the other hand, there was an observed increased incidence of infection, prolonged mechanical ventilation and prolonged ICU stay in the early PN cohort compared to the delayed PN cohort. A Canadian-led observational study using a similar approach documented an improvement in calorie provision but also failed to show any clinical benefit with the adoption of this strategy [58]. In the face of the data it would appear that supplemental PN is not recommended.

No discussion of PN is complete without considering the potential serious (and life-threatening) complications associated with its use. These include development of catheter-related infection, metabolic complications such as refeeding syndrome, and hyperglycemia. Given the risk of complications, and the complexity of ordering a therapy with 72 active ingredients, clinicians involved in the ordering, compounding, and administration should be very familiar with published safe practices guidelines intended to provide protocols for reducing risk [59].

Patients receiving PN are at increased risk of catheter-related blood stream infections (especially fungal), compared to patients who have central venous catheters (CVCs) but do not receive PN [60]. Moreover, an observational study demonstrated that PN can increase not only the risk of blood stream infection but also pneumonia, surgical site and urinary tract infection [61]. Minimization or reduction of this complication can best be achieved by utilizing strategies to reduce the overall use of PN. When PN is required, best practices to minimize catheter-related blood stream infection should be adhered to strictly. Aseptic technique should be used for central catheter placement, and proper hand hygiene and maximal barrier precautions should also be used during the procedure. Introduction of care bundles has been shown to be effective in implementing these changes [62]. Single lumen catheters are preferred to multilumen catheters, and the subclavian approach is a preferred location for central catheter placement. After central catheter placement, the single lumen of the catheter should be dedicated, and used solely, for PN [63].

Refeeding Syndrome

Refeeding syndrome was first reported in soldiers who developed fatal diarrhea, heart failure, and neurological complications, including coma and convulsions, when released from Japanese prisoner of war camps at the end of the Second World War [64]. Any type of malnutrition and prolonged calorie deficit can be a major risk

Table 7.2 Potential
complications of parenteral
feeding

Bacteremia/blood stream infection
Refeeding syndrome
Hyperglycemia
Specific nutrient deficiencies due to shortages

factor for refeeding syndrome. It may be triggered by initiation of either enteral or parenteral nutrition, and may even be caused by intravenous solutions containing 5 % dextrose in the most severe of cases.

Refeeding syndrome occurs in approximately 0.8 % of hospitalized adult patients [65]. The incidence appears to be higher in critically ill patients. It is common because nutritional support is often delayed for patients in the ICU as a consequence of enteral intolerance and bowel hypomotility. A prospective study showed that 34 % of ICU patients who did not receive nutrition for at least 48 h experienced hypophosphatemia after initiation of enteral or parenteral nutrition [66]. Therefore, it is important to identify patients at risk. Initiation of enteral or parenteral feeding should be done slowly and carefully in at-risk patients to help prevent refeeding syndrome [67] (Table 7.2).

The hallmark feature of refeeding syndrome is hypophosphatemia, however, other biochemical abnormalities are common including hypokalemia, disorder of sodium and fluid balance, changes in glucose, protein and fat metabolism, thiamine deficiency, and hypomagnesemia [68]. Stores of phosphate can be depleted by prolonged starvation. When carbohydrate is introduced into the body, insulin levels rise, causing decreases in extracellular phosphate levels by several mechanisms. Glycolysis, which requires phosphorylation, as well as increased production of ATP are both induced and consume phosphorus. Moreover, as nutrients are administered, tissue anabolism increases demand for production of high-energy phosphate bonds, which further depletes phosphorus stores. Synthesis of ATP, 2-3-diphosphoglycerate (DPG), and creatine phosphokinase (CPK) are increased and may also contribute to hypophosphatemia [69].

The results of hypophosphatemia induced by refeeding syndrome may be very serious and even fatal. They include cardiac dysfunction and respiratory failure [70]. Severe hypophosphatemia (< 1.0 mmol/L) may cause respiratory failure and refractory weaning from the ventilator, which can be improved if hypophosphatemia is corrected [71, 72]. Severe hypophosphatemia is also associated with rhabdomyolysis, cardiac arrhythmias, altered mental status, seizures, hemolysis, impaired hepatic function, and depressed white cell function [69].

In a similar fashion to phosphate, potassium levels can precipitously shift intracellularly as a result of increased anabolism and insulin release. Potassium and magnesium are co-factors in the Na–K-ATPase pump that is responsible for driving these changes. Potassium has many physiological functions including regulation of cellular membrane potential, cellular metabolism, and glycogen and protein synthesis. Mild changes (e.g., serum concentrations 2.5–3.5 mEq/L) in potassium can cause nausea, vomiting and weakness. If left untreated severe hypokalemia (i.e., <2.5 mEq/L) can lead to paralysis, respiratory compromise, rhabdomyolysis, and life-threatening cardiac arrhythmias.

In the ICU, patients should be screened for high risk of developing refeeding syndrome prior to the initiation of enteral or parenteral nutrition. Empiric supplementation of thiamine should precede initiation of artificial nutrition, and even as dextrose-containing intravenous fluids are started in these patients [73]. Electrolytes should be closely monitored when enteral or parenteral nutrition is initiated. If the patient develops refeeding syndrome, caloric intake levels should be restricted to as little as 10 kcal/kg/day and aggressive repletion of electrolytes (phosphate, potassium, and magnesium) should be initiated and continued until the electrolytes are stabilized. In extreme cases, (BMI <14 kg/m^2, negligible intake for more than 2 weeks), it may be advisable to restrict initial calorie provision to a maximum of 5 kcal/kg/day with the addition of continuous monitoring of cardiac rhythm.

Endocrine Complications

Hyperglycemia

Hyperglycemia is a common complication for critically ill patients with or without a personal history of diabetes (Table 7.3). This is thought to be due to increases in stress-related hormones such as cortisol, catecholamines, and glucagon with critical illness. Hyperglycemia is associated with increased mortality and morbidity in the critically ill [74]. Parenteral nutrition is also associated with higher glucose levels than enteral feeding [75].

There are two major approaches to the management of hyperglycemia in the ICU: conventional insulin therapy and intensive insulin therapy. Several large randomized control trials on these approaches have been published over the past 15 years.

In the landmark 2001 Leuven surgical trial, Van den Berghe and colleagues found that intensive insulin therapy improved morbidity and mortality in the surgical ICU. It was the first major randomized control trial to address this important issue. A total of 1,548 critically ill surgical patients were enrolled in this trial. Patients received either intensive insulin therapy to maintain blood glucose levels between 80 and 110 mg/dL or conventional insulin therapy to maintain blood glucose between 180 and 200 mg/dL [76]. Mortality rate was significantly lower in the intensive insulin therapy group, although hypoglycemia was seen more frequently in the intensive insulin therapy group. Subsequent post-hoc subgroup analyses have

Table 7.3 Endocrine complications in the ICU

Hyperglycemia
Hypoglycemia
Thyroid storm
Myxedema coma
Adrenal insufficiency

identified potential confounders within this work. Specifically, a disproportionate number of patients had undergone cardiothoracic surgery (approximately 70 %) and while the observed effect was true for this large subgroup, it was not applicable to the remaining groups of patients (i.e., vascular, trauma and general surgery patients), raising the obvious question: Are subsequent outcomes related to the precipitating illness rather than just being a factor of "critical illness" per se?

In 2006, a second prospective randomized control trial, this time in critically ill medical patients, was conducted by Van Den Berghe et al. (the Leuven medical trial). Twelve hundred medical ICU patients received either intensive insulin therapy or conventional insulin therapy. In contrast to their first trial, a higher mortality rate was observed during the first 3 days of ICU admission in the intensive insulin therapy group.

The Normoglycemia in Intensive Care Evaluation Survival Using Glucose Algorithm Regulation (NICESUGAR) trial was published in 2009 [78]. The 6,104 patients recruited to this trial were a mixed population of both critically ill medical and surgical patients. Intensive insulin therapy significantly increased the incidence of severe hypoglycemia and 90-day mortality. Several meta-analyses, published after the NICESUGAR trial, have also concluded that intensive insulin therapy is not beneficial.

Currently, conventional insulin therapy (blood glucose target of 140–180 mg/dL) rather than intensive insulin therapy target (blood glucose target 80–110 mg/dL) is recommended in both surgical and medical ICUs [79].

It should be noted that in the two studies which failed to show the benefit of intensive insulin therapy (i.e., the Leuven medical trial and the NICESUGAR trial), the majority of patients received enteral nutrition. In contrast, in the Leuven surgical trial (which showed reduction of mortality in intensive insulin therapy) 81 % of patients received parenteral nutrition (with or without enteral nutrition) [77]. While parenteral nutrition increases blood sugar more than enteral nutrition on a calorie for calorie basis, enteral nutrition has the potential to be associated with more blood glucose fluctuations than that which would be typically seen with a continuous PN infusion. Enteral feeding is more likely to be interrupted in the ICU, theoretically exposing the patient to increased risk for sudden drops in blood glucose. This is also compounded by the variable intestinal absorption rates of nutrients seen in critical illness. Further studies may be warranted to compare intensive insulin therapy and conventional insulin therapy dependent on mode of nutritional support, especially with respect to PN.

Hypoglycemia

Severe hypoglycemia is an infrequent complication for critically ill patients (less than 1.5 % of patients in ICUs) [80]. Moderate or severe hypoglycemia in the ICU is independently associated with an increased risk of mortality [81]. Because patients in the ICU are commonly sedated, it is difficult to detect warning signs of hypoglycemia such as tremor, palpitations, anxiety, sweating, cognitive dysfunction, and so on.

History of diabetes, septic shock, mechanical ventilation, intensive insulin therapy, liver failure and severity of illness itself are risk factors for development of severe hypoglycemia [82]. Malnutrition can also cause hypoglycemia. For critically ill malnourished patients, hypoglycemia can be associated with increased mortality, longer length of ICU stay, and prolonged ventilator requirement [83].

Diagnosis of hypoglycemia, especially from capillary blood samples, is associated with increased frequency of falsely elevated glucose readings [80, 84]. It is therefore not recommended to use finger stick measurements to diagnose hypoglycemia. Hypoglycemia detected with finger stick measurements must be corroborated in the laboratory. However, the treatment should not be delayed. A 50 % dextrose intravenous solution should be administered if a high suspicion of hypoglycemia exists. If intravenous access cannot be established, patients can be given 1–2 mg of glucagon by intramuscular injection.

Thyroid Disease

Clinicians should be sensitive to the possibility, albeit unusual, for critically ill patients to develop thyroid-related syndromes. Signs may be subtle and non-specific. Severe thyroid disorders, related to both hypo- and hyperthyroid, can be triggered by critical illness.

Thyroid Storm

Thyroid storm is a life-threatening manifestation of hyperthyroidism. The incidence of thyroid storm is less than 10 % of patients hospitalized for thyrotoxicosis and it is more common in women than men [85]. Mortality of thyroid storm is reported between 10 and 30 % [86]. Grave's disease is the most common underlying cause of thyrotoxicosis in cases of thyroid storm. Other causes of thyroid storm are a solitary toxic adenoma, toxic multinodular goiter, hypersecretory thyroid carcinoma, thyrotropin-secreting pituitary adenoma, struma ovarii/teratoma, and human chorionic gonadotropin-secreting hydatidiform mole [85]. There is usually a precipitating event such as trauma, severe infection, or diabetic ketoacidosis. Thyroid storm has also been reported to be precipitated by sudden withdrawal of antithyroid medication and administration of medications which contain iodine such as contrast dye or amiodarone.

The clinical symptoms and presentation include high-grade fever, altered mental status, respiratory distress, cardiac arrhythmias, congestive heart failure, diffuse muscle weakness, tremor, anxiety, agitation, confusion, psychosis, coma, and gastrointestinal symptoms (nausea, vomiting, and abdominal pain).

The diagnosis of thyroid storm in critically ill patients is based on clinical presentation followed by laboratory confirmatory tests. Total and free thyroxine (T4) and triiodothyronine (T3) are increased while thyrotropin (TSH) levels are reduced. However, during critical illness, patients can have non-thyroidal illness syndrome, which is characterized by low serum levels of T3, normal or low serum levels of thyroxine (T4), and normal or low serum levels of thyroid-stimulating hormone TSH [87]. Thus, levels of T4 and T3 do not always correlate with presentation and severity.

Treatment of thyroid storm should be initiated first with supportive therapy, then symptomatic treatment that includes respiratory and hemodynamic support and measures to control hyperthermia, and lastly antithyroid drug therapy [88]. Beta-blockers such as propanolol or esmolol can be administered to control heart rate and blood pressure. Beta-blockade is essential in controlling the peripheral actions of thyroid hormone. Oxygen therapy, fluid and electrolyte replacement, antipyretics (acetaminophen is preferred to aspirin), and environmental cooling should be considered based on patients' clinical presentation [89]. Antithyroid drug therapy with thionamides (propylthiouracil and methimazole) interferes with the thyroperoxidase-catalyzed coupling process and has inhibitory effect on thyroid follicular cell function. The dosing of propylthiouracil for the treatment of thyroid storm is 600–1,000 mg as a loading dose, followed by 200–400 mg every 4–6 h. Methimazole, which has a longer half-life than propylthiouracil, can also be used for the treatment of thyroid storm. The dosing for methimazole is 20–25 mg every 6 h.

Iodine therapy can be considered in severe thyrotoxicosis after administration of thioamides. Iodine therapy blocks the release of pre-stored hormone, and decreases iodide transport and oxidation in follicular cells. If iodine is administered prior to thioamide therapy, it can be used for new thyroid hormone synthesis. Therefore, thionamides should be given first and iodine given at least 1 h after starting antithyroid drug therapy.

Glucocorticoids have an inhibitory effect on peripheral conversion of T4 to T3 and so may also be used for treatment of thyroid storm (i.e., hydrocortisone 100 mg every 6–8 h). Lithium has been used to inhibit thyroid hormone release. Due to various side-effects (renal and neurologic toxicity) and its limited efficacy, it should only be used when thioamide therapy is contraindicated.

Myxedema Coma

Myxedema coma is a severe form of hypothyroidism. It is very rare but has high mortality rate (50–60 %) [90]. It usually develops in previously hypothyroid patients with precipitating factors such as hypothermia, infection, congestive heart failure, trauma, metabolic disturbances (acidosis, hypoglycemia, hyponatremia), medications (narcotics, amiodarone, lithium), gastrointestinal bleeding, and withdrawal of levothyroxine [90, 91].

Typical clinical findings are lethargy, which progresses to stupor and then coma, respiratory failure, and severe hypothermia. Hypothermia and decreased mental status are the hallmarks of myxedema coma. The degree of hypothermia is correlated with prognosis of the disease. Patients with a core body temperature less than 90 F have the worst prognosis [90]. Cardiovascular manifestations include arrhythmias and conduction disturbances such as bradycardia, varying degrees of block, low voltage, flattened or inverted T waves, prolonged Q–T interval, and torsades de pointes ventricular tachycardia. Depressed hypoxic respiratory drive and ventilatory response to hypercapnia can lead to respiratory failure. Hyponatremia is a very common electrolyte disturbance in myxedema coma. It is associated with inappropriate antidiuretic hormone (ADH) secretion or coexisting conditions such as adrenal insufficiency. Severe hyponatremia in myxedema coma can contribute to generalized seizure.

The diagnosis of myxedema coma should be based on history and clinical manifestations. It can be confirmed by laboratory tests, which are markedly elevated TSH with low T3 and T4 levels. Hyponatremia, hypoglycemia, hypercapnia and respiratory acidosis can coexist. Thyroid hormone therapy should be initiated in the presence of highly suspicious clinical findings before confirmation of laboratory test results [90].

The method of thyroid hormone replacement (dose, frequency, and route of administration) is controversial. Occurrence of myxedema is rare and so evidence to support any practice is limited. High dose thyroid hormone replacement can cause serious side-effects such as tachyarrhythmias or myocardial infarction. On the other hand, without thyroid hormone replacement myxedema coma has a very high mortality rate.

A prior trial for parenteral T4 replacement in 2004 randomized a total of 11 patients who were to receive either high loading dose of T4 (500 mg) followed by daily maintenance dose (100 mg), or only the maintenance dose (100 mg) [92]. The high loading dose group had a lower mortality rate, but given the small sample size this difference was not statistically significant.

In critical illness, the rate of conversion of T4 to T3 is reduced and T3 is a more active and effective form of thyroid hormone than T4. Therefore, intravenous T3 administration can be considered. It may be given as an initial bolus dose of 10 mcg, followed by 10 mcg every 4 h for the first 24 h, followed by 10 mcg every 6 h. However, T3 replacement has a greater risk of adverse cardiovascular side-effects.

All patients with myxedema should have continuous electrocardiogram (ECG) monitoring during thyroid hormone replacement. Given the association with adrenal insufficiency, hydrocortisone replacement (50–100 mg every 6–8 h for 7–10 days) is also recommended [90]. The treatment of precipitating causes and supportive therapy are also very important.

Critical-Illness-Related Corticosteroid Insufficiency

Critical-illness-related corticosteroid insufficiency (CIRCI) occurs in patients without previous adrenal dysfunction in whom cortisol production is not sufficiently increased in critical illness [93]. This syndrome is also known as "relative adrenal insufficiency." Pathophysiology of CIRCI is different from primary adrenal insufficiency, which is caused by destruction of adrenal glands (e.g., autoimmunity, infection, ischemia, hemorrhage, etc.). CIRCI is caused by reversible hypothalamic-pituitary dysfunction, although the mechanism of this dysfunction during critical illness remains poorly understood. The prevalence of CIRCI varies widely but has been reported in as much as 75 % of patients in one intensive care setting [94].

Common symptoms and signs suggestive of CIRCI are hypotension resistant to volume resuscitation, eosinophilia, hypoglycemia (usually mild), hyponatremia, hyperkalemia, and pituitary deficiencies. Hypotension resistant to volume resuscitation is the most common sign that suggests CIRCI. Other typical signs of adrenal insufficiency are weakness, weight loss, anorexia, lethargy, nausea, vomiting, abdominal pain, and diarrhea [93].

Laboratory assays of plasma cortisol and response to adrenocorticotrophic hormone (ACTH) are unreliable in critically ill patients. Similarly, they appear to be of limited use as a stratification tool to decide who would best benefit from treatment with glucocorticoid replacement. Meta-analyses have attempted to answer the question as to whether or not empiric administration of corticosteroids may be of benefit in critical illness [95, 96]. These analyses suggest decreased mortality, particularly in the sickest patients. In patients without shock or less severe forms of shock, steroids appear to be of limited use. Thus most experts reserve steroids for patients with refractory shock, although data to support this approach is lacking in quality. There are trials currently recruiting to clarify the role of steroids in these patients.

References

1. Norman K, Pichard C, Lochs H, Pirlich M. Prognostic impact of disease-related malnutrition. Clin Nutr. 2008;27:5.
2. Manzanares W, Dhaliwal R, Jiang X, Murch L, Heyland DK. Antioxidant micronutrients in the critically ill: a systematic review and meta-analysis. Crit Care. 2012;16(2):R66.
3. Singer P, Berger MM, Van den Berghe G, Biolo G, Calder P, Forbes A, et al. ESPEN guidelines on parenteral nutrition: intensive care. Clin Nutr. 2009;28(4):387–400.
4. Manzanares W, Hardy G. Thiamine supplementation in the critically ill. Curr Opin Clin Nutr Metab Care. 2011;14(6):610–7.
5. NCGCACC 2010 National Clinical Guideline Centre for Acute and Chronic Conditions. Clinical guideline 100. London: Royal College of Physicians; 2010.
6. Ambrose ML, Bowden SC, Whelan G. Thiamin treatment and working memory function of alcohol-dependent people: preliminary findings. Alcohol Clin Exp Res. 2001;25(1):112–6.
7. Agay D, Sandre C, Ducros V, et al. Optimization of selenium status by a single intra-peritoneal injection of Se in Se deficient rat: possible application to burned patient treatment. Free Radic Biol Med. 2005;39:762–8.
8. Angstwurm MW, Schottdorf J, Schopohl J, Gaertner R. Selenium replacement in patients with severe systemic inflammatory response syndrome improves clinical outcome. Crit Care Med. 1999;27(9):1807–13.
9. Angstwurm MW, Engelmann L, Zimmermann T, Lehmann C, Spes CH, Abel P, et al. Selenium in intensive care (SIC): results of a prospective randomized, placebo-controlled, multiple-center study in patients with severe systemic inflammatory response syndrome, sepsis, and septic shock. Crit Care Med. 2007;35(1):118–26.
10. Manzanares W, Biestro A, Torre MH, Galusso F, Facchin G, Hardy G. High-dose selenium reduces ventilator-associated pneumonia and illness severity in critically ill patients with systemic inflammation. Intensive Care Med. 2011;37(7):1120–7.

11. Forceville X, Laviolle B, Annane D, Vitoux D, Bleichner G, Korach JM, et al. Effects of high doses of selenium, as sodium selenite, in septic shock: a placebo-controlled, randomized, double-blind, phase II study. Crit Care. 2007;11(4):R73.

12. Andrews PJ, Avenell A, Noble DW, Campbell MK, Croal BL, Simpson WG, et al. Randomised trial of glutamine, selenium, or both, to supplement parenteral nutrition for critically ill patients. BMJ. 2011;342:d1542.

13. Heyland D, Muscedere J, Wischmeyer PE, Cook D, Jones G, Albert M, et al. A randomized trial of glutamine and antioxidants in critically ill patients. N Engl J Med. 2013;368(16): 1489–97.

14. Hardy G, Hardy I, Manzanares W. Selenium supplementation in the critically ill. Nutr Clin Pract. 2012;27(1):21–33.

15. Rayman MP. Selenium and human health. Lancet. 2012;379(9822):1256–68.

16. Jackson NC, Carroll PV, Russell-Jones DL, Sönksen PH, Treacher DF, Umpleby AM. The metabolic consequences of critical illness: acute effects on glutamine and protein metabolism. Am J Physiol. 1999;276(1 Pt 1):E163–70.

17. Bongers T, Griffiths RD, McArdle A. Exogenous glutamine: the clinical evidence. Crit Care Med. 2007;35(9 Suppl):S545–52.

18. Novak F, Heyland DK, Avenell A, Drover JW, Su X. Glutamine supplementation in serious illness: a systematic review of the evidence. Crit Care Med. 2002;30(9):2022–9.

19. Lee P, Eisman JA, Center JR. Vitamin D deficiency in critically ill patients. N Engl J Med. 2009;360(18):1912–4.

20. Nathens AB, Neff MJ, Jurkovich GJ, Klotz P, Farver K, Ruzinski JT, et al. Randomized, prospective trial of antioxidant supplementation in critically ill surgical patients. Ann Surg. 2002;236(6):814–22.

21. McClave SA, Martindale RG, Vanek VW, McCarthy M, Roberts P, Taylor B, et al. Guidelines for the Provision and Assessment of Nutrition Support Therapy in the Adult Critically Ill Patient: Society of Critical Care Medicine (SCCM) and American Society for Parenteral and Enteral Nutrition (A.S.P.E.N.). JPEN J Parenter Enteral Nutr. 2009;33(3):277–316.

22. Seres DS, Valcarcel M, Guillaume A. Advantages of enteral nutrition over parenteral nutrition. Therap Adv Gastroenterol. 2013;6(2):157–67.

23. Harper CG, Giles M, Finlay-Jones R. Clinical signs in the Wernicke–Korsakoff complex: a retrospective analysis of 131 cases diagnosed at necropsy. J Neurol Neurosurg Psychiatry. 1986;49:341–5.

24. Sorokin R, Gottlieb JE. Enhancing patient safety during feeding-tube insertion: a review of more than 2,000 insertions. JPEN J Parenter Enteral Nutr. 2006;30(5):440–5.

25. Amorosa JK, Bramwit MP, Mohammed TL, Reddy GP, Brown K, Dyer DS, et al. ACR appropriateness criteria routine chest radiographs in intensive care unit patients. J Am Coll Radiol. 2013;10(3):170–4.

26. Seguin P, Le Bouquin V, Aguillon D, Maurice A, Laviolle B, Mallédant Y. Testing nasogastric tube placement: evaluation of three different methods in intensive care unit. Ann Fr Anesth Reanim. 2005;24(6):594–9.

27. Hensel M, Marnitz R. Pneumothorax following nasogastric feeding tube insertion: case report and review of the literature. Anaesthesist. 2010;59(3):229–32. 234.

28. Genú PR, de Oliveira DM, Vasconcellos RJ, Nogueira RV, Vasconcelos BC. Inadvertent intracranial placement of a nasogastric tube in a patient with severe craniofacial trauma: a case report. J Oral Maxillofac Surg. 2004;62(11):1435–8.

29. Safdar N, Dezfulian C, Collard H, et al. Clinical and economic consequences of ventilator-associated pneumonia: a systematic review. Crit Care Med. 2005;33:2184–93.

30. Bonten MJ, Gaillard CA, de Leeuw PW, Stobberingh EE. Role of colonization of the upper intestinal tract in the pathogenesis of ventilator associated pneumonia. Clin Infect Dis. 1997;24:309–19.

31. Torres A, Serra-Batlles J, Ros E, Piera C, Puig de la Bellacasa J, Cobos A, et al. Pulmonary aspiration of gastric contents in patients receiving mechanical ventilation: the effect of body position. Ann Intern Med. 1992;116:540–3.

32. Carrilho CM, Grion CM, Bonametti AM, Medeiros EA, Matsuo T. Multivariate analysis of the factors associated with the risk of pneumonia in intensive care units. Braz J Infect Dis. 2007;11(3):339–44.
33. Tejada Artigas A, Bello Dronda S, Chacón Vallés E, Muñoz Marco J, Villuendas Usón MC, Figueras P, et al. Risk factors for nosocomial pneumonia in critically ill trauma patients. Crit Care Med. 2001;29(2):304–9.
34. Wolkewitz M, Vonberg RP, Grundmann H, Beyersmann J, Gastmeier P, Bärwolff S, et al. Risk factors for the development of nosocomial pneumonia and mortality on intensive care units: application of competing risks models. Crit Care. 2008;12(2):R44.
35. Reignier J, Mercier E, Le Gouge A, Boulain T, Desachy A, Bellec F, et al. Effect of not monitoring residual gastric volume on risk of ventilator-associated pneumonia in adults receiving mechanical ventilation and early enteral feeding: a randomized controlled trial. JAMA. 2013;309(3):249–56.
36. Muscedere J, Rewa O, McKechnie K, Jiang X, Laporta D, Heyland DK. Subglottic secretion drainage for the prevention of ventilator associated pneumonia: a systematic review and meta-analysis. Crit Care Med. 2011;39:1985–91.
37. Chan EY, Ruest A, Meade MO, Cook DJ. Oral decontamination for prevention of pneumonia in mechanically ventilated adults: systematic review and meta-analysis. BMJ. 2007;334(7599): 889.
38. Alhazzani W, Smith O, Muscedere J, Medd J, Cook D. Toothbrushing for critically ill mechanically ventilated patients: a systematic review and meta-analysis of randomized trials evaluating ventilator-associated pneumonia. Crit Care Med. 2013;41(2):646–55.
39. Hsu CW, Sun SF, Lin SL, Kang SP, Chu KA, Lin CH, et al. Duodenal versus gastric feeding in medical intensive care unit patients: a prospective, randomized, clinical study. Crit Care Med. 2009;37(6):1866–72.
40. Heyland DK, Drover JW, MacDonald S, Novak F, Lam M. Effect of postpyloric feeding on gastroesophageal regurgitation and pulmonary microaspiration: results of a randomized controlled trial. Crit Care Med. 2001;29:1495–501.
41. Ho KM, Dobb GJ, Webb SA. A comparison of early gastric and post-pyloric feeding in critically ill patients: a meta-analysis. Intensive Care Med. 2006;32:639–49.
42. Marik PE, Zaloga GP. Gastric versus post-pyloric feeding: a systematic review. Crit Care. 2003;7:R46–51.
43. Rhoney DH, Parker Jr D, Formea CM, Yap C, Coplin WM. Tolerability of bolus versus continuous gastric feeding in brain-injured patients. Neurol Res. 2002;24(6):613–20.
44. Bowling TE, Cliff B, Wright JW, Blackshaw PE, Perkins AC, Lobo DN. The effects of bolus and continuous nasogastric feeding on gastro-oesophageal reflux and gastric emptying in healthy volunteers: a randomised three-way crossover pilot study. Clin Nutr. 2008;27(4):608–13.
45. Serpa LF, Kimura M, Faintuch J, Ceconello I. Effects of continuous versus bolus infusion of enteral nutrition in critical patients. Rev Hosp Clin Fac Med Sao Paulo. 2003;58(1):9–14.
46. Booth CM, Heyland DK, Paterson WG. Gastrointestinal promotility drugs in the critical care setting: a systematic review of the evidence. Crit Care Med. 2002;30:1429–35.
47. Deehan S, Dobb GJ. Metoclopramide-induced raised intracranial pressure after head injury. J Neurosurg Anesthesiol. 2002;14(2):157–60.
48. Luft VC, Beghetto MG, de Mello ED, Polanczyk CA. Role of enteral nutrition in the incidence of diarrhea among hospitalized adult patients. Nutrition. 2008;24(6):528–35.
49. Whelan K, Schneider SM. Mechanisms, prevention, and management of diarrhea in enteral nutrition. Curr Opin Gastroenterol. 2011;27(2):152–9.
50. McIvor AC, Meguid MM, Curtas S, Warren J, Kaplan DS. Intestinal obstruction from cecal bezoar; a complication of fiber-containing tube feedings. Nutrition. 1990;6(1):115–7.
51. Scaife CL, Saffle JR, Morris SE. Intestinal obstruction secondary to enteral feedings in burn trauma patients. J Trauma. 1999;47(5):859–63.
52. Cangelosi MJ, Auerbach HR, Cohen JT. A clinical and economic evaluation of enteral nutrition. Curr Med Res Opin. 2011;27(2):413–22.

53. Simpson F, Doig GS. Parenteral vs. enteral nutrition in the critically ill patient: a meta-analysis of trials using the intention to treat principle. Intensive Care Med. 2005;31(1): 12–23.

54. Doig GS, Simpson F, Sweetman EA, Finfer SR, Cooper DJ, Heighes PT, et al. Early parenteral nutrition in critically ill patients with short-term relative contraindications to early enteral nutrition: a randomized controlled trial. JAMA. 2013;309(20):2130–8.

55. Casaer MP, Mesotten D, Hermans G, Wouters PJ, Schetz M, Meyfroidt G, et al. Early versus late parenteral nutrition in critically ill adults. N Engl J Med. 2011;365(6):506–17. doi:10.1056/NEJMoa1102662.

56. Binnekade JM, Tepaske R, Bruynzeel P, Mathus-Vliegen EM, de Hann RJ. Daily enteral feeding practice on the ICU: attainment of goals and interfering factors. Crit Care. 2005; 9(3):R218–25.

57. Martins JR, Shiroma GM, Horie LM, Logullo L, Silva Mde L, Waitzberg DL. Factors leading to discrepancies between prescription and intake of enteral nutrition therapy in hospitalized patients. Nutrition. 2012;28(9):864–7.

58. Kutsogiannis J, Alberda C, Gramlich L, Cahill NE, Wang M, Day AG, et al. Early use of supplemental parenteral nutrition in critically ill patients: results of an international multi-center observational study. Crit Care Med. 2011;39(12):2691–9.

59. Mirtallo J, Canada T, Johnson D, Kumpf V, Petersen C, Sacks G, et al. Safe practices for parenteral nutrition task force for the revision of safe practices for parenteral nutrition. JPEN J Parenter Enteral Nutr. 2004;28:S39.

60. Kritchevsky SB, Braun BI, Kusek L, Wong ES, Solomon SL, Parry MF, et al. The impact of hospital practice on central venous catheter associated bloodstream infection rates at the patient and unit level: a multicenter study. Am J Med Qual. 2008;23(1):24–38.

61. Yang SP, Chen YY, Hsu HS, Wang FD, Chen LY, Fung CP. A risk factor analysis of healthcare-associated fungal infections in an intensive care unit: a retrospective cohort study. BMC Infect Dis. 2013;13:10.

62. Pronovost P, Needham D, Berenholtz S, Sinopoli D, Chu H, Cosgrove S, et al. An intervention to decrease catheter-related bloodstream infections in the ICU. N Engl J Med. 2006;355(26):2725–32.

63. Dimick JB, Swoboda S, Talamini MA, Pelz RK, Hendrix CW, Lipsett PA. Risk of colonization of central venous catheters: catheters for total parenteral nutrition vs other catheters. Am J Crit Care. 2003;12(4):328–35.

64. Schnitker MA, Mattman PE, Bliss TL. A clinical study of malnutrition in Japanese prisoners of war. Ann Intern Med. 1951;35:69–96.

65. Afzal NA, Addai S, Fagbemi A, Murch S, Thomson M, Heuschkel R. Refeeding syndrome with enteral nutrition in children: a case report, literature review and clinical guidelines. Clin Nutr. 2002;21:515–20.

66. Marik PE, Bedigan MK. Refeeding hypophosphatemia in an intensive care unit: a prospective study. Arch Surg. 1996;131:1043–7.

67. Stanga Z, Brunner A, Leuenberger M, Grimble RF, Shenkin A, Allison SP, et al. Nutrition in clinical practice-the refeeding syndrome: illustrative cases and guidelines for prevention and treatment. Eur J Clin Nutr. 2008;62(6):687–94.

68. Crook MA, Hally V, Panteli JV. The importance of the refeeding syndrome. Nutrition. 2001;17:632–7.

69. Marinella MA. The refeeding syndrome and hypophosphatemia. Nutr Rev. 2003;61(9): 320–3.

70. Kohn MR, Golden NH, Shenker IR. Cardiac arrest and delirium: presentations of the refeeding syndrome in severely malnourished adolescents with anorexia nervosa. J Adolesc Health. 1998;22:239–43.

71. Gustavsson CG, Eriksson L. Acute respiratory failure in anorexia nervosa with hypophosphatemia. J Intern Med. 1989;225:63–4.

72. Liu PY, Jeng CY. Severe hypophosphatemia in a patient with diabetic ketoacidosis and acute respiratory failure. J Chin Med Assoc. 2004;67:355–9.

73. Mehanna H, Nankivell PC, Moledina J, Travis J. Refeeding syndrome – awareness, prevention and management. Head Neck Oncol. 2009;1(1):4.

74. Falciglia M, Freyberg RW, Almenoff PL, D'Alessio DA, Render ML. Hyperglycemia-related mortality in critically ill patients varies with admission diagnosis. Crit Care Med. 2009;37(12): 3001–9.
75. Lee H, Koh SO, Park MS. Higher dextrose delivery via TPN related to the development of hyperglycemia in non-diabetic critically ill patients. Nutr Res Pract. 2011;5(5):450–4.
76. Van den Berghe G, Wouters P, Weekers F, Verwaest C, Bruyninckx F, Schetz M, et al. Intensive insulin therapy in critically ill patients. N Engl J Med. 2001;345(19):1359–67.
77. Van den Berghe G, Wilmer A, Hermans G, Meersseman W, Wouters PJ, Milants I, et al. Intensive insulin therapy in the medical ICU. N Engl J Med. 2006;354(5):449–61.
78. NICE-SUGAR Study Investigators, Finfer S, Chittock DR, Su SY, Blair D, Foster D, et al. Intensive versus conventional glucose control in critically ill patients. N Engl J Med. 2009;360(13):1283–97.
79. Egi M, Finfer S, Bellomo R. Glycemic control in the ICU. Chest. 2011;140(1):212–20.
80. Lacherade JC, Jacquemet S, Preiser JC. An overview of hypoglycemia in the critically ill. J Diabetes Sci Technol. 2009;3(6):1242–9.
81. NICE-SUGAR Study Investigators, Finfer S, Liu B, Chittock DR, Norton R, Myburgh JA, et al. Hypoglycemia and risk of death in critically ill patients. N Engl J Med. 2012;367(12):1108–18.
82. Krinsley JS, Grover A. Severe hypoglycemia in critically ill patients: risk factors and outcomes. Crit Care Med. 2007;35(10):2262–7.
83. Leite HP, de Lima LF, de Oliveira Iglesias SB, Pacheco JC, de Carvalho WB. Malnutrition may worsen the prognosis of critically ill children with hyperglycemia and hypoglycemia. JPEN J Parenter Enteral Nutr. 2013;37(3):335–41.
84. Critchell CD, Savarese V, Callahan A, Aboud C, Jabbour S, Marik P. Accuracy of bedside capillary blood glucose measurements in critically ill patients. Intensive Care Med. 2007;33(12):2079–84.
85. Nayak B, Burman K. Thyrotoxicosis and thyroid storm. Endocrinol Metab Clin North Am. 2006;35(4):663–86. vii.
86. Chong HW, See KC, Phua J. Thyroid storm with multiorgan failure. Thyroid. 2010;20(3): 333–6.
87. Bello G, Ceaichisciuc I, Silva S, Antonelli M. The role of thyroid dysfunction in the critically ill: a review of the literature. Minerva Anestesiol. 2010;76(11):919–28.
88. Ringel MD. Management of hypothyroidism and hyperthyroidism in the intensive care unit. Crit Care Clin. 2001;17(1):59–74.
89. Bajwa SJ, Jindal R. Endocrine emergencies in critically ill patients: challenges in diagnosis and management. Indian J Endocrinol Metab. 2012;16(5):722–7.
90. Wartofsky L. Myxedema coma. Endocrinol Metab Clin North Am. 2006;35(4):687–98. vii–viii.
91. Klubo-Gwiezdzinska J, Wartofsky L. Thyroid emergencies. Med Clin North Am. 2012;96(2): 385–403.
92. Rodríguez I, Fluiters E, Pérez-Méndez LF, Luna R, Páramo C, García-Mayor RV. Factors associated with mortality of patients with myxoedema coma: prospective study in 11 cases treated in a single institution. J Endocrinol. 2004;180(2):347–50.
93. Marik PE. Mechanisms and clinical consequences of critical illness associated adrenal insufficiency. Curr Opin Crit Care. 2007;13(4):363–9.
94. Bouachour G, Tirot P, Gouello JP, Mathieu E, Vincent JF, Alquier P. Adrenocortical function during septic shock. Intensive Care Med. 1995;21(1):57–62.
95. Annane D, Bellissant E, Bollaert PE, Briegel J, Confalonieri M, De Gaudio R, et al. Corticosteroids in the treatment of severe sepsis and septic shock in adults: a systematic review. JAMA. 2009;301(22):2362.
96. Sligl WI, Milner Jr DA, Sundar S, Mphatswe W, Majumdar SR. Safety and efficacy of corticosteroids for the treatment of septic shock: a systematic review and meta-analysis. Clin Infect Dis. 2009;49(1):93–101.

Chapter 8
Procedural Complications

Başak Çoruh, Amy E. Morris, and Patricia A. Kritek

Abstract Procedures are frequently performed in the intensive care unit with the potential for complications. In this chapter, we review system-based efforts to reduce non-pulmonary procedural complications, including procedural check-lists and pre-procedure time-outs. Several commonly performed critical care procedures including central venous and pulmonary artery catheter placement, arterial cannulation, lumbar puncture, paracentesis, and gastroesophageal balloon tamponade are reviewed. Evidence-based and practical recommendations are provided for clinicians in practice to reduce procedural complications.

Keywords Procedure • Complication • ICU • Critical care • Paracentesis • Central venous catheter • Gastroesophageal balloon tamponade • Lumbar puncture • Arterial catheter • Pulmonary artery catheter

Background

Critically ill patients often undergo invasive procedures during a stay in the intensive care unit (ICU). These procedures may be performed for diagnostic or therapeutic purposes, and the risk profile ranges from low (e.g., phlebotomy) to relatively high (e.g., placement of a pulmonary artery catheter). All procedures pose some risk of complications, even if performed by a skilled, experienced clinician under optimal circumstances. In this chapter we will review general principles of risk reduction for procedures in the ICU (Table 8.1) and discuss specific complications and

B. Çoruh, M.D. (✉) • A.E. Morris, M.D. • P.A. Kritek, M.D., Ed.M.
Division of Pulmonary and Critical Care Medicine, University of Washington,
1959 NE Pacific Street, Box 356522, Seattle, WA 98195, USA
e-mail: bcoruh@u.washington.edu; ammo@u.washington.edu; pkritek@u.washington.edu

J.B. Richards and R.D. Stapleton (eds.), *Non-Pulmonary Complications of Critical Care:*   187
A Clinical Guide, Respiratory Medicine, DOI 10.1007/978-1-4939-0873-8_8,
© Springer Science+Business Media New York 2014

Table 8.1 Strategies for reducing procedural risk in the ICU

Strategy	Examples
System-based	Promotion of a "Culture of Safety"
	Standardized equipment for common procedures
	Adverse event tracking systems
	Procedural checklists and "time-out" procedures
Educational	Simulation training
	Online education including just-in-time modules and videos
At the bedside	Appropriate timing and use of back-up resources
	Identification of a back-up plan if the procedure cannot be successfully completed or if a major complication occurs
	Proper positioning of patient and equipment
	Use of ultrasound for procedural guidance
	Appropriate supervision, when indicated

strategies for preventing them for some of the most commonly performed and highest risk procedures in this population.

Procedural complication rates published in the literature vary widely. The incidence of complications following procedures in the ICU will vary depending on the expertise of the practitioner and the underlying co-morbidities of the patient. Additionally, in each clinical scenario, the individual patient's risk-benefit profile should be assessed before proceeding with any procedure. Throughout this chapter, we provide the reader with a general sense of the frequency with which a given complication occurs, the specific clinical conditions that may increase the risk of a complication, and strategies to minimize the risk of complications.

System-Based Efforts to Reduce Procedural Complications

Over the last decade, the Institute for Healthcare Improvement (IHI) has worked to increase the emphasis on a "culture of safety" throughout the hospital and, in particular, in the ICU. A culture of safety implies an environment in which there is increased awareness of patient safety as a goal, and both individual practitioners and the institution itself are aligned toward this goal. In this environment there is a shared sense of responsibility among all the members of the care team to address problems that may affect patient safety, and providers actively participate in efforts to improve care and optimize patient safety. Institutions with a strong safety culture have demonstrated improved patient outcomes [1]. Many strategies exist to promote a culture of safety, from individual efforts to teach trainees that it is not only acceptable but expected that they call a senior provider if they have difficulty with a procedure, to large system-wide initiatives. The latter category might include vigorous error reporting systems, a policy encouraging interdisciplinary rounds, and equipment standardization for commonly performed procedures. We will focus on two system-based tools to improve patient safety that are particularly applicable to

BEFORE PROCEDURE

- Consent form completed (unless emergent)
- Patient's allergies assessed
- Operator hand hygiene
- Avoid femoral site; choose optimal insertion site based on:
  - Anatomy
  - Coagulopathy
  - Overlying burns or infection
  - Lung disease
- Ultrasound examination if internal jugular site is selected
- Skin preparation with chlorhexidine
- Maximum barrier precautions
  - Operator wears hat, mask, sterile gloves, sterile gown
  - Others in room wear hat and mask
  - Patient covered with full body drape
- Procedural "time-out" performed
  - Patient ID x 2 (including name, date of birth, and/or medical record number)
  - Procedure to be performed announced
  - Insertion site marked
  - Patient positioned correctly for procedure
  - Needed equipment and supplies available
  - Labels placed on all medications and syringes

DURING PROCEDURE

- Ultrasound guidance used for elective internal jugular insertions
- Second operator to complete procedure if > 3 needle passes
- Confirmation of venous placement via manometry, pressure transduction, ultrasound, and/or blood gas analysis
- Confirmation of venous placement of the guidewire
- Confirmation of final catheter in venous system prior to use
- Aspiration of blood from all catheter lumens
- Catheter secured in place

AFTER PROCEDURE

- Bio-occlusive dressing applied
- Sterile technique maintained while applying dressing
- Dressing timed/dated
- Catheter tip confirmed by chest radiograph

Fig. 8.1 Sample CVC checklist

bedside procedures and are often under-utilized: procedural checklists and pre-procedure time-outs.

Procedural checklists have been used for decades in other high-risk professions such as the aviation industry, where checklists were first adopted in response to high-profile disasters in which variations in standard practice and communication errors contributed to passenger deaths. Checklists are now ubiquitous in hospitals and are commonly accepted as a way to reduce errors of omission during commonly performed procedures (Fig. 8.1). Several studies have demonstrated improved patient outcomes when checklists are employed for procedures such as central venous catheter (CVC) placement and thoracentesis [2].

The practice of taking a few minutes prior to beginning a procedure for a team huddle or "time-out" has migrated from surgical safety checklists in the operating room (OR) to broader use before bedside procedures throughout the hospital. A time-out is an important communication tool in which all members of the care team introduce themselves and their roles, confirm that they are caring for the correct patient, and review key aspects of the procedure about to be performed. Although evidence is lacking that time-outs alone have a direct effect on patient outcomes, there are compelling data suggesting that implementation of a surgical safety checklist, which includes a time-out, can significantly reduce patient morbidity and mortality in the OR. It is plausible that these beneficial outcomes extend to bedside procedures.

A key component of a standardized approach to procedures, including the use of time-outs and checklists, is that these efforts tend to put team members on an equal footing, empowering nurses and other staff to voice safety concerns and even stop the procedure if they recognize a potential error that could put a patient at risk. Good communication between providers is a central element in fostering a culture of safety in the ICU in general, and is particularly important when performing higher risk invasive procedures.

Procedural Training

Experts debate the best approach to procedural training for physicians and other health care providers. With the increased availability of interventional radiology at many centers, and in the age of duty hour restrictions, some medical education experts have raised concern that current trainees lack confidence and expertise in the performance of common procedures by the time they complete their training programs.

In this environment it is crucial that providers move away from the "see one, do one, teach one" approach to procedural education and take advantage of the range of instructional methods that can minimize procedural complications. Online tools for medical education are increasingly available, moving procedural training away from the bedside to anywhere trainees have access to training websites and videos. Smart phones and tablet computers allow for "just-in-time" education with brief refresher modules for operators. Many training programs are developing their own curricula, but the abundance of freely available material online should encourage every program to at least direct their trainees to high-quality resources they can explore on their own.

Simulation is another powerful tool in procedural training. While much of simulator-based procedural training uses high-fidelity mannequins often specially created for a specific procedure, simulation does not necessarily require such expensive support tools to provide useful practice for trainees. For example, a banana can be used to teach the Seldinger technique in CVC placement. Trainees report greater confidence after simulation experiences and rate these sessions as having high educational impact. Patients have more confidence in providers who have had simulation practice, and most importantly, the use of simulation has been demonstrated to improve subsequent procedural performance on live patients [3].

Reducing Risk at the Bedside

In addition to improving the training for providers who perform procedures on critically ill patients, there are a number of tools that individual providers and care teams can employ at the bedside to minimize the occurrence of procedural complications. Checklists and time-outs are useful safety tools, but the importance of accurate medical decision-making cannot be overstated. Every proposed procedure should be carefully considered to ensure it is necessary, and that it is being performed at the appropriate time. Unless it is urgent, a procedure should generally be deferred when staffing is low or operators are fatigued (e.g., after a long shift or late at night). The care team should also ensure that performing the procedure at the bedside is the most appropriate setting, rather than referral to an interventional radiology suite or operating room. Finally, operators should have sufficient experience and a back-up plan in place if they encounter difficulty, including a specific individual who has agreed to supervise or be available for immediate assistance if needed.

Patient and operator positioning is often overlooked in bedside procedures. Patients should be positioned to ensure that anatomic landmarks are well-visualized and that they are physically comfortable. This applies to the operators as well; a provider hunched over a bed that is too low may be inappropriately rushed due to discomfort, may not have easy access to her equipment, or may not have good visualization of the ultrasound screen.

Point-of-Care Ultrasound

As ultrasound machines have become smaller and less expensive, critical care providers are increasingly using them at the point-of-care (POC) for diagnostic and procedural guidance. Ultrasound may be used before a procedure to confirm external landmarks and physical exam findings and to plan the procedure. For example, prior to a paracentesis, the operator can use ultrasound to confirm the presence of ascites and the absence of subcutaneous vessels at the intended insertion site, and anticipate the depth of needle insertion where ascitic fluid will be reached. Ultrasound may also be used for direct visualization of the needle in invasive procedures, as is commonly done in CVC placement. Ultrasound guidance has been demonstrated to decrease the incidence of complications in a variety of procedures, including CVC placement, thoracentesis, paracentesis and lumbar puncture [4–7].

Table 8.2 Common ICU procedures and associated complications

Procedure	Complications
Central venous catheter placement	Arterial puncture or cannulation
	Hematoma
	Pneumothorax
	Catheter malposition
	Air embolism
	Central line-associated bloodstream infection
	Catheter-associated thrombosis
Pulmonary artery catheter placement	Dysrhythmia
	Complete heart block in patients with a left bundle branch block
	Advancing catheter through PFO, ASD or VSD
	Pulmonary hemorrhage
	Pulmonary infarction
	Pulmonary artery rupture
	Knotting of catheter
Arterial catheter placement	Vascular occlusion and thrombosis
	Infection
	Bleeding
Lumbar puncture	Back pain
	Bleeding
	Infection
	Post-LP headache
	Neurologic complications
Paracentesis	Bleeding
	Fluid leak
	Infection
	Solid organ injury
	Bowel perforation and peritonitis
	Intravascular volume shifts causing hypovolemia and renal dysfunction
Gastroesophageal balloon tamponade	Tissue ischemia/necrosis
	Esophageal rupture
	Aspiration

Appropriate use of bedside ultrasound requires that practitioners also use their knowledge of external landmarks to plan a procedure and correlate their physical examination with their ultrasound findings. Providers should have sufficient ultrasound-specific training to interpret the images they are seeing on the screen and "know what they don't know." That is, POC ultrasound practitioners must be able to identify when a procedure is not appropriate for bedside ultrasound guidance and when someone with more experience, such as a procedural or interventional radiologist, should assist with the case.

The subsequent sections of this chapter address specific complications of commonly performed bedside procedures in the ICU. Discussion will include strategies to prevent complications as well as approaches to early identification and initiation of treatment of common complications. Table 8.2 is a summary of all of the procedures discussed below, and the associated common complications. There are complications that are seen in almost all procedures (e.g., bleeding and infection) as well as those that are unique to specific conditions and interventions. Patient discomfort and pain is a potential complication of all of the procedures discussed below and should be anticipated, recognized and addressed in a timely fashion.

Central Venous Catheters

Over five million CVCs are inserted annually in the USA and these devices are frequently used in the critical care setting [8]. All CVCs are placed in a deep central vein, but catheters may differ in size, material, and number of lumens. Further, catheters are differentiated by their intended duration of use. Some catheters are ideal for short-term use over days to weeks and include non-tunneled catheters placed in the internal jugular, subclavian, or femoral vein, and peripherally inserted central catheters (PICC) inserted into the basilic, brachial, or cephalic vein. Other catheters are designed for long-term access and may be left in place for weeks, months, or even years. These include catheters that are surgically tunneled under the skin and implanted ports. Non-tunneled catheters are the most frequently used CVCs in critical care and are the most likely to be placed by the critical care practitioner.

Indications for the use of non-tunneled CVCs include lack of adequate peripheral IV access, need for frequent phlebotomy, rapid volume resuscitation and infusion of certain irritant medications. CVCs are preferred for delivery of vesicant medications such as vasopressors (e.g., norepinephrine), chemotherapy, and hyperosmotic therapy, including parenteral nutrition. Depending on their type, CVCs may also provide access for hemodynamic monitoring and transvenous pacing, or for temporary hemodialysis and plasmapheresis. CVCs are ubiquitous in the critical care setting, but their placement is associated with complication rates are as high as 15 % [8]. Complications due to CVCs may be related to the procedure itself and occur during or shortly after placement, or complications may present in a delayed fashion (Table 8.3). A figure demonstrating several CVC complications is shown in Fig. 8.2.

Early Complications

Early complications of CVC placement are frequently mechanical in nature and include arterial puncture or cannulation, hematoma, pneumothorax, catheter malposition, and/or air embolism. The rate of these mechanical complications correlates with the operator's experience; clinicians who have placed more CVCs have lower complication rates than less experienced practitioners. Early complications also increase significantly with the number of attempts at venous access. The frequency of arterial puncture or pneumothorax after three attempts is six-fold greater than after one attempt at cannulation [9]. Therefore, after three failed needle passes, operators should seek help from a more experienced clinician. Other risk factors for early mechanical complications include the extremes of body mass index, previous

Table 8.3 Complications of central venous catheters and recommendations to minimize risk

Timing	Complication	Tips to minimize risk of complication
Early	Arterial puncture or cannulation	Position patients properly during CVC placement
		Identify anatomic landmarks
		Use ultrasound guidance
		Confirm venous access with pressure transduction
	Hematoma	Consider blood product transfusion in coagulopathic patients
		Select insertion site that minimizes risk
		Position patient properly during CVC placement
		Identify anatomic landmarks
		Use ultrasound guidance
	Pneumothorax	Use internal jugular vein site
		Identify anatomic landmarks
		Use ultrasound guidance
	Catheter malposition	Choose right internal jugular vein site
		Identify anatomic landmarks
		Monitor for arrhythmias during and following CVC placement
	Air embolism	Place patient in the Trendelenburg position for CVC placement
		Occlude needle hub prior to insertion of guidewire
		Ensure that catheter hubs are sealed
		Secure CVC to prevent accidental removal
Late	Central line-associated bloodstream infection (CLABSI)	Use a checklist for CVC insertion
		Perform a daily assessment of whether catheter is indicated
		Consider using antibiotic-impregnated catheters
		Avoid routine exchange of catheters
		Avoid antibiotic prophylaxis for CLABSI
	Catheter-associated thrombosis	Perform a daily assessment of whether catheter is indicated
		Use venous thromboembolism prophylaxis in hospitalized patients without a contraindication

catheterizations and larger catheter size. The use of ultrasound guidance for CVC placement has been shown to reduce several of the complications discussed below as well as increase the chance of successful venous cannulation [4].

Arterial Puncture or Cannulation

Inadvertent arterial puncture occurs most commonly during attempts at femoral CVCs, and least commonly with the subclavian approach. Arterial puncture is best prevented by proper patient positioning and ultrasound-assisted insertion, in addition to using known anatomic landmarks. The artery can readily be distinguished from the adjacent target vein by its anatomic location and lack of compressibility. Ultrasound should be used not only to visualize the needle tip entering the artery in real time but also to visualize the guidewire in the vein, as the operator may inadvertently advance the needle into the artery prior to guidewire insertion. Arterial puncture is often recognized due to the presence of bright red, pulsatile blood return, though these findings are less reliable in a patient with hypotension and hypoxemia.

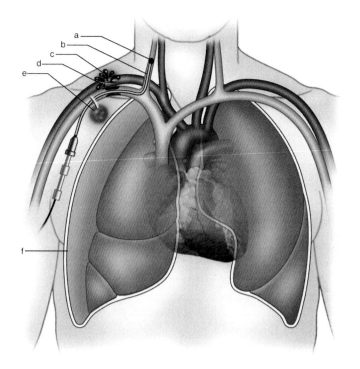

Fig. 8.2 Image demonstrating several possible complications of CVC placement. (**a**) catheter-associated thrombosis, (**b**) catheter malposition, (**c**) arterial hematoma, (**d**) subclavian vein stenosis, (**e**) exit site infection, (**f**) pneumothorax

Venous access can be confirmed with pressure transduction, simple manometry, or concurrent blood gas sampling (i.e., sending a blood gas from the CVC and an arterial catheter at the same time) to document a difference in oxygen tension. Unfortunately these methods are often not employed until after dilation of the tract and potentially the vessel, such that arterial injury has already occurred prior to verifying whether the CVC is in an artery or vein. A new commercially available device allows for measurement of intravascular pressure during CVC placement. Specifically, a disposable, sterile pressure transducer can be placed between the needle and syringe to allow for measurement of intravascular pressure during cannulation. The device has a side port to allow passage of the guidewire, thus allowing pressure transduction after wire placement. Currently there is inadequate evidence that this device results in fewer complications than the standard procedure for placing a CVC, but it has the potential to further decrease the risk of arterial cannulation.

If arterial puncture occurs, further management is dictated by the size of the vascular defect. Arterial puncture with a small gauge needle can be managed by withdrawing the needle and placing manual pressure on the site for five to ten minutes. If the artery is cannulated and the complication is not recognized until after artery dilation, the catheter should be left in place. Vascular surgery and/or interventional radiology consultation should be immediately obtained for open or endovascular repair of the vessel.

Hematoma

The presence of a hematoma after attempted CVC placement is often a result of inadvertent arterial puncture, occurring most frequently during attempted femoral venous cannulation. Hematoma formation is more common in patients with disorders of hemostasis. Most experts recommend transfusion of appropriate blood products in coagulopathic patients to achieve a platelet count of 50,000/μL and international normalized ratio (INR) of less than or equal to 1.5. While these thresholds are generally agreed upon, there are no data to support these cutoffs and these goals are often unattainable in certain clinical conditions (e.g., liver failure, autoimmune thrombocytopenias). CVCs may need to be inserted emergently and attempts to meet these thresholds should not delay the procedure. In such cases, insertion site selection may decrease the risk of causing a hematoma, as large hematomas are less common with internal jugular CVC placement due to blood vessels in the neck being easily accessible for compression if bleeding occurs. Mediastinal hematoma with the subclavian approach and retroperitoneal hematoma with the femoral approach are rare complications associated with high morbidity and even increased mortality.

Pneumothorax

Pneumothorax is one of the most feared early complications of CVC placement with the internal jugular or subclavian approach, but is relatively rare. Pneumothorax occurs if there is violation of the pleural cavity, resulting in a collection of air within the pleural space. The risk of pneumothorax increases with the number of cannulation attempts, larger catheters and during emergent CVC placement [9]. Pneumothorax is less common with the internal jugular approach and can be further minimized by the use of ultrasound during the procedure.

Aspiration of air into the needle during the CVC placement should raise concern for the presence of a pneumothorax and if air is aspirated, the procedure should be aborted. Patients who are awake and alert who develop a pneumothorax may complain of dyspnea, cough or chest pain. Signs of pneumothorax include diminished breath sounds on the affected side, hypoxemia and hypotension if tension pneumothorax physiology develops. Pneumothorax may be identified on a post-procedure chest radiograph but can also be quickly and accurately diagnosed with bedside ultrasonography. With an experienced operator, bedside ultrasonography has a higher sensitivity for pneumothorax than an anterior–posterior chest radiograph and similar sensitivity to chest computed tomography [10]. Management of a procedural pneumothorax depends on its size and the patient's clinical status. Management of small pneumothoraces may simply include observation, supplemental oxygen, and serial chest radiographs, while larger pneumothoraces require tube thoracostomy or immediate needle decompression in the setting of tension pneumothorax.

Catheter Malposition

A chest radiograph is often obtained to verify CVC position after placement in the internal jugular or subclavian vein. The tip of the catheter should be at the junction of the superior vena cava and right atrium. At least one small study suggests that routine post-procedure radiographs may not be necessary in uncomplicated right internal jugular vein CVC placement [11]. Although only demonstrated to occur in approximately 3 % of CVC placements [12], catheter tip malposition is defined as extrathoracic or intracardiac placement and may result in additional complications. Catheters that are advanced into the right atrium or right ventricle may result in arrhythmias. As such, if arrhythmias do occur, the catheter should be withdrawn such that the distal tip of the catheter is located outside of the heart.

Catheters may also be advanced into the wrong vessel. In general, the internal jugular approach provides more direct access to the heart, and is less likely to result in catheter placement in the innominate or azygos vein. A subclavian approach may result in cannulation of the ipsilateral jugular vein if the guidewire and catheter extend cephalad into the internal jugular vein rather than tracking towards the heart. Catheter malposition is difficult to identify during the procedure itself and is usually diagnosed post-procedure with chest radiography. Anatomic variants such as a persistent left-sided superior vena cava may also be identified in this manner.

Air Embolism

Intravascular air embolism may occur when there is a connection between a blood vessel and the ambient air with a pressure gradient that favors air entry into the bloodstream. Although more common during CVC removal, an air embolism can also occur during insertion. Air may be inadvertently injected directly into the blood vessel, or may be pulled into the vessel due to significantly negative intrathoracic pressure, such as during inspiration in a spontaneously breathing patient. The incidence of air embolism with CVC insertion is rare and is most likely to occur with tunneled catheter placement.

Signs and symptoms of an air embolism depend on the volume of air, and whether the air is present in the venous or arterial system. A large volume of venous air can occlude pulmonary blood flow, cause an acute increase in pulmonary vascular resistance, and precipitate acute cardiocirculatory collapse. Small volumes of air in the arterial circulation can cause catastrophic neurological events such as seizure or stroke.

Air embolism is best prevented by placing the patient in the Trendelenburg position during CVC placement, occluding the needle hub prior to insertion of the guidewire, and ensuring that all catheter hubs are sealed. Catheters should be well-secured after placement to minimize the risk of accidental CVC removal and resultant air embolism. Treatment of a suspected air embolus includes placing the patient in the left lateral decubitus and Trendelenburg position to trap the air in the right heart, application of 100 % oxygen to facilitate absorption of the air, catheter air aspiration, and possibly hyperbaric oxygen therapy if arterial air embolism is suspected.

Late Complications

Delayed complications of CVC placement include catheter-related bloodstream infection and catheter-associated thrombosis. Both of these complications increase with the duration of time that a catheter is left in a patient's vein. These complications are best minimized by a daily assessment of whether the catheter is still indicated, and removal of the catheter if it is not needed.

Central Line Associated Bloodstream Infection

Infections are a common complication of CVCs, with approximately 250,000 central line associated bloodstream infections (CLABSI) occurring annually in the USA [13]. Catheter-related bloodstream infections may originate from the catheter hub or from the skin insertion site, leading to perpetuation along the external catheter site. These infections increase morbidity and healthcare costs substantially.

Consistent use of clinical practice guidelines can drastically reduce the incidence of CLABSI [2]. Evidence supports the use of hand hygiene, chlorhexidine skin preparation, full barrier precautions during catheter insertion, avoidance of the femoral site, and prompt removal of the CVC when possible (Fig. 8.1). As previously discussed, using checklists before and during placement of a CVC improves adherence to clinical practice guidelines. Antibiotic-impregnated catheters may be used in select patients when rates of CLABSI remain high despite successful implementation of a checklist program. Clinicians should avoid routine exchange of catheters to minimize CLABSI, and systemic antibiotic prophylaxis is not appropriate to prevent catheter colonization [14].

Signs and symptoms of infection in a patient with a CVC in place for three or more days should raise concern for the presence of a CLABSI, and two sets of blood cultures should be obtained. One culture should be obtained from the suspected catheter and one should be drawn from a peripheral vein. If the catheter exit site appears infected, the catheter should immediately be removed; if a CVC is still needed, it should be placed in a new site. There are three accepted criteria for diagnosing a CLABSI. First, quantitative blood cultures may be obtained to demonstrate a three-fold greater colony count from the catheter hub than from a peripheral vein. Second, differential time to positivity of cultures can be compared. Growth from the catheter blood culture at least two hours before bacterial growth is detected in the peripheral blood is diagnostic of a CLABSI. Third, growth of more than 15 colony forming units of bacteria from the catheter tip after catheter removal suggests colonization; however, if the same organism is then isolated from a peripheral blood culture, CLABSI is confirmed. Any one of these three criteria is diagnostic of a CLABSI. Patients with a suspected CLABSI should be treated with antibiotics and the catheter must be removed [15].

Catheter-Associated Thrombosis

Thrombosis can be induced by any indwelling CVC. Catheter-associated thrombosis occurs commonly in patients with CVCs, and the rate of thrombosis increases with the duration that the catheter is left in place. Thrombosis occurs most commonly in the femoral vein and least commonly with subclavian catheters. Other risk factors for catheter-associated thrombosis include increasing patient age, thrombophilia, malignancy, and the use of certain infusates (e.g., amphotericin, parenteral nutrition). Catheter-associated thrombosis may also result from the catheter mechanically impeding blood flow, resulting in hemostasis.

Importantly, catheter-associated thrombi can cause significant morbidity and even mortality. Up to 15 % of patients with upper extremity venous thromboembolism may develop pulmonary emboli [16]. Prevention of catheter-associated thrombi is best accomplished by prophylactic dosing of heparin or low-molecular weight heparin, as is used to prevent other venous thromboembolic complications in hospitalized patients, and removal of the CVC when it is no longer needed. There is little specific evidence to guide management of catheter-related thrombosis, and practice is essentially extrapolated from management practices for other forms of venous thromboembolism [17].

Pulmonary Artery Catheters

Pulmonary artery catheters (PACs) require placement of an introducer sheath in a large central vein, followed by the introduction of a long catheter that traverses through the right atrium and right ventricle to a pulmonary artery. The PAC has a small balloon at its tip, which when inflated allows the catheter to follow blood flow until it "wedges" into a small pulmonary artery. Transduction of pressure from the PAC's most distal port, which is distal to the balloon, measures the intravascular pressure of the pulmonary arterial pressure when the balloon is deflated, and estimates the left atrial pressure when the balloon is inflated. The PAC's more proximal ports allow for the transduction of the central venous pressure as well as infusion of medications. While PACs can provide detailed data regarding a patient's cardiac output and hemodynamic parameters, several studies have shown that their routine use in critically ill patients does not affect mortality or length of stay [18].

In addition to the potential complications associated with introducer sheath placement (see the above section on "Central Venous Catheters"), PACs are associated with several unique complications. In contrast to CVCs, PACs frequently cause arrhythmias, with the majority of these being ventricular dysrhythmias (most frequently premature ventricular contractions) during placement. Most of these dysrhythmias are self-terminating upon withdrawal of the catheter, although a small proportion will require urgent medical intervention, including cardioversion.

An electrocardiogram should be performed in all patients prior to PAC placement to assess for a left bundle branch block (LBBB). As transient right bundle branch block may occur during PAC placement, a patient with a pre-existing LBBB may develop complete heart block. Preventing complete heart block in patients with LBBB includes avoiding placing PACs in these patients. If the clinical determination is that the risk of potentially precipitating complete heart block is outweighed by the benefit of placing a PAC, it is critical to minimize the time during which the catheter tip is in the right ventricle. In addition, transcutaneous pacing pads should be placed on the patient prior to placing the PAC, in case complete heart block develops during the procedure and persists despite promptly withdrawing the catheter.

Pulmonary hemorrhage and infarction are both rare complications of PAC placement, but are associated with significant mortality. Risk factors for both include older age, pulmonary hypertension, and systemic anticoagulation. Most cases, however, are thought to be related to improper catheter balloon inflation. Pulmonary artery rupture presents with hemoptysis and is managed with endotracheal intubation and emergent surgical management. The prognosis of pulmonary artery rupture is extremely poor.

Due to their long length and flexibility, PACs can loop into a knot during insertion. While rare, this complication is more likely to occur in patients with an enlarged right ventricle, as the catheter can coil while advancing through a large ventricular chamber. While advancing the PAC, the operator should monitor the transduced waveforms as well as the distance that the catheter is being advanced. If the waveforms indicate that the catheter tip is in and is remaining in the right ventricle while advancing >10 cm, there is increased likelihood that the catheter is looping in the ventricle rather than exiting to the pulmonary artery, and this is associated with increased risk of coiling and knotting. Catheter coiling can be observed and more quickly corrected with fluoroscopic guidance during PAC placement. Catheters that are kinked or knotted require interventional endovascular management for removal.

Finally, PACs should not be placed at the bedside in patients with a known large arterial septal defect, patent foramen ovale, or ventricular septal defect. In patients with these deficits, a PAC may be inadvertently advanced from the right heart to the left heart and the arterial circulation. While this would be noted on the transduced waveforms as a marked increase in pressure, there is increased risk of causing arterial emboli (i.e., from mechanically disrupting an atherosclerotic plaque or thrombus). If a PAC is felt to be clinically necessary in such patients, the catheter should be placed with fluoroscopic guidance.

Arterial Catheters

Arterial catheters are commonly used in the ICU for both blood pressure monitoring and blood gas sampling. Most catheters are placed in the radial artery although alternative sites include brachial, axillary, femoral and dorsalis pedis arteries. While generally well tolerated with a low rate of complications, arterial catheters carry several important risks including vascular injury, thrombosis, infection, and bleeding. Alternate sites carry higher and/or additional risk as compared to the radial artery.

Vascular Injury

One of the most serious injuries related to arterial catheterization is vascular occlusion. Arterial occlusion can result in ischemia distal to the site of cannulation and, if not recognized in a timely fashion, permanent tissue damage and loss of function. For this reason, the catheter should be placed in an artery where there is collateral circulation to protect the tissue from ischemia when possible.

There is no convincing evidence that performing an Allen's test prior to placement of a radial arterial catheter decreases the likelihood of ischemic complications [19]. Despite this, many institutions recommend performing this maneuver to assess for collateral flow before placing a radial artery catheter. To perform the modified Allen test:

1. Palpate both the radial and ulnar pulses
2. Hold pressure over both pulses to occlude flow while the patient clenches and unclenches hand multiple times until hand blanches
3. Patient unclenches fist
4. Release pressure on ulnar artery
5. Assess blood flow by observing for return of color to the hand

The clinical utility of Allen's test is limited, as assessing circulation is subjective (i.e., return to normal hand color) and it cannot be done in a sedated or unresponsive patient.

Because of limited collateral circulation, the brachial artery should be avoided if at all possible. Occlusion of this artery can have catastrophic results if not recognized immediately. Cannulation of the axillary artery poses similar risks.

Vascular occlusion most commonly occurs due to thrombosis at the site of the catheter. This is more likely to occur in small vessels with larger catheters. Additionally, the longer a catheter is in place, the greater the risk of thrombus formation. For this reason, it is essential that after placement the need for an arterial catheter is assessed daily with prompt removal when no longer necessary for patient care. Other risk factors for thrombosis include low cardiac output (due to low circulatory flow), underlying peripheral vascular disease, and vasospasm (e.g., patients with Raynaud's).

Emboli that are released from a catheter-associated thrombus can cause distal ischemia. This more commonly occurs with femoral arterial catheters. Knowledge about underlying peripheral vascular disease and careful monitoring of distal pulses is essential in all patients with arterial catheters.

Studies have shown that heparin flushes can reduce the risk of thrombus formation on arterial catheter tips. When heparin is contraindicated, sodium citrate flushes are a reasonable alternative [20].

In rare cases, an arteriovenous fistula can form after arterial cannulation. Fistula formation results from inadvertent puncture of both artery and vein during placement. Fistulae occur more frequently with femoral artery cannulation as compared to other sites. Ultrasound guidance of femoral artery catheter placement may reduce the risk of this complication.

Bleeding

Placement of any vascular catheter is associated with a risk of bleeding. As compared to CVCs, there is a greater risk of significant bleeding with arterial cannulation due to higher intravascular pressures in arteries as compared to veins. Unsuccessful attempts, particularly attempts during which both a needle and a catheter are introduced, require the provider to compress the vessel for a prolonged period of time to decrease the risk of significant bleeding. Coagulopathy and thrombocytopenia create a greater risk for significant bleeding and are often associated with hematoma formation.

Inadvertent removal of an arterial catheter confers a significant risk of bleeding. With a vessel under systemic pressure, more bleeding can occur in a shorter period of time as compared to inadvertent removal of a venous catheter. For this reason, arterial catheters are ideally placed in easily compressible vessels (e.g., radial artery). The femoral artery can be difficult to adequately compress, particularly in obese patients, and carries the greatest risk of large volume blood loss. In rare circumstances, compression or closure devices are necessary to adequately stop bleeding from a femoral artery puncture or catheter removal.

Infection

Patients with arterial catheters are at risk for catheter-associated blood-stream infections. The risk appears to be less than that seen with CVCs but there are limited studies describing arterial line infection rates. Infection may be more likely with femoral artery catheters than with radial ones, although the data from studies are not complete. Similar to CVCs, the risk of infection increases with the duration of use, once again mandating a daily assessment of need. Similar approaches as those described for CLABSI are used for diagnosis of arterial catheter-related blood stream infection.

Should a site become erythematous, painful or indurated, the arterial catheter should be removed.

Care should be taken to place arterial lines under sterile conditions and maintain them with sterile dressings. There is no convincing evidence that there is a benefit to full-body draping as is routinely employed for CVC placement. Many institutions require only a small, local drape for arterial line placement in addition to mask and sterile gloves. Eye protection is particularly important during placement of arterial catheters as the high-pressure arterial flow confers greater risk of exposure to the operator.

Lumbar Puncture

Critical care providers often perform lumbar puncture (LP) to sample the cerebro-spinal fluid (CSF) of patients with suspected neurologic infection, bleeding or inflammation. This procedure involves inserting a needle through the meninges to reach CSF in the subarachnoid space surrounding the spinal cord, and is associated with potential procedural complications. Spinal injections into the subarachnoid space and epidural catheters (placed outside the meninges) are distinct procedures that are subject to some of the same complications as LP.

Back Pain

Back pain is a common complaint after LP, even if the procedure itself was uncom-plicated. Unsuccessful LP attempts are more likely to cause pain and stress for patients. Obese patients or those with abnormal anatomy (e.g., scoliosis), prior trauma or spinal surgery are at increased risk for unsuccessful LP attempts. In these patients, providers should consider using fluoroscopy or ultrasound to guide the procedure. Both fluoroscopy and ultrasound increase the success rate and reduce the incidence of traumatic LP [7].

Bleeding

Bleeding at the site of needle puncture is usually minimal. However, bleeding can occur in deeper tissues with little external evidence. Hematomas large enough to cause spinal cord compromise occur rarely, with an estimated incidence of 0.1 % of all LP [21]. However, it is important for the provider to be aware of this complica-tion and to evaluate for it when clinically indicated. Patients with persistent or pro-gressive abnormal neurologic findings should undergo imaging of the lumbar spine, ideally magnetic resonance imaging (MRI). Patients with thrombocytopenia, intrin-sic coagulopathies, or those taking anticoagulant or antiplatelet medications other than aspirin are at highest risk of peri-spinal hematomas. Most guidelines recommend ensuring a platelet count of at least 50,000/μL and INR of less than or equal to 1.5 prior to LP.

Infection

Severe pain or tenderness, purulence and expanding erythema at the procedural site all suggest possible infection. Although a superficial infection could potentially spread to deeper tissues, the incidence of serious infection, particularly meningitis, is low and has most often been reported following the administration of spinal anesthesia. Meningitis due to the procedure is very rare after diagnostic LP. The organisms most commonly isolated are oral flora such as *Streptococcus* and *Staphylococcus* species. For this reason, in addition to general aseptic techniques, most experts and the Center for Disease Control and Prevention (CDC) recommend that practitioners wear a face mask while performing this procedure [22].

Post-Lumbar Puncture Headache

Post-LP headache is a common phenomenon, typically developing within 48 h of the procedure and lasting anywhere from 2 days to 2 weeks. Headache is often worse when sitting up, improved when supine, and may be associated with dizziness, nausea or vomiting. Occasionally, post-LP headache can be associated with neck stiffness and visual changes, making it difficult to distinguish this benign complication from more serious processes. The headache is thought to be caused by leakage of CSF from the dura following LP, resulting in pressure fluctuations within the meningeal space and traction on cerebral structures.

Younger patients, women and those with a history of headaches are more susceptible to developing post-LP headache. Several studies have shown that using smaller needles and orienting the bevel longitudinally, parallel to the dural fibers, can reduce the incidence of headache. Many experts recommend a 22-gauge atraumatic (as opposed to cutting) needle. Most patients respond to pain medication and supine positioning, although prophylactic bed rest has not been shown to decrease the incidence of headache [23].

More severe or refractory headaches may be successfully treated using intravenous caffeine or an epidural blood patch, which closes the dural leak. When considering these therapies for post-LP headache, however, one should also consider alternative diagnoses, particularly if the headache is severe, progressive, and not exacerbated by upright positioning. Though rare, cerebral venous thrombosis has been reported after LP. Diagnosis requires neuroimaging, and neurologic consultation should be considered.

Neurologic Complications

Neurologic complications of LP are very rare. Spinal cord injury due to spinal hematoma is discussed above. Of even greater concern is the risk of cerebral hernia-tion when LP is performed in the setting of elevated intracranial pressure (ICP). Historically, physicians have obtained a thorough history and performed a complete neurologic and ophthalmologic exam to exclude unilateral brain lesions or intracra-nial hypertension prior to performing LP. As computed tomography (CT) has become faster and easier to perform, it is routine practice in many institutions to obtain a head CT prior to performing LP. However, this practice is problematic because it may delay diagnosis and treatment of meningitis in patients at low risk of having increased ICP. Therefore, most experts recommend a combination of history and judicious use of head CT only in patients who are felt to be at increased risk of having an elevated ICP. One large study of patients suspected of having meningitis unearthed the following risk factors that are associated with increased risk of having increased ICP [24]:

- Altered mentation
- Focal neurologic signs
- Papilledema
- Seizure within the past week
- Impaired cellular immunity (most commonly human immunodeficiency virus [HIV] with low CD4 count)

Patients without any of these risk factors or other specific reasons to suspect increased ICP should proceed directly to LP without reflexively performing a pre-procedural head CT.

Paracentesis

Paracentesis is a common invasive procedure performed on hospitalized patients. Paracentesis may be diagnostic or therapeutic (i.e., large volume) in nature. This is an important distinction as a smaller needle is used in a diagnostic procedure, mini-mizing some of the potential complications.

Bleeding

Many patients undergoing paracentesis have underlying chronic liver disease with associated coagulopathy. A small amount of bleeding at the puncture site is not unexpected during this procedure, particularly when a larger gauge needle or cath-eter is used. Severe subcutaneous or intraperitoneal bleeding can occur if the needle pierces a blood vessel. While this is a relatively rare complication, it can be potentially avoided altogether by pre-procedural physical examination and ultrasound guidance. Of note, routine administration of fresh frozen plasma to reduce coagulopathy does not decrease the rate of hemorrhagic complications.

It is crucial for providers to understand the vascular anatomy of the abdominal wall in order to avoid large subcutaneous vessels. The greatest risks of arterial puncture are the inferior epigastric arteries which run posterior to the rectus abdominis muscles and are not easily compressed. The left lower quadrant, lateral to the rectus abdominis muscles, is considered by many to be the safest site to perform paracentesis. In addition, there is some evidence that the use of ultrasound to determine the needle insertion site can reduce the risk of hemorrhagic and other complications [6]. Specifically, the operator must have an ultrasound machine with color Doppler capability and the ability to interpret the resulting images. In addition, as in all procedures for which ultrasound guidance is used, the operator must have an understanding of the use of two-dimensional images to reveal three-dimensional structures. Many interventional radiologists advocate for real-time guidance of the needle tip during paracentesis, rather than simple site selection or "marking."

If a hematoma does occur, serial ultrasound exams may be adequate to track the progress of small subcutaneous hematomas, which will likely tamponade over time. Large volume bleeding may require urgent abdominal imaging to assess the size and location of the bleed, interventional radiology to embolize the injured vessel, or surgery for an urgent laparotomy. In patients with severe coagulation disturbances, appropriate blood products should be transfused.

Ascites Fluid Leak

Patients with large volume ascites are at risk for a persistent fluid leak at the site of a paracentesis. This is the most commonly reported complication of paracentesis and is often a self-limited phenomenon, but in rare cases patients can develop ongoing, large volume leaks that result in significant fluid shifts and protein loss. The risk of this complication can be minimized by using a smaller gauge needle and using a "Z-track" approach (Fig. 8.3).

Infection

Infectious complications of paracentesis may be local—confined to the skin and soft tissue—or infection may extend to the peritoneal space with potentially serious consequences. Paracentesis should never be performed through an area of infected skin, or in areas at high risk for infection, such as a colostomy site or between skin folds in a morbidly obese patient. Sterile technique should be practiced during the procedure; however, there is uncertainty regarding what personal sterile equipment

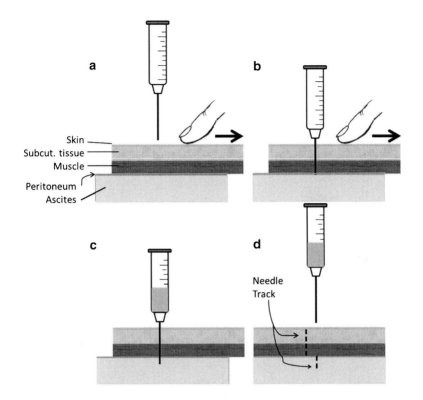

Fig. 8.3 The Z-track technique to prevent ascites fluid leak after paracentesis. (**a**) Application of downward traction on the skin just below the point of needle insertion moves the skin and subcutaneous tissues; the peritoneum will not move. (**b**) The needle is inserted into the peritoneal cavity while downward traction is applied. (**c**) Once the peritoneal cavity is entered, skin traction may be released and the procedure completed. (**d**) When the needle is removed, the subcutaneous tissues will slide back to their original position, effectively sealing the peritoneal defect to decrease the risk of leakage of ascitic fluid

the operator should use during the procedure. In the absence of compelling evidence, we recommend operators wear a sterile gown, particularly while performing a therapeutic paracentesis as this can be a prolonged procedure and therefore represent an extended opportunity for contamination of the procedural site.

Solid Organ or Bowel Wall Injury

Laceration of an intra-abdominal structure is a very rare complication of paracentesis, but if it occurs it can result in catastrophic hemorrhage from solid organ injury or severe intraperitoneal infection from penetrating bowel wall injury. Occasionally, patients may require surgical repair after suffering a lacerated organ or bowel.

Providers can minimize the risk of this complication by performing a thorough pre-procedural physical examination to confirm the presence of large ascites and verifying the presence and location of ascites with bedside ultrasound guidance. Ultrasound can confirm a fluid pocket of sufficient size and depth, absence of adhesions tethering the bowel to the peritoneum, and absence of unexpected structures such as an enlarged spleen or intra-abdominal mass.

If bleeding occurs as a result of solid organ injury, patients may develop pain as well as hypotension if the hemorrhage is massive. Urgent abdominal CT can clarify the location and size of the bleed, and guide interventional radiology or surgical repair efforts. In the case of a bowel wall injury, patients rarely develop overt peritonitis. If infection does develop, symptoms and signs may develop with a variable time course over hours or days. Repeat paracentesis may be required to diagnose peritonitis, and imaging with abdominal CT may be warranted to identify the site of bowel injury. Timely surgical consultation is obligatory.

Intravascular Volume Shifts

Patients with tense ascites often require therapeutic paracentesis to remove large volumes of fluid and to alleviate symptoms. In the ICU, large volume paracentesis may be employed as a strategy to increase mobility or improve respiratory mechanics. Five liters is commonly considered the maximum volume to be removed with one procedure, as most patients can tolerate having this volume removed without significant hemodynamic consequences [25]. Hypotension and renal dysfunction have been reported in patients undergoing paracentesis with removal of more than 5 liters. Hypotension and renal failure are thought to be due to fluid shifts, as volume shifts from the intravascular space to the peritoneal cavity after removing a large volume of ascites. To minimize such fluid shifts, it is common practice to infuse a colloid solution (e.g., 25 % albumin) at the time of paracentesis. There is some evidence from small randomized studies that this is effective, but larger confirmatory trials are lacking [26]. In this context, we recommend that an albumin infusion be considered in patients undergoing paracentesis in the ICU if more than 5 liters are to be removed, to potentially decrease the risk of post-procedural hemodynamic and renal impairment.

Gastroesophageal Balloon Tamponade

Gastroesophageal balloon tamponade is a procedure used to temporarily slow or stop severe variceal bleeding. This is not a definitive treatment and should only be used when other interventions (e.g., endoscopic banding) have been ineffective and the patient is at risk of exsanguination.

There are two types of balloon tamponade devices. One has only a large gastric balloon (i.e., Linton–Nachlas) while the other has both a gastric and an esophageal balloon (i.e., Sengstaken–Blakemore and Minnesota tubes). To place a gastroesoph-ageal balloon, the tube is threaded through the nose or mouth and advanced at least 50 cm to reach the stomach. The gastric balloon is then inflated with air and a chest radiograph is obtained to demonstrate that the balloon has been successfully and completely advanced into the stomach. Once gastric placement has been verified, the tube is pulled proximally until resistance is felt and traction is placed on the tube such that the gastric balloon is pulled up tightly against the lower esophageal sphincter at the gastroesophageal junction. This alone may stop variceal bleeding. If bleeding continues, and a two-balloon system has been used, the esophageal bal-loon can then be inflated for further tamponade. The tube is then tethered to a hel-met or weighted with a pulley system to maintain tension on the system, keeping the gastric balloon pulled up against the lower esophageal sphincter.

Ischemia and Rupture

The main complications associated with balloon tamponade are related to direct pressure on the esophagus from the esophageal balloon. Pressure of the balloon on the esophageal mucosa can result in local ischemia with tissue necrosis and ulcer-ation. Frank rupture of the esophageal wall occurs when the balloon's pressure exceeds esophageal wall tension. Given these potential complications, pressures in the esophageal balloon should not exceed 45 mmHg on initial inflation. Once bleed-ing has been controlled, pressure in the balloon should be decreased to 25 mmHg as long as the patient tolerates the lower pressure without further bleeding [27].

To minimize the risk of necrosis and rupture, attempts should be made to deflate the esophageal balloon as soon as possible. The balloon tamponade device may be kept in place, with balloons deflated, to confirm that bleeding has stopped but the balloons should not remain inflated for more than 24 h.

Aspiration

Patients with balloon tamponade devices in place are at high risk of aspiration. To minimize this risk, all patients should be intubated prior to gastroesophageal tube placement. The head of the patient's bed should be kept elevated. Most importantly, the device should be removed as soon as it is safe to do so.

Rebleeding

The most common issue related to balloon tamponade is that patients commonly rebleed when the balloon(s) is deflated. While this is not truly a procedural complica-tion, as it is a result of the patient's underlying disease, rebleeding is a common challenge faced by practitioners. The only solution to rebleeding with balloon deflation is more definitive interventions to achieve hemostasis, such as repeat endoscopic evaluation and intervention or transjugular intrahepatic portosystemic shunt (i.e., TIPS).

Recommendations

- Use procedural checklists which include a time-out for procedures performed in the ICU.
- Consider ultrasound guidance for many, if not all, procedures occurring in the ICU.
- When possible, correct coagulopathy and thrombocytopenia prior to lumbar puncture or placement of a central venous or arterial catheter.
- For all procedures, appropriately position the patient and identify anatomic landmarks prior to beginning the procedure.
- After placement, review the need for all CVCs and arterial catheters daily. Catheters should be removed if no longer clinically indicated to reduce the risk of infection and thrombosis.
- If new neurologic findings (e.g., decreased motor or sensory function) are seen following an LP, evaluate further with imaging of the lumbar spine, preferably with MRI.
- Use a "Z-track" approach (Fig. 8.3) for large volume paracentesis to minimize the risk of persistent ascites leak.
- Consider the infusion of albumin when performing therapeutic paracentesis of more than 5 liters.
- To avoid esophageal ischemia and rupture, deflate the esophageal balloon of a gastroesophageal balloon tamponade device as soon as hemostasis has been obtained.

References

1. Institute for Healthcare Improvement [Internet]. Available at http://www.ihi.org/Pages/default.aspx
2. Pronovost P, Needham D, Berenholtz S, Sinopoli D, Chu H, Cosgrove S, et al. An intervention to decrease catheter-related bloodstream infections in the ICU. N Engl J Med. 2006;355(26): 2725–32.
3. Ma IW, Brindle ME, Ronksley PE, Lorenzetti DL, Sauve RS, Ghali WA. Use of simulation-based education to improve outcomes of central venous catheterization: a systematic review and meta-analysis. Acad Med. 2011;86(9):1137–47.
4. Wu SY, Ling Q, Cao LH, Wang J, Xu MX, Zeng WA. Real-time two-dimensional ultrasound guidance for central venous cannulation: a meta-analysis. Anesthesiology. 2013;118(2):361–75.
5. Gordon CE, Feller-Kopman D, Balk EM, Smetana GW. Pneumothorax following thoracentesis: a systematic review and meta-analysis. Arch Intern Med. 2010;170(4):332–9.
6. Mercaldi CJ, Lanes SF. Ultrasound guidance decreases complications and improves the cost of care among patients undergoing thoracentesis and paracentesis. Chest. 2013;143(2):532–8.

7. Shaikh F, Brzezinski J, Alexander S, Arzola C, Carvalho JC, Beyene J, et al. Ultrasound imaging for lumbar punctures and epidural catheterisations: systematic review and meta-analysis. BMJ. 2013;346:f1720.
8. McGee DC, Gould MK. Preventing complications of central venous catheterization. N Engl J Med. 2003;348(12):1123–33.
9. Mansfield PF, Hohn DC, Fornage BD, Gregurich MA, Ota DM. Complications and failures of subclavian-vein catheterization. N Engl J Med. 1994;331(26):1735–8.
10. Volpicelli G. Sonographic diagnosis of pneumothorax. Intensive Care Med. 2011;37(2):224–32.
11. Lessnau KD. Is chest radiography necessary after uncomplicated insertion of a triple-lumen catheter in the right internal jugular vein, using the anterior approach? Chest. 2005;127(1):220–3.
12. Pikwer A, Baath L, Davidson B, Perstoft I, Akeson J. The incidence and risk of central venous catheter malpositioning: a prospective cohort study in 1619 patients. Anaesth Intensive Care. 2008;36(1):30–7.
13. Crnich CJ, Maki DG. Infections caused by intravascular devices: epidemiology, pathogenesis, diagnosis, prevention, and treatment. In: APIC text of infection control and epidemiology. vol 1. 2nd ed. Washington: Association for Professionals in Infection Control and Epidemiology, Inc.; 2005. p. 24.21–24.26
14. O'Grady NP, Alexander M, Burns LA, Dellinger EP, Garland J, Heard SO, et al. Guidelines for the prevention of intravascular catheter-related infections. Clin Infect Dis. 2011;52(9):e162–93.
15. Mermel LA, Allon M, Bouza E, Craven DE, Flynn P, O'Grady NP, et al. Clinical practice guidelines for the diagnosis and management of intravascular catheter-related infection: 2009 update by the Infectious Diseases Society of America. Clin Infect Dis. 2009;49(1):1–45.
16. Burns KE, McLaren A. A critical review of thromboembolic complications associated with central venous catheters. Can J Anaesth. 2008;55(8):532–41.
17. Guyatt GH, Akl EA, Crowther M, Gutterman DD, Schuünemann HJ, American College of Chest Physicians Antithrombotic Therapy and Prevention of Thrombosis Panel. Executive summary: antithrombotic therapy and prevention of thrombosis, 9th ed: American College of Chest Physicians Evidence-Based Clinical Practice Guidelines. Chest. 2012;141(2 Suppl):7S–47S.
18. Rajaram SS, Desai NK, Kalra A, Gajera M, Cavanaugh SK, Brampton W, et al. Pulmonary artery catheters for adult patients in intensive care. Cochrane Database Syst Rev. 2013;2, CD003408.
19. Brzezinski M, Luisetti T, London MJ. Radial artery cannulation: a comprehensive review of recent anatomic and physiologic investigations. Anesth Analg. 2009;109(6):1763–81.
20. Randolph AG, Cook DJ, Gonzales CA, Andrew M. Benefit of heparin in peripheral venous and arterial catheters: systematic review and meta-analysis of randomised controlled trials. BMJ. 1998;316(7136):969–75.
21. Lawton MT, Porter RW, Heiserman JE, Jacobowitz R, Sonntag VK, Dickman CA. Surgical management of spinal epidural hematoma: relationship between surgical timing and neurologic outcome. J Neurosurg. 1995;83(1):1–7.
22. Siegel JD, Rhinehart E, Jackson M, Chiarello L, Health Care Infection Control Practices Advisory Committee. 2007 guideline for isolation precautions: preventing transmission of infectious agents in health care settings. Am J Infect Control. 2007;35(10 Suppl 2):S65–164.
23. Sudlow C, Warlow C. Posture and fluids for preventing post-dural puncture headache. Cochrane Database Syst Rev. 2002;2, CD001790.
24. Hasbun R, Abrahams J, Jekel J, Quagliarello VJ. Computed tomography of the head before lumbar puncture in adults with suspected meningitis. N Engl J Med. 2001;345(24):1727–33.
25. European Association for the Study of the Liver. EASL clinical practice guidelines on the management of ascites, spontaneous bacterial peritonitis, and hepatorenal syndrome in cirrhosis. J Hepatol. 2010;53(3):397–417.
26. Bernardi M, Caraceni P, Navickis RJ, Wilkes MM. Albumin infusion in patients undergoing large-volume paracentesis: a meta-analysis of randomized trials. Hepatology. 2012;55(4):1172–81.
27. Lata J, Hulek P, Vanasek T. Management of acute variceal bleeding. Dig Dis. 2003;21(1):6–15.

Chapter 9
Preventing Complications: Consistent Meticulous Supportive Care in the ICU

Benjamin A. Bonneton, Serkan Senkal, and Ognjen Gajic

Abstract The intensive care process is an error-prone context where the conjunction of organ failures, complex life support interventions, pharmacologic interactions and frequent invasive procedures increase the risk of complications. Impairment, errors and omissions within daily supportive care delivery further complicate the prognosis. Although most of the prevention measures recommended by evidence-based guidelines require simple protocols and little specialized equipment, their implementation is inconsistent and defective. Checklists, decision support tools, interfaces, ergonomics and computer applications in particular have been proven to reduce medical error within complex care process. The objective of this chapter is to describe important barriers and potential solutions for improving critical care delivery in order to optimize patient safety and outcome.

Keywords ICU • Preventing complications • Supportive care • Safety culture • Decision support • Checklists • Daily routine • Plan of care • Teamwork

Scope of the Problem

It is estimated that 100,000 people die in US hospitals each year because of preventable medical errors [1]. Due to organ failures and complex life support interventions, critically ill patients are particularly prone to complications. Multiple pharmacologic interactions and frequent invasive procedures heighten the risk of adverse events [2]. Data overload, interruptions, multitasking, and the interdisciplinary nature of the intensive care unit (ICU) further complicate care delivery

B.A. Bonneton, M.D. (✉) • S. Senkal, M.D. • O. Gajic, M.D.
Division of Pulmonary and Critical Care Medicine, Mayo Clinic,
200 First Street SW, Rochester, MN 55905, USA
e-mail: bonneton.benjamin@mayo.edu; senkal.serkan@mayo.edu; gajic.ognjen@mayo.edu

J.B. Richards and R.D. Stapleton (eds.), *Non-Pulmonary Complications of Critical Care:*   213
A Clinical Guide, Respiratory Medicine, DOI 10.1007/978-1-4939-0873-8_9,
© Springer Science+Business Media New York 2014

increasing the chance for error and omission. Clinicians may focus on immediate life-threatening issues, but ignore or miss subtle but important "housekeeping" issues necessary to prevent all too common hospital-acquired complications.

The vulnerability of this error-prone delivery process is particularly high early in the course of critical illness (golden hours), but remains constant during the ICU stay. Avoiding diagnostic errors and therapeutic delays is essential to reduce costly complications, preventable death and disability [3, 4].

Irrespective of underlying critical illness or therapeutic and technologic advancements, the final outcome of critically ill patients still largely depends on the quality of daily supportive care and preventing potential complications. Most of the prevention measures recommended by evidence-based guidelines require simple protocols and little specialized equipment. They are well-described and have been proven effective in reducing complications, yet their implementation is inconsistent and defective in the vast majority of ICUs worldwide, and could be facilitated by checklists, decision support tools, interfaces and computer applications.

In this context, in this chapter we describe important barriers and potential solutions for improving critical care delivery in order to optimize patient safety and outcomes.

Common Complications of Critical Illness

Most health care-acquired complications develop through complex interactions between underlying patient characteristics and unintended or adverse effects of diagnostic and therapeutic interventions. Immobilization, sedation, adverse drug reactions and invasive procedures all increase the risks of adverse events and complications. Table 9.1 provides the definitions of common and important complications of critical illness with related potential strategies for preventing these complications. In addition to the complications noted in the table, any intervention or organ support system used in the ICU may cause procedural complications.

Why Are Complications So Common in the ICU?

Despite the advancements in medical knowledge and technologies, the current process of critical care delivery remains a significant source of errors and harms. Multiple barriers limit potential improvements of current care delivery processes, among which human factors hold a central position.

Complex process of care delivery may drastically increase the likelihood of error (Fig. 9.1). *Poorly designed care processes* often contain an excessive number of steps, ambiguous information and lack of prioritization. Fragmented provider-centered care delivery, inadequate safety culture and shift work impair communication

Table 9.1 Critical care-related complications and preventive measures

Complication	Potential prevention strategies
Neurological	
Delirium	Sleep enhancement, minimize use of benzodiazepines and opioids, correct electrolyte disturbances, early mobilization or passive exercise, family presence, orient to time, location, and key individuals, provide glasses and hearing aids, encourage participation in self-care
Coma	Limit continuous infusions of benzodiazepines and opioids, correct specific electrolyte disturbances
Ischemic stroke	Systemic anticoagulation in patients at high risk of thromboemboli
Brain edema/herniation	Head of bed elevation, maintain adequate cerebral perfusion pressure
Intracranial hemorrhage	Monitor anticoagulation and adjusting medication doses appropriately
Seizures	Seizure prophylaxis (head trauma, alcohol withdrawal), correct electrolyte abnormalities, avoid neurotoxic medications
Central pontine myelinolysis	Avoid overly rapid correction of hyponatremia
Cardiovascular	
Acute coronary syndrome	Beta blockers, aspirin, statin use in high-risk patients, optimize hemodynamics
Arrhythmias/cardiac arrest	Maintain airway, oxygenation, acid–base balance; monitor hemodynamics and cardiovascular medications; correct electrolyte disturbances; assess and document resuscitation status
Venous Thromboembolism (VTE)	Early mobilization, chemical and mechanical thromboprophylaxis
Pulmonary	
Atelectasis	Early mobilization, chest physical therapy, incentive spirometry, positive pressure ventilation as needed, head of bed elevation
Pulmonary edema	Pursue a conservative volume resuscitation strategy when possible
Pneumothorax	Lung-protective mechanical ventilation, ultrasound-guided central line placement and thoracocentesis
Acute Respiratory Distress Syndrome	Lung-protective mechanical ventilation, restrictive transfusion, male-predominant fresh frozen plasma, prevention of aspiration
Renal	
Acute kidney injury	Identify patients at high risk, avoid nephrotoxic agents, optimize hemodynamics, limit fluid overload and intra-abdominal hypertension
Infection	
Ventilator-Associated Pneumonia	Head of bed elevation, liberation from mechanical ventilation as soon as possible, protocol for sedation break, hand washing, oral hygiene
Central Line-Associated Bloodstream Infection	Central line bundle: hand washing, barrier precautions, chlorhexidine skin antisepsis, daily assessment for removal of devices that are no longer needed
Catheter-Associated Urinary Tract Infection	Assess if urinary catheter is still needed on a daily basis
Clostridium difficile infection	Wash hands, use barrier precautions, de-escalation broad spectrum antibiotics in a timely manner, limit duration of antibiotic treatment, consider probiotics

(continued)

Table 9.1 (continued)

Gastrointestinal	
Diarrhea	Limit medication triggers and adhere to nutritional triggers
Ileus/constipation	Limit medication triggers, correction of electrolyte abnormalities, provide bowel regimen
Vomiting/aspiration	Bedside swallowing evaluation, head of the bed position, caution with endotracheal and gastric tube placement, prokinetic agents
Gastrointestinal bleeding	Pharmacological stress ulcer prophylaxis, early enteral nutrition
Abdominal compartment syndrome	Monitor bladder pressure, minimize fluid overload, provide gastric and rectal decompression, perform paracentesis as needed, optimize sedation and paralysis, provide lung-protective ventilation, optimize hemodynamic support
Hematological	
Anemia	Minimize unnecessary blood draws
Transfusion complications	Restrictive transfusion strategy
Bleeding	Monitor anticoagulation
Endocrine	
Hyperglycemia/hypoglycemia	Monitor glucose with insulin as needed to maintain blood glucose level between 80 and 180 mg/dL
Adrenal insufficiency	Corticosteroid replacement when clinically appropriate
Skin	
Pressure ulcers	Frequent turning, special mattresses, manage bladder and/or bowel incontinence, adequate nutrition
Medication	
Adverse drug reactions	Pharmacist presence during ICU rounds, medication reconciliation, active monitoring for adverse drug reactions and drug–drug interactions, electronic medical record decision support tools
Long-term complications	
Critical illness polyneuromyopathy	Early mobilization, avoid hyperglycemia, minimize neuromuscular blockade and corticosteroid use
Neurocognitive complications	Delirium treatment and prevention, avoid cerebral hypoperfusion and avoid adverse drug reactions
Neuropsychologic complications	ICU diary, early recognition and treatment of depression and posttraumatic stress disorder

	Probability of Success for Each Step in the Process			
Number of Steps	0.95	0.990	0.999	0.999999
1	0.95	0.990	0.999	0.9999
25	0.28	0.78	0.98	0.998
50	0.08	0.61	0.95	0.995
100	0.006	0.37	0.90	0.990

Fig. 9.1 Probability of success of multistep interventions in complex care processes. Reprinted from Botwinick L, Bisognano M, Haraden C. Leadership Guide to Patient Safety. IHI Innovation Series white paper. Cambridge, Massachusetts: Institute for Healthcare Improvement; 2006. Available at www.IHI.org

and coordination particularly during the vulnerable period of care transitions (hand-offs at the change of shift or patient transfer). As multiple sources of failures may compromise each step of the multistep complex care process, the cumulative effect may quickly encumber the patient's outcome (Fig. 9.1).

Health professionals in the ICU also face significant *information overload*: exponential proliferation of medical literature and the implementation of electronic medical records decrease the signal-to-noise ratio making the relevant clinical information more difficult to find, therefore slowing or misleading the diagnostic and therapeutic process. Frequent interruptions (pagers, alarms) and noise contribute to the chaotic physical environment of the ICU, and directly limit clinicians' ability to focus cognitive effort on a single task or to coordinate complex critical care processes.

Of course, inadequate *ICU structure* (lack of room space or patient-staff visibility, excessive number of beds, inadequate lighting) and *staffing issues* (insufficient pool, nursing shortages, work stress and burnout, poor communication, high turnover, inadequate safety culture) may cumulatively impair the daily care process. Similarly, inadequate attention to human factor *ergonomics* potentiates both errors and adverse events. Inadequate *organizational* ergonomics (defect in multidisciplinary team staffing, bed availability, adverse events reporting, double-checking, teamwork), *cognitive* ergonomics (information overload, not user-friendly computer interfaces, multitasking, failing to prioritize human knowledge or safety goals) and/or *physical* ergonomics (non-convenient room size, technical or equipment issues) all contribute to poor clinician performance [5]. Often, stakeholders may be prone to conflict when motivated by *wrong incentives*, which pervert the clinical process to serve narrow interests, away from high-quality patient-centered care.

Suggested Solutions to Improve Critical Care Delivery and Prevent ICU Complications

Safe and error-free critical care delivery can only be achieved through a systems approach based on the implementation of science and engineering. The "science of health care delivery" uses scientific methods to study practical application of medical knowledge and technology. Emerging concepts that should frame the systems in which critical care is provided to maximize the value of critical care are described below.

Safety Culture

Potential human error must be addressed and minimized within the health care delivery process. Providers ought to adopt safe practice tools with the greatest compliance to successfully minimize medical errors [6]. All members of the team (regardless of rank or role) ought to be able to speak freely and potential adverse events and near-misses have to be discussed openly focusing on systems solutions (such as root cause analyses) rather than focusing on individual blame.

Human Factor Engineering and Ergonomics

Applying human factor engineering concepts is essential for studying and reducing medical error in the ICU [6]. Human factor ergonomics provides a bundle of various tools intended to limit the conditions of error emergence (duty hours, simulation, smart alarms), to systematize routine control (double-checking, daily goals-of-care list, checklists, decision support systems, standardized team communication), to analyze errors (report, identification, root cause analysis and correction). Cognitive ergonomics can be enhanced by easy-to-use, context-appropriate electronic monitoring and interfaces (see below), designed for a standardized and disciplined approach to critical care delivery.

Ambient Intelligence

The current generation of electronic information systems in the ICU largely failed to improve care delivery. Specifically, the available electronic medical records introduce information overload, which complicates and disrupts already complex care processes [7]. A new generation of health information technologies aims to assist safe critical care delivery by creating smart environments including decision support at the time of decision making [8]. Decision support works best when integrated with charting or an order entry system, is capable of smart alerts, tracking and feedback, is adapted to the structure and specialty of the unit, and is available on mobile devices (tablets, smartphones) [9]. An adequate use of electronic environment may help clinicians to deliver safer and more efficient care [10], by assisting them during the task completion. Recently introduced novel electronic tools are designed to highlight relevant clinical data (rather than present unfiltered data and contribute to information overload.) Highlighting pertinent clinical data within the complex decision-making environment can be performed by task-specific dashboards and smart alerts. These tools can decrease cognitive load and error [11].

Prompting Prioritized Information

In order to be useful at the point-of-care (POC), critical care decision support tools are best presented in the form of checklists or algorithms emphasizing prioritized information, such as those designed for use in an operating room [12]. Real-time, evidence-based checklists facilitate knowledge translation at the POC [13], and help provide timely, reliable and optimized patient care. Furthermore, real-time, evidence-based checklists can decrease time to decision making and assure optimal compliance with current evidence and recommendations [14]. Rigorous checklist implementation facilitated by complementary verbal prompting during ICU rounds (for missed items) was associated with dramatic improvement in efficiency and safety of care delivery and improved patient outcomes in a tertiary care teaching institution [3].

"Less Is More"

Daily practice and intensive care management needs to eliminate iatrogenic waste and minimize patients' exposure to the risks of unnecessary complications. Strategies to minimize iatrogenic waste and decrease unnecessary risk include minimizing sedation, prompt weaning of mechanical ventilation, restrictive blood transfusion practices, minimizing exposure to unnecessary laboratory and diagnostic tests and invasive interventions (i.e., early removal of intravascular devices and urinary catheters, foregoing daily routine laboratory tests and portable chest X-rays). Similarly, invasive and complex hemodynamic monitoring devices are largely being replaced with non-invasive POC clinical tools.

Furthermore, judicious test ordering can also decrease the cognitive "noise" that clinicians are required to process each day. Not ordering a relatively low yield test means that the clinician doesn't have to spend time or mental energy on following-up and interpreting that test result. This reduction in performing low yield cognitive processing is another example of the value of "less is more" strategies, and results in increased time and cognitive availability for focusing on higher-level problems, thereby facilitating high-quality clinical reasoning.

Staffing, Regionalization, Telemedicine and Physician Extenders

Intensive care is ideally provided by a multidisciplinary team led by a trained intensivist within a dedicated closed ICU [15], where inter-provider communication is promoted as a critical component of teamwork efficiency [16]. Recently, staffing models include an increasing number of physician extenders (e.g., nurse practitioners and/or physician assistants) specifically trained to optimize ICU care delivery [17]. Adequate 24-h availability of a critical care specialist is not available, access to their expertise can be facilitated by remote technology (telemedicine) [18].

Patient/Family-Centered Care

Decision-making and goals-of-care elaboration should remain guided by patient and family goals and beliefs, particularly with regard to end-of-life issues. The consistency of supportive care improves when a unified approach is adopted and when

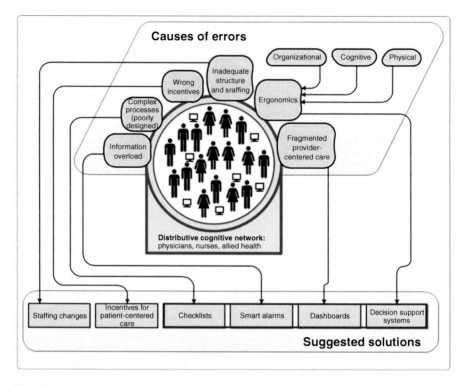

Fig. 9.2 Challenges and opportunities for improving critical care delivery. Reprinted from Pickering BW, Litell JM, Herasevich V, Gajic O. Clinical review: the hospital of the future—building intelligent environments to facilitate safe and effective acute care delivery. Crit Care. 2012;16(2):220

collaboration between the patient or family and clinicians is emphasized. The goal of patient or family and clinician collaboration is to ensure shared understanding of common explicit goals and identify specific individualized goals. Figure 9.2 summarizes the main causes of errors and suggested solutions for improved critical care delivery.

Many tools and processes have been recently developed, tested, and validated for critical care delivery improvement. These tools include multidisciplinary rounds, ICU care bundles, checklists, rounding support tools and daily goals of care sheets, smart alarms, dashboards and real-time decision support tools. These tools are specifically designed to enhance both efficiency and reliability of critical care delivery [7].

Intensive care may particularly benefit from crisis management checklists. Displayed by an appropriate decision support tool (i.e., the electronic medical record), crisis management checklists may serve to insure the effective and timely treatment delivery at bedside during critical events, avoiding omission of critical clinical steps and thereby preventing medical errors [18]. Crisis management checklists result in standardization of the clinical care provided by different providers dealing with similar clinical issues, and ultimately improve outcomes for critically ill patients. As the introduction of simple surgical checklists improved outcomes across three continents [13], crisis management checklists during ICU care may be particularly helpful to itemize and control (even verbally) the most important steps of care plans [19, 20].

Bundled Evidence-Based Practice Interventions

Bundles of ICU evidence-based practices such as ABCDE bundle (Awakening and Breathing Coordination, Delirium Monitoring and Management, and Early Mobility) [21], may improve a patient's outcome by combining several interventions during daily clinical practice. In addition to improving sedation management and shortening mechanical ventilation, bundles can spur intra-team communication and further standardization of care processes. These strategies are best implemented by a coordinated multidisciplinary team of care providers (physicians, nurses, respiratory therapist, physical therapist, social worker, and others as necessary.) Each member of the multidisciplinary team ensures the best compliance to their domain-specific item of the bundle [22].

Daily assessment must include the utilization of valid and reliable tools (Confusion Assessment Method for the Intensive Care Unit [CAM-ICU], Intensive Care Delirium Screening Checklist, Sedation-Agitation Scale, Motor Activity Assessment Scale), assessment protocols (spontaneous awakening trials, spontaneous breathing trials) as well as the communication and coordination of the various health care professionals involved in the patient's care [23].

In the same way, the identification and implementation of *daily goal-directed measures* has been shown to significantly improve understanding of the goals of an individual patient's care plan among providers, as well as facilitate accurate handoff [24]. The transmission of individual information between professionals is likewise promoted by the integration of *interdisciplinary daily rounding* which improves effective teamwork, collaboration and *inter-provider* communication in ICUs [25].

Combining various tools in a *multidimensional approach* should help mitigate errors and consequently improve clinical and economic effectiveness of an ICU [26].

Despite overwhelming evidence for the clinical benefit of these interventions, adherence in real-life practice is grossly suboptimal [27]. Promising results have been reported by using both real-time verbal prompting by a specifically assigned team member [3] and novel *electronic decision support tools* (Fig. 9.3) [7]. Verbal prompting or electronic decision support tools are intended to enable more efficient assessment of a patient's clinical data by specifically addressing the key components of best clinical practice (Fig. 9.2).

Sedation break indicated	☐ N/A	☐ Yes	☐ No
			  ☐ appropriately awake
			  ☐ seizure control
			  ☐ elevated ICP
			  ☐ neuromuscular blockade
			  ☐ facilitate supportive care
			  ☐ other

Treat delirium	☐ N/A	☐ Yes
		  ☐ sleep enhancement
		  ☐ minimize benzodiazepine
		  ☐ start neuroleptic
		  ☐ other
			☐ No
			  ☐ delirium resolved
			  ☐ other

Treat pain	☐ N/A	☐ Yes
		  ☐ adjust pain medication
		  ☐ pain consult
			☐ No
			  ☐ pain resolved
			  ☐ other

Continue vasoactive medication	☐ N/A	☐ Yes	☐ No
			  ☐ stop
			  ☐ wean
			  ☐ change medication order
			  ☐ other

Review cardiac medication	☐ N/A	☐ Yes	☐ No
			  ☐ stop
			  ☐ wean
			  ☐ change medication order
			  ☐ other

Remove vascular device	☐ N/A	☐ Yes
		Device:
			☐ No
			  ☐ monitoring
			  ☐ IV medication
			  ☐ parenteral nutrition
			  ☐ other

Lung protective ventilation	☐ N/A	☐ Yes	☐ No ☐ other

Spontaneous breathing trial	☐ N/A	☐ Yes	☐ No
			  ☐ severe hypoxemia
			  ☐ neuromuscular blockade
			  ☐ hemodynamic instability
			  ☐ other

HOB elevated to 30 degrees	☐ N/A	☐ Yes	☐ No
			  ☐ spinal drain or surgery
			  ☐ other

Even or negative fluid goal today	☐ N/A	☐ Yes Fluid target:	☐ No ☐ other

Review and correct electrolyte	☐ N/A	☐ Yes	☐ No
			  ☐ electrolyte check not indicated today
			  ☐ other

Fig. 9.3 AWARE screen capture—an incentive checklist for daily rounds. Care items are displayed according to patient's condition and risk factors. User-friendly interface enables various professionals to update the checklist anytime and promotes an efficient patient-centered daily rounds tool

Remove urinary catheter	☐ N/A	☐ Yes	☐ No
			☐ strict I/O
			☐ sedation /ventilation
			☐ wound
			☐ CC hospice
			☐ chronic
			☐ immobilized
			☐ other
Chemical DVT prophylaxis	☐ N/A	☐ Yes	☐ No
			☐ bleeding risk
			☐ auto anticoagulated
			☐ systemic anticoagulation
			☐ therapeutic anticoagulated for other indication
			☐ other
Stress ulcer prophylaxis	☐ N/A	☐ Yes	☐ No
			☐ no indication
			☐ other
Glucose control appropriate	☐ N/A	☐ Yes	☐ No
			☐ DCS consult ☐ Insulin drip
			☐ other
Enteral nutrition today	☐ N/A	☐ Yes	☐ No
			☐ ileus
			☐ aspiration risk
			☐ surgical contraindication
			☐ other
Need for antimicrobial reviewed	☐ N/A	☐ Yes	☐ No
		☐ continue	☐ other
		☐ de-escalate	
		☐ change coverage	
		☐ ID consult	
Adequate source control	☐ N/A	☐ Yes	☐ No
			☐ imaging
			☐ surgical consult
			☐ IR consult
			☐ ID consult
Physical therapy	☐ N/A	☐ Yes	☐ No
		☐ mobilized as tolerated	☐ mobilization contraindicated
		☐ PT/OT consult	☐ other
		☐ passive range of motion	
		☐ other	

Fig. 9.3 (continued)

Summary of Recommendations and Conclusion

In conclusion, meticulous supportive care is a critical component of critical care delivery. Novel processes and tools have been developed to enhance the reliability and efficiency of ICU care. Standardization of care across unique health care providers may be achieved as these electronic tools are designed to optimize the process of health care delivery, cognitive processing, and the organization of the ICU. The literature demonstrates that POC implementation of these tools has invariably demonstrated benefit with regard to minimizing diagnostic error and waste, therapeutic harm, preventable death, disability and cost.

Summary of Key Points

- Safety culture
- Decision support justified by recommendation and based on medical research evidence
- Human factor engineering and ergonomics: decision support at time of decision making
- Ambient intelligence
- "Less is more"
- Non-invasive monitoring/testing
- Staffing/regionalization/telemedicine/physician extenders: Intensivist team and unit
- Checklists and prompters: Ensure the effective and timely treatments delivery at bedside: Patient/family-centered care
- In-patient services primarily ICU, intermediate, and rehabilitation
- Identify goal-directed plan of care, facilitating accurate handover
- Interdisciplinary daily round to improve effective teamwork, collaboration and communication
- Daily routine: systematic implementation and update for each patient

References

1. Kohn LT, Corrigan J, Donaldson MS. To err is human: building a safer health system. Washington: National Academy Press; 2000.
2. Weiss CH, Amaral LA. Moving the science of quality improvement in critical care medicine forward. Am J Respir Crit Care Med. 2010;182(12):1461–2.
3. Weiss CH, Moazed F, McEvoy CA, Singer BD, Szleifer I, Amaral LA, et al. Prompting physicians to address a daily checklist and process of care and clinical outcomes: a single-site study. Am J Respir Crit Care Med. 2011;184(6):680–6.
4. Pronovost PJ, Berenholtz SM, Needham DM. Translating evidence into practice: a model for large scale knowledge translation. BMJ. 2008;337:a1714.
5. Schutz AL, Counte MA, Meurer S. Assessment of patient safety research from an organizational ergonomics and structural perspective. Ergonomics. 2007;50(9):1451–84.
6. Moreno RP, Rhodes A, Donchin Y. Patient safety in intensive care medicine: the declaration of Vienna. Intensive Care Med. 2009;35(10):1667–72.
7. Pickering BW, Litell JM, Herasevich V, Gajic O. Clinical review: the hospital of the future – building intelligent environments to facilitate safe and effective acute care delivery. Crit Care. 2012;16(2):220.
8. Lobach D, Sanders GD, Bright TJ, Wong A, Dhurjati R, Bristow E, et al. Enabling Health Care Decisionmaking Through Clinical Decision Support and Knowledge Management. Evidence Report No. 203. (Prepared by the Duke Evidence-based Practice Center under Contract

No. 290-2007-10066-I.) AHRQ Publication No. 12-E001-EF. Rockville, MD: Agency for Healthcare Research and Quality. April 2012

9. Ahmed A, Chandra S, Herasevich V, Gajic O, Pickering BW. The effect of two different electronic health record user interfaces on intensive care provider task load, errors of cognition, and performance. Crit Care Med. 2011;39(7):1626–34.

10. Buntin MB, Burke MF, Hoaglin MC, Blumenthal D. The benefits of health information technology: a review of the recent literature shows predominantly positive results. Health Aff. 2011;30(3):464–71.

11. Pickering BW, Gajic O, Ahmed A, Herasevich V, Keegan MT. Data utilization for medical decision making at the time of patient admission to ICU*. Crit Care Med. 2013;41(6):1502–10.

12. Haynes AB, Weiser TG, Berry WR, Lipsitz SR, Breizat A-HS, Dellinger EP, et al. A surgical safety checklist to reduce morbidity and mortality in a global population. N Engl J Med. 2009;360(5):491–9.

13. Gawande A. The checklist: if something so simple can transform intensive care, what else can it do? New Yorker. 2007;10:86–101.

14. Byrnes MC, Schuerer DJ, Schallom ME, Sona CS, Mazuski JE, Taylor BE, et al. Implementation of a mandatory checklist of protocols and objectives improves compliance with a wide range of evidence-based intensive care unit practices. Crit Care Med. 2009;37(10):2775–81.

15. Pronovost PJ, Angus DC, Dorman T, Robinson KA, Dremsizov TT, Young TL. Physician staffing patterns and clinical outcomes in critically ill patients: a systematic review. JAMA. 2002;288(17):2151–62.

16. Baggs JG, Schmitt MH, Mushlin AI, Mitchell PH, Eldredge DH, Oakes D, et al. Association between nurse–physician collaboration and patient outcomes in three intensive care units. Crit Care Med. 1999;27(9):1991–8.

17. Gershengorn HB, Wunsch H, Wahab R, Leaf DE, Brodie D, Li G, et al. Impact of nonphysician staffing on outcomes in a medical ICU. Chest. 2011;139(6):1347–53.

18. Lilly CM, Cody S, Zhao H, Landry K, Baker SP, McIlwaine J, et al. Hospital mortality, length of stay, and preventable complications among critically ill patients before and after tele-ICU reengineering of critical care processes. JAMA. 2011;305(21):2175–83.

19. Myung JL, Hayley BG, Michael D, Peter H, Daniel ST, Ognjen G, et al. Checklist for lung injury prevention (CLIP): a pilot study on implementation across multiple hospitals and multiple clinical areas. D102 Quality Improvement in Critical Care Medicine: American Thoracic Society. p. A6567-A.

20. DuBose JJ, Inaba K, Shiflett A, Trankiem C, Teixeira PG, Salim A, et al. Measurable outcomes of quality improvement in a trauma intensive care unit: the impact of a daily quality rounding checklist. J Trauma. 2008;64(1):22–7.

21. Balas MC, Vasilevskis EE, Burke WJ, Boehm L, Pun BT, Olsen KM, et al. Critical care nurses' role in implementing the "ABCDE bundle" into practice. Crit Care Nurse. 2012;32(2):35–8. 40–7.

22. Resar R, Pronovost P, Haraden C, Simmonds T, Rainey T, Nolan T. Using a bundle approach to improve ventilator care processes and reduce ventilator-associated pneumonia. Jt Comm J Qual Patient Saf. 2005;31(5):243–8.

23. Pronovost P, Berenholtz S, Dorman T, Lipsett PA, Simmonds T, Haraden C. Improving communication in the ICU using daily goals. J Crit Care. 2003;18(2):71–5.

24. Narasimhan M, Eisen LA, Mahoney CD, Acerra FL, Rosen MJ. Improving nurse–physician communication and satisfaction in the intensive care unit with a daily goals worksheet. Am J Crit Care. 2006;15(2):217–22.

25. Philpin S. 'Handing over': transmission of information between nurses in an intensive therapy unit. Nurs Crit Care. 2006;11(2):86–93.

26. Donchin Y, Gopher D, Olin M, Badihi Y, Biesky M, Sprung CL, et al. A look into the nature and causes of human errors in the intensive care unit. 1995. Qual Saf Health Care. 2003;12(2):143–7.

27. Cabana MD, Rand CS, Powe NR, Wu AW, Wilson MH, Abboud PA, et al. Why don't physicians follow clinical practice guidelines? A framework for improvement. JAMA. 1999;282(15): 1458–65.

Index

A

Abdominal compartment syndrome (ACS),
106–108
Acute acalculous cholecystitis (AAC)
diagnosis, 159–160
epidemiology, 158
pathophysiology of, 158–159
preventive measures, 160
risk factors, 158–159
signs and symptoms, 159
treatment, 160
Acute glomerulonephritis, 33
Acute interstitial nephritis (AIN), 32–33
Acute kidney injury (AKI)
acid–base balance, 39–40
acute interstitial nephritis, 32–33
biomarkers, 26
blood tests, 24
complications of
bleeding, 35–36
cardiovascular, 36
nephrogenic systemic fibrosis, 36
contrast-induced nephropathy, 29–30
definition of, 20–21
epidemiology, 20
fluid resuscitation
adequate nutrition, 38
crystalloids and colloids, 37–38
vasopressors, 38
glomerulonephritis and vasculitis, 33
hepatorenal syndrome, 35
imaging studies, 26
intravascular volume assessment, 22
intrinsic, 27, 28
ischemic injury, 28–29
metabolic acidosis, 40–41

nephrotoxic drugs
aminoglycosides, 31–32
NSAIDs, 32
vancomycin, 30–31
oliguria, urine output, 24
patient's history, 22
postrenal, 27–28
prerenal, 26–27
renal replacement therapy
continuous renal replacement
therapy, 39
indications, 38–39
intermittent hemodialysis, 39
peritoneal dialysis, 39
rhabdomyolysis, 33–34
serum creatinine, 23, 24
signs and symptoms, 22
urea nitrogen, 23, 24
urinary sediment examination, 25
urine electrolytes and osmolality, 25
vascular causes
large-vessel disease, 34–35
small-vessel disease, 34
Acute mesenteric ischemia, 124–125
Acute oliguria, 24
Acute renal failure (ARF). *See* Acute kidney
injury (AKI)
Acute upper GI bleeding (AUGIB),
120–123
Adaptation to the Intensive Care Environment
(ATICE) instrument, 50
Adrenal insufficiency, 180–181
American Society for Parenteral and Enteral
Nutrition (ASPEN), 166, 168,
172–173
Aminoglycosides, AKI, 31–32

Anemia
    blood loss, 62, 63
    blood transfusion
        allergic reactions, 98
        bacterial infections, 96
        blood loss minimization, 67
        blood substitutes/oxygen carrying
            agents, 67
        coagulopathic complications,
            100–101
        delayed hemolytic transfusion
            reactions, 97
        erythropoietin, 67
        febrile non-hemolytic transfusion
            reactions, 98
        goals, 65
        hyperhemolytic reactions, 97
        immune-mediated NISHOT, 97–99
        iron supplementation, 67
        leukoreduction, 66
        metabolic derangements, 100
        non-immune hemolytic reactions, 100
        non-immune-mediated NISHOT,
            99–100
        PRBC storage, 66
        PRBC alloimmunization, 99
        PRBC storage lesion, 101
        transfusion-associated circulatory
            overload, 99–100
        transfusion-related immunomodulation,
            99
        transfusion-related lung injury,
            98–99
        transfusion thresholds, 66
        viral infections, 96
    decreased RBC production, 63
    evaluation
        hemoglobin level, 64
        serum iron, 64
        transferrin saturation, 65
    increased RBC destruction, 63, 64
    RBCs life span, 62
Arterial catheters
    bleeding, 202
    infection, 202–203
    vascular injury, 201–202
Asymptomatic bacteriuria (ASB), 136
Asystole, 9, 11
Atrial fibrillation (A fib), 2–3
Autonomic nerve dysfunction, 115
Awakening and Breathing Coordination,
        Delirium Monitoring, Early
        Mobility, and Exercise (ABCDE)
        approach, 57

B
Bleeding
    AKI, 35–36
    arterial catheters, 202
    lumbar puncture, 203–204
    paracentesis, 205–206

C
Cardiac arrest
    asystole, 11
    PEA arrest, 9–10
    V tach and V fib, 7–9
Cardiovascular complications
    atrial fibrillation, 2–3
    cardiac arrest
        asystole, 11
        PEA arrest, 9–10
        V tach and V fib, 7–9
    myocardial infarction
        NSTEMI, 3–5
        STEMI, 5–6
    pericardial tamponade, 14–15
    post-resuscitation syndrome, 11–12
    reperfusion injury, 11–12
    targeted temperature management,
        12–14
Catheter-associated urinary tract infection
        (CAUTI)
    definition of, 136
    diagnosis of, 138–139
    epidemiology, 136
    pathophysiology, 137
    preventive measures, 139–140
    risk factors, 137–138
    signs and symptoms, 138
    treatment, 139
Catheter-related bloodstream infections
        (CRBSIs)
    colonization and biofilm formation,
        141–142
    definitive diagnosis, 143
    epidemiology, 140–141
    prevention of
        aseptic techniques, 144
        chlorhexidine silver sulfadiazine, 146
        education and training, 144
        hand washing, 144
        needleless connectors, 146
    risk factors, 142
    signs and symptoms, 142–143
    treatment of, 143–144
Central line associated bloodstream infection
        (CLABSI), 198–199

Central venous catheters
    air embolism, 197–198
    arterial puncture or cannulation, 194–196
    catheter-associated thrombosis, 199
    catheter malposition, 197
    central line associated bloodstream
        infection, 198–199
    early complications, 193–194
    hematoma, 196
    pneumothorax, 196–197
Cholestasis, 119, 120
Chronic lymphocytic leukemia (CLL), 77
Chronic myelogenous leukemia (CML), 77
Clostridium difficile colitis
    diagnosis of, 150–151
    epidemiology, 147
    pathophysiology, 147–148
    prevention, 153
    risk factors, 148–149
    signs and symptoms, 149
    stool tests for, 150
    treatment, 151–153
Confusion Assessment Method for the ICU
        (CAM-ICU), 55
Continuous renal replacement therapy
        (CRRT), 39
Contrast-induced nephropathy (CIN), 29–30
Critical care delivery
    care related complications, 214–216
    improvements
        challenges and opportunities, 220
        daily assessment, 221
        daily goal-directed measures, 221
        decision support, 218
        human factor engineering concepts, 218
        human factor ergonomics, 218
        interdisciplinary daily rounding, 221
        "less is more" strategies, 219
        multidimensional approach, 221
        patient/family-centered
            care, 219–221
        point-of-care, 218–219
        safety culture, 217
        staffing models, 219
        teamwork, 219
        verbal prompting, 221
    poorly designed care processes, 214, 217
Critical-illness-related corticosteroid
        insufficiency (CIRCI), 180–181
Cystatin-C, 26

D
Deep vein thrombosis
    diagnosis of, 85–86
    treatment of, 90

Delayed gastric emptying (DGE), 114–116
Delirium
    alpha-2 agonists, 56
    Confusion Assessment Method
        (CAM-ICU), 55
    long-term cognitive impairment, 57
    pathophysiological mechanisms, 55–56
    post traumatic stress disorder, 57
    risk factors, 55
    screening checklist, 55
    SEDCOM trial, 56–57
Diaphragmatic hiatus dysfunction, 111
Disseminated intravascular coagulation, 91–92
Duodenogastroesophageal reflux, 112

E
Early Parenteral Nutrition to Supplement
        Insufficient Enteral Nutrition in
        Intensive Care (EPaNIC) study, 173
Electrical muscle stimulation, 54–55
Endocrine complications
    adrenal insufficiency, 180–181
    hyperglycemia, 176–177
    hypoglycemia, 177–178
    myxedema coma, 179–180
    thyroid storm, 178–179
Enteral nutrition
    aspiration, 171–172
    diarrhea, 172–173
    nasogastric sump tubes, 170
    nosocomial pneumonia, 170
    potential complications, 172
Enteric nerve dysfunction, 115
Erythrocytosis/polycythemia
    absolute polycythemia, 68
    etiologies, 68, 69
    evaluation, 69
    management, 69
    relative polycythemia, 68
Erythropoietin (EPO) therapy, 67
Esophagus, GI complications
    duodenogastroesophageal reflux, 112
    esophagitis, 110–111
    gastroesophageal reflux, 111–112

F
Fluids and Catheters Treatment Trial
        (FACTT), 37

G
Gastroesophageal balloon tamponade
    aspiration, 209
    balloon tamponade devices, 208–209

Gastroesophageal balloon tamponade (*cont.*)
 ischemia and rupture, 209
 rebleeding, 209–210
Gastrointestinal (GI) complications, 124–127
 abdominal compartment syndrome, 106–108
 esophagus
  duodenogastroesophageal reflux, 112
  esophagitis, 110–111
  gastroesophageal reflux, 111–112
 hepatobiliary
  acute acalculous cholecystitis, 117–118
  cholestasis, 119, 120
  ischemic hepatopathy, 118–119
 intestinal
  diarrhea, 127–131
  hemorrhage, 120–124
  ischemic intestinal injury, 124–127
 intra-abdominal hypertension, 106–108
 pneumoperitoneum
  intra-abdominal causes, 109
  post-cardiopulmonary resuscitation, 109
  thoracic causes, 109
 retroperitoneal-based complications, 131
 stomach
  dysmotility and feeding intolerance, 114–116
  stress ulcers, 112–114

H
HELLP syndrome, 94
Hematologic complications
 anemia (*see* Anemia)
 erythrocytosis/polycythemia
  absolute polycythemia, 68
  etiologies, 68, 69
  evaluation, 69
  management, 69
  relative polycythemia, 68
 leukocytosis
  etiologies of, 76
  hematologic malignancies, 77
  infectious causes, 77–78
  non-infectious causes, 78
 neutropenia
  antibiotic regimen, 73–74
  antibiotic therapy, 73
  catheter-related infections, 75
  causes of, 70
  cytomegalovirus, 71
  empiric antifungal therapy, 74
  environmental precautions, 75
  etiologies of, 70–71
  hematologic malignancies, 72
  hematopoietic growth factors, 74

 human herpes virus 6 and measles, 71
 human immunodeficiency virus, 71
 mechanisms, 70
 medication-induced neutropenia, 70
 physical examination, 72
 sepsis, 72
 treatment duration, 74
 treatment guidelines, cancer, 73
 viral treatment, 74
 zoonoses, 72
 thrombocytopenia
  complications, 79
  etiologies of, 79–81
  evaluation, 81
  management, 81–82
 thrombocytosis
  disseminated intravascular coagulation, 91–92
  evaluation, 83
  HELLP syndrome, 94
  hemoytic uremic syndrome, 93
  heparin-induced thrombocytopenia, 92–93
  iatrogenic coagulopathy, 94
  liver failure, 94
  management, 83–84
  primary thrombocytosis, 82–83
  secondary (reactive) thrombocytosis, 83
  thrombotic/thrombocytopenic purpura, 93
  venous thromboembolism (*see* Venous thromboembolism (VTE))
Hemoytic uremic syndrome, 93
Heparin-induced thrombocytopenia, 92–93
Hepatorenal syndrome (HRS), 35
Human herpes virus 6 and measles, 71
Human immunodeficiency virus (HIV), 71
Hyperglycemia, 176–177
Hypoglycemia, 177–178

I
ICU-acquired weakness
 critical illness myopathy, 48
 critical illness polyneuropathy, 48
 differential diagnosis, 48–49
 immobilization, 46
 MRC scale, 49
 risk factors, 49
Intestinal complications
 diarrhea
  Clostridium difficile infection, 127–130
  enteral feeding, 130
  medications, 131

hemorrhage
    Upper GI bleed, 120–123
    Lower GI bleed, 123–124
    ischemic intestinal injury
        acute mesenteric ischemia, 124–125
        large bowel ischemia, 125–126
        pseudo-obstruction, 126–127
Intra-abdominal hypertension (IAH)
    fluid balance management, 108
    invasive interventions, 107
    primary ACS, 106
    risk factors, 107
    secondary ACS, 106
    trans-bladder measurement, 108
Ischemic injury
    AKI, 28–29
    intestine
        acute mesenteric ischemia, 124–125
        large bowel ischemia, 125–126
        pseudo-obstruction, 126–127

K
Kidney Disease Improving Global Outcomes
    (KDIGO) group, 20, 21

L
Large bowel ischemia, 125–126
Large vessel renovascular disease, 34–35
Leukocytosis
    etiologies of, 76
    hematologic malignancies, 77
    infectious causes, 77–78
    non-infectious causes, 78
Lower esophageal sphincter (LES)
    dysfunction, 111
Lower GI bleeding (LGIB), 123–124
Lumbar puncture
    back pain, 203
    bleeding, 203–204
    infection, 204
    neurologic complications, 205
    post-lumbar puncture headache, 204

M
Malnutrition
    acute disease-related malnutrition, 166
    classifications, 166
    definition, 166
    enteral nutrition
        aspiration, 171–172
        diarrhea, 172–173
        nasogastric sump tubes, 170
        nosocomial pneumonia, 170

        potential complications, 172
    micronutrient deficiencies
        glutamine, 168–169
        selenium, 168
        signs and symptoms, 167
        thiamine, 167
        vitamin D, 169
        vitamins E and C, 169
    parenteral nutrition, 173–175
    refeeding syndrome, 174–176
Maximizing Efficacy of Targeted Sedation and
    Reducing Neurological Dysfunction
    (MENDS) trial, 56
Medical Research Council (MRC) scale, 49
Medication-induced neutropenia, 70–71
Metabolic acidosis, AKI, 40–41
Micronutrient deficiencies
    glutamine, 168–169
    selenium, 168
    signs and symptoms, 167
    thiamine, 167
    vitamin D, 169
    vitamins E and C, 169
Multinational Association for Supportive Care
    in Cancer (MASCC) scoring
    system, 73
Myocardial infarction
    NSTEMI, 3–5
    STEMI, 5–6
Myxedema coma
    cardiovascular manifestations, 179
    clinical findings, 179
    diagnosis of, 180
    hyponatremia, 180
    treatment of, 180

N
Nephrogenic systemic fibrosis
    (NSF), 36
Nephrotoxic drugs, AKI
    aminoglycosides, 31–32
    NSAIDs, 32
    vancomycin, 30–31
Neurological complications
    ICU-acquired weakness
        critical illness myopathy, 48
        critical illness polyneuropathy, 48
        differential diagnosis, 48–49
        immobilization, 46
        MRC scale, 49
        risk factors, 49
    ICU delirium
        alpha-2 agonists, 56
        Confusion Assessment Method
        (CAM-ICU), 55

Neurological complications (*cont.*)
    long-term cognitive impairment, 57
    pathophysiological mechanisms, 55–56
    post traumatic stress disorder, 57
    risk factors, 55
    screening checklist, 55
    SEDCOM trial, 56–57
  mobilization strategy
    bedside bicycle ergometer, 51
    clinical parameters, 50
    electrical muscle stimulation, 54–55
    in mechanically ventilated patients, 51
    mobilization protocols, 50–51
    multi-disciplinary approach, 52–54
Neutropenia
  causes of, 70
  cytomegalovirus, 71
  etiologies of, 70–71
  hematologic malignancies, 72
  human herpes virus 6 and measles, 71
  human immunodeficiency virus, 71
  management
    antibiotic regimen, 73–74
    antibiotic therapy, 73
    catheter-related infections, 75
    empiric antifungal therapy, 74
    environmental precautions, 75
    hematopoietic growth factors, 74
    treatment duration, 74
    treatment guidelines, cancer, 73
    viral treatment, 74
  mechanisms, 70
  medication-induced neutropenia, 70
  physical examination, 72
  sepsis, 72
  zoonoses, 72
Non-ST elevation myocardial infarction
    (NSTEMI)
  clinical signs and symptoms, 3
  coronary artery vasospasm, 4
  demand-related ischemia, 4
  diagnostic workup, 3–4
  potential causes, 4
  treatment of, 4–5
Nonsteroidal anti-inflammatory drugs
    (NSAIDs), 32
Normoglycemia in Intensive Care Evaluation
    Survival Using Glucose Algorithm
    Regulation (NICESUGAR) trial,
    177
Nosocomial sinusitis
  diagnosis, 156–157
  epidemiology, 154

  pathophysiology of, 154–155
  preventive measures, 157
  risk factors, 155
  signs and symptoms, 156
  treatment, 157

P
Paracentesis
  ascites fluid leak, 206
  bleeding, 205–206
  infection, 206–207
  intravascular volume shifts, 208
  solid organ or bowel wall injury,
    207–208
  Z-track technique, 207
Pericardial tamponade, 14–15
Peritoneal dialysis, 39
Pneumoperitoneum, GI complications
  intra-abdominal causes, 109
  post-cardiopulmonary resuscitation, 109
  thoracic causes, 109
Post-resuscitation syndrome, 11–12
Post traumatic stress disorder (PTSD), 57
Primary polycythemias, 68, 69
Procedural complications
  arterial catheters
    bleeding, 202
    infection, 202–203
    vascular injury, 201–202
  bedside, 191–193
  central venous catheters
    air embolism, 197–198
    arterial puncture or cannulation,
      194–196
    catheter-associated thrombosis, 199
    catheter malposition, 197
    central line associated bloodstream
      infection, 198–199
    early complications, 193–194
    hematoma, 196
    pneumothorax, 196–197
  gastroesophageal balloon tamponade
    aspiration, 209
    balloon tamponade devices,
      208–209
    ischemia and rupture, 209
    rebleeding, 209–210
  incidence of, 188
  lumbar puncture
    back pain, 203
    bleeding, 203–204
    infection, 204

neurologic complications, 205
post-lumbar puncture headache, 204
paracentesis
    ascites fluid leak, 206
    bleeding, 205–206
    infection, 206–207
    intravascular volume shifts, 208
    solid organ or bowel wall injury,
        207–208
    Z-track technique, 207
procedural training
    medical education, 190
    simulation, 190–191
pulmonary artery catheters (PACs),
    199–200
recommendations, 210
system-based efforts
    culture of safety, 188
    pre-procedure time-outs, 190
    procedural checklists, 189–190
Protein-calorie malnutrition, 166
Pseudo-obstruction, 126–127
Pulmonary artery catheters (PACs),
    199–200
Pulmonary embolism
    bedside echocardiography, 88
    computed tomography pulmonary
        angiography, 87
    magnetic resonance angiography, 88
    pulmonary angiography, 88
    treatment of, 90–91
    ventilation perfusion lung scanning,
        87–88
Pulseless electrical activity (PEA), 9–10

R
Refeeding syndrome, 174–176
Renal artery stenosis (RAS), 34–35
Renal complications. See Acute kidney injury
    (AKI)
Renal Insufficiency Following Contrast Media
    Administration (REMEDIAL)
    study, 29–30
Renal replacement therapy (RRT)
    continuous renal replacement therapy, 39
    indications, 38–39
    intermittent hemodialysis, 39
    peritoneal dialysis, 39
Reperfusion injury, 11–12
Rhabdomyolysis, AKI, 33–34
Risk, Injury, Failure, Loss and End-stage
    kidney (RIFLE) criteria, 21

S
Safety and Efficacy of Dexmedetomidine
    Compared with Midazolam
    (SEDCOM) trial, 56
Saline versus Albumin Fluid Evaluation
    (SAFE) Study, 37
Secondary polycythemia, 68, 69
Small vessel renovascular disease, 34
Spontaneous retroperitoneal bleeding
    (SRB), 131
ST elevation myocardial infarction (STEMI),
    5–6
    causes, 5
    signs and symptoms, 6
    treatment of, 6
Stomach, GI complications
    dysmotility and feeding intolerance,
        114–116
    stress ulcers, 112–114
Stress ulcers, 112–114

T
Targeted temperature management (TTM),
    12–14
Thrombocytopenia
    complications, 79
    decreased platelet production, 81
    dilutional thrombocytopenia, 80–81
    evaluation, 81
    increased platelet destruction
        immune-mediated mechanisms,
            79–80
        non-immune-mediated, 79
    management, 81–82
    splenomegaly, 81
    spurious thrombocytopenia, 79
Thrombocytosis
    disseminated intravascular coagulation,
        91–92
    evaluation, 83
    HELLP syndrome, 94
    hemoytic uremic syndrome, 93
    heparin-induced thrombocytopenia,
        92–93
    iatrogenic coagulopathy, 94
    liver failure, 94
    management, 83–84
    primary thrombocytosis, 82–83
    secondary (reactive) thrombocytosis, 83
    thrombotic/thrombocytopenic purpura, 93
    venous thromboembolism (see Venous
        thromboembolism (VTE))

Thyroid storm
    diagnosis of, 178–179
    Grave's disease, 178
    incidence of, 178
    signs and symptoms, 178
    treatment of, 179
Transfusion Requirements in Critical Care
    (TRICC) trial, 66
Transient lower esophageal sphincter
    relaxations (TLERs), 111

V
Vasculitis, 33
Venous thromboembolism (VTE)
    anticoagulation, 89–90
    clinical presentation, 85

    deep vein thrombosis
        diagnosis of, 85–86
        treatment of, 90
    pulmonary embolism
        bedside echocardiography, 88
        computed tomography pulmonary
          angiography, 87
        magnetic resonance angiography, 88
        pulmonary angiography, 88
        treatment of, 90–91
        ventilation perfusion lung scanning,
          87–88
    risk factors, 84
    risk stratification and prognosis, 89
Ventricular fibrillation (V fib), 7–9
Ventricular tachycardia (V tach),
    7–9